Editors/Academic Advisory Board

Members of the Academic Advisory Board are instrumental in the final selection of articles for each edition of TAKING SIDES. Their review of articles for content, level, and appropriateness provides critical direction to the editors and staff. We think that you will find their careful consideration well reflected in this volume.

TAKING SIDES: Clashing Views on

Bioethical Issues

Fourteenth Edition

EDITOR

Carol Levine
United Hospital Fund

ACADEMIC ADVISORY BOARD MEMBERS

Editors/Academic Advisory Board continued

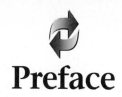

Preface

This is a book about choices—hard and tragic choices. The choices are hard not only because they often involve life and death but also because there are convincing arguments on both sides of the issues. An ethical dilemma, by definition, is one that poses a conflict not between good and evil but between one good principle and another that is equally good. The choices are hard because the decisions that are made—by individuals, groups, and public policymakers—will influence the kind of society we have today and the one we will have in the future.

Although the views expressed in the selections in this volume are strong—even passionate—they are also subtle, concerned with the nuances of the particular debate. *How* one argues matters in bioethics; you will see and have to weigh the significance of varying rhetorical styles and appeals throughout this volume.

Although there are no easy answers to any of the issues in the book, the questions will be answered in some fashion—partly by individual choices and partly by decisions that are made by professionals and government. We must make them the best answers possible, and that can only be done by informed and thoughtful consideration. This book, then, can serve as a beginning for what ideally will become an ongoing process of examination and reflection.

In approaching each new edition, the editor must make some hard choices of her own. In trying to keep the selections up-to-date, sometimes older ones must be replaced. In other instances, newer articles are just that—newer, but not necessarily better. Striking a balance between timeliness and timelessness is challenging. For each issue, additional points of view are noted in the postscripts, and readers are encouraged to pursue these references.

Changes to this edition Many popular issues and the basic structure of the book remain from the previous edition. There are seven units: Medical Decision Making; End-of-Life Dilemmas (formerly Death and Dying); Choices in Reproduction; Children, Adolescents, and Bioethics; Genetics; Human Experimentation (formerly Human and Animal Experimentation); and Bioethics and Public Policy. There are four completely new issues: "Is 'Palliative Sedation' Ethically Different from Active Euthanasia? (Issue 5); "Do the Potential Benefits of Synthetic Biology Outweigh the Possible Risks?" (Issue 13); "Does Community Consultation in Research Protect Vulnerable Groups?" (Issue 15); and "Is It Fair to Require Individuals to Purchase Health Insurance?" (Issue 16). In addition, one issue from a previous edition has been restored: "Should There Be a Market in Human Organs?" (Issue 17), with a new "Yes" selection. There are two new selections for Issue 4 ("Have Advance Directives Failed?"). There are new "Yes" selections in Issue 11 ("Should Vaccination for HPV Be Mandated for Teenage Girls?", Issue 14 ("Should New Drugs Be Given to Patients Outside Clinical Trials?"), and Issue 19 ("Should Performance-Enhancing Drugs Be Banned from Sports?"). In all there are 17 new selections. Unit introductions, issue introductions, and postscripts have been updated as necessary. Also, the *Internet References* page that begins each unit offers relevant Internet site addresses (URLs) that should prove useful as starting points for further research.

A word to the instructor   An *Instructor's Resource Guide with Test Questions* (multiple choice and essay) is available through the publisher, and a general guidebook, *Using Taking Sides in the Classroom,* which discusses methods and techniques for using the pro–con approach in any classroom setting, is also available. An online version of *Using Taking Sides in the Classroom* and a correspondence service for *Taking Sides* adopters can be found at http://www.mhcls .com/usingts/.

Taking Sides: Clashing Views on Bioethical Issues is only one title in the *Taking Sides* series. If you are interested in seeing the table of contents for any of the other titles, please visit the *Taking Sides* Web site at http://www.mhcls .com/takingsides/.

Many people have helped on previous editions, chief among them Alexis Kuerbis, Dillan Siegler, Ben Munisteri, and Lauri Posner. Paul Homer, Eric Feldman, and Arthur Caplan were generously helpful at earlier stages of the series. Daniel Callahan and Willard Gaylin, cofounders of The Hastings Center, were instrumental in encouraging me to take on this project.

Carol Levine
United Hospital Fund

For Hannah, Amy, Asher, Maddy, and Max

Contents In Brief

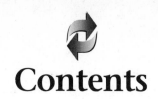

Contents

Physician Robert M. Arnold and professor of psychiatry and sociology Charles W. Lidz assert that informed consent in clinical care is an essential process that promotes good communication and patient autonomy despite the obstacles of implementation. Philosopher Onora O'Neill argues that the most evident change in medical practice in recent decades may be a loss of trust in physicians rather than any growth of patient autonomy. Informed consent in practice, she says, often amounts simply to a right to choose or refuse treatments, not a deeper and more meaningful expression of self-mastery.

Leslie J. Blackhall, Gelya Frank, and Sheila Murphy, from the University of Southern California, and Vicki Michel, from the Loyola Law School, advise clinical and bioethics professionals facing truth-telling dilemmas to make room for the diverse ethical views of the populations they serve. Philosopher Mark Kuczewski and bioethicist Patrick J. McCruden argue that by insisting on informed consent or an appropriate waiver process, the health care system respects cultural differences rather than stereotyping them.

Paul Antony, Chief Medical Officer of Pharmaceutical Research and Manufacturers of America (PhRMA), asserts that direct-to-consumer advertising can be a powerful tool in educating millions of people and improving their health through better communication with physicians, better adherence to medication regimens, and more active involvement in their own health care. Physicians David A. Kessler and Douglas A. Levy contend that as a result of direct-to-consumer advertising, consumers ultimately take medicines they may not need, spend money on brand medicines that may be no better than alternatives, or avoid healthy behaviors.

UNIT 2   END-OF-LIFE DILEMMAS   61

Psychologist Angela Fagerlin and law professor Carl E. Schneider believe not only that living wills have failed to live up to their advocates' expectations but also that these expectations were unrealistic from the start. Susan E. Hickman, Bernard J. Hammes, Alvin H. Moss, and Susan W. Tolle, multidisciplinary specialists in end-of-life care, recognize the limitations of traditional advance directives but argue that newer processes of introducing advance directives can achieve their original aims.

The American Medical Association affirms that in cases of extreme suffering the physician's duty to relieve pain and suffering includes palliative sedation—using drugs that result in unconsciousness and may hasten death. Philosopher Margaret P. Battin believes that palliative or terminal sedation is an unsatisfying compromise that offers no greater protection against abuse than do institutional safeguards established for direct physician aid in dying.

Physician Marcia Angell asserts that a physician's main duties are to respect patient autonomy and to relieve suffering, even if that sometimes means assisting in a patient's death. Physician Kathleen M. Foley counters that if physician-assisted suicide becomes legal, it will begin to substitute for interventions that otherwise might enhance the quality of life for dying patients.

Philosopher Patrick Lee and professor of jurisprudence Robert P. George assert that human embryos and fetuses are complete (though immature) human beings and that intentional abortion is unjust and objectively immoral. Philosopher Margaret Olivia Little believes that the moral status of the fetus is only one aspect of the morality of abortion. She points to gestation as an intimacy, motherhood as a relationship, and creation as a process to advance a more nuanced approach.

Jean Toal states the Majority Opinion in a case involving a pregnant woman's use of crack cocaine, the Supreme Court of South Carolina

Physician Emil J. Freireich believes that patients with advanced cancer and limited life expectancy should have the same privilege as all individuals in a free society. Law professor George J. Annas argues that there is no constitutional right to demand experimental interventions, and that fully open access would undermine the FDA's ability to protect the public from unsafe drugs.

Neal Dickert and Jeremy Sugarman, physicians and ethicists, propose ethical goals for evaluating community consultation in research, which they believe will protect communities as well as individuals from harm. Philosopher Eric T. Juengst asserts that community consultation can provide researchers with cultural insights and assist in recruiting participants but not offer protection for communities.

UNIT 7   BIOETHICS AND PUBLIC POLICY   285

Law professor Sara Rosenbaum and economist Jonathan Gruber contend that the provision of the health reform legislation requiring individuals who are not covered by an employer health plan to pay a penalty if they do not buy health insurance is constitutional and the only way that access to health care can be assured for all. Economics professor Glen Whitman argues that the individual tax mandate is based on false assumptions about the level of uncompensated care and is likely to drive up costs rather than result in savings.

Law student Donald W. Herbe asserts that pharmacists' moral beliefs concerning abortion and emergency contraception are genuinely fundamental and deserve respect. He proposes that professional pharmaceutical organizations lead the way to recognizing a true right of conscience, which would eventually result in universal legislation protecting against all potential ramifications of choosing conscience. Julie Cantor, a lawyer, and Ken Baum, a physician and lawyer, reject an absolute right to object, as well as no right to object, to these prescriptions but assert that pharmacists who cannot or will not dispense a drug have a professional obligation to meet the needs of their customers by referring them elsewhere.

Correlation Guide

The *Taking Sides* series presents current issues in a debate-style format designed to stimulate student interest and develop critical thinking skills. Each issue is thoughtfully framed with an issue summary, an issue introduction, and a postscript. The pro and con essays—selected for their liveliness and substance—represent the arguments of leading scholars and commentators in their fields.

Taking Sides: Clashing Views on Bioethical Issues, 14/e is an easy-to-use reader that presents issues on important topics such as *Advance Directives*, *HPV Vaccination*, and *Synthetic Biology*. For more information on *Taking Sides* and other *McGraw-Hill Contemporary Learning Series* titles, visit http://www.mhhe.com/cls.

This convenient guide matches the issues in **Taking Sides: Bioethical Issues, 14/e** with the corresponding chapters in one of our best-selling McGraw-Hill Ethics textbooks by DeGrazia et al.

Taking Sides: Bioethical Issues, 14/e	Biomedical Ethics, 7/e by DeGrazia et al.
Issue 1: Is Informed Consent Still Central to Medical Ethics?	**Chapter 1:** General Introduction
Issue 2: Should Truth-Telling Depend on the Patient's Culture?	**Chapter 2:** The Professional-Patient Relationship
Issue 3: Does Direct-to-Consumer Drug Advertising Enhance Patient Choice?	**Chapter 13:** Contested Therapies and Biomedical Enhancement **Chapter 9:** Social Justice and Health-Care Policy
Issue 4: Have Advance Directives Failed?	**Chapter 5:** Death and Decisions Regarding Life-Sustaining Treatment
Issue 5: Is "Palliative Sedation" Ethically Different from Active Euthanasia?	**Chapter 6:** Suicide, Physician-Assisted Suicide, and Active Euthanasia
Issue 6: Should Physicians Be Allowed to Assist in Patient Suicide?	**Chapter 6:** Suicide, Physician-Assisted Suicide, and Active Euthanasia
Issue 7: Is Abortion Immoral?	**Chapter 7:** Abortion and Embryonic Stem-Cell Research
Issue 8: Should a Pregnant Woman Be Punished for Exposing Her Fetus to Risk?	**Chapter 8:** Genetics and Human Reproduction
Issue 9: Should Adolescents Be Allowed to Make Their Own Life-and-Death Decisions?	**Chapter 5:** Death and Decisions Regarding Life-Sustaining Treatment
Issue 10: Is It Ethical to Use Steroids and Surgery to Stunt Disabled Children's Growth?	**Chapter 4:** Human and Animal Research
Issue 11: Should Vaccination for HPV Be Mandated for Teenage Girls?	**Chapter 9:** Social Justice and Health-Care Policy

(continued)

Taking Sides: Bioethical Issues, 14/e	Biomedical Ethics, 7/e by DeGrazia et al.
Issue 12: Is Genetic Enhancement an Unacceptable Use of Technology?	**Chapter 8:** Genetics and Human Reproduction
Issue 13: Do the Potential Benefits of Synthetic Biology Outweigh the Possible Risks?	**Chapter 13:** Contested Therapies and Biomedical Enhancement
Issue 14: Should New Drugs Be Given to Patients Outside Clinical Trials?	**Chapter 4:** Human and Animal Research
Issue 15: Does Community Consultation in Research Protect Vulnerable Groups?	**Chapter 2:** The Professional-Patient Relationship
Issue 16: Is It Fair to Require Individuals to Purchase Health Insurance?	**Chapter 9:** Social Justice and Health-Care Policy
Issue 17: Should There Be a Market in Human Organs?	**Chapter 9:** Social Justice and Health-Care Policy
Issue 18: Does Military Necessity Override Medical Ethics?	**Chapter 1:** General Introduction
Issue 19: Should Performance-Enhancing Drugs Be Banned from Sports?	**Chapter 13:** Contested Therapies and Biomedical Enhancement
Issue 20: Should Pharmacists Be Allowed to Deny Prescriptions on Grounds of Conscience?	**Chapter 2:** The Professional-Patient Relationship

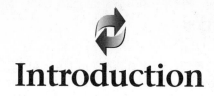

Introduction

Medicine and Moral Arguments

Carol Levine

In the fall of 1975 a 21-year-old woman lay in a New Jersey hospital—as she had for months—in a coma, the victim of a toxic combination of barbiturates and alcohol. Doctors agreed that her brain was irreversibly damaged and that she would never recover. Her parents, after anguished consultation with their priest, asked the doctors and hospital to disconnect the respirator that was artificially maintaining their daughter's life. When the doctors and hospital refused, the parents petitioned the court to be made her legal guardian so that they could authorize the withdrawal of treatment. After hearing all the arguments, the court sided with the parents, and the respirator was removed. Contrary to everyone's expectations, however, the young woman did not die but began to breathe on her own (perhaps because, in anticipation of the court order, the nursing staff had gradually weaned her from total dependence on the respirator). She lived for 10 years until her death in June 1985—comatose, lying in a fetal position, and fed with tubes—in a New Jersey nursing home.

The young woman's name was Karen Ann Quinlan, and her case brought national attention to the thorny ethical questions raised by modern medical technology: When, if ever, should life-sustaining technology be withdrawn? Is the sanctity of life an absolute value? What kinds of treatment are really beneficial to a patient in a "chronic vegetative state" like Karen's? And, perhaps the most troubling question, who shall decide? These and similar questions are at the heart of the growing field of biomedical ethics, or (as it is usually called) *bioethics*.

Ethical dilemmas in medicine are, of course, nothing new. They have been recognized and discussed in Western medicine since a small group of physicians—led by Hippocrates—on the Isle of Cos in Greece, around the fourth century BC subscribed to a code of practice that newly graduated physicians still swear to uphold today. But unlike earlier times, when physicians and scientists had only limited abilities to change the course of disease, today they can intervene in profound ways in the most fundamental processes of life and death. Moreover, ethical dilemmas in medicine are no longer considered the sole province of professionals. Professional codes of ethics, to be sure, offer some guidance, but they are usually unclear and ambiguous about what to do in specific situations. More important, these codes assume that whatever decision is to be made is up to the professional, not the patient. Today, to an ever-greater degree, laypeople—patients, families, lawyers, clergy, and others—want to and have become involved in ethical decision making not only in individual cases, such as the Quinlan case, but also in large societal decisions, such as how to allocate scarce medical resources, including high-technology machinery, newborn intensive care units, and the expertise of physicians. While questions about the physician–patient relationship and individual cases are still prominent in bioethics (see, for example, the issues on truth telling and assisting dying patients in suicide), today the field covers a broad range of other decisions as well, such as the use of genetic technology, the harvesting and transplantation of organs, equity in access to health care and medication, and experimentation involving human subjects.

This involvement is part of broader social trends: a general disenchantment with the authority of all professionals and, hence, a greater readiness to challenge the traditional belief that "doctor knows best"; the growth of various civil rights movements among women, the aged, and minorities—of which the patients' rights movement is a spin-off; the enormous size and complexity of the health care delivery system, in which patients and families often feel alienated from the professionals; the increasing cost of medical care, much of it at public expense; and the growth of the "medical model," in which conditions that used to be considered outside the scope of physicians' control, such as alcoholism and behavioral problems, have come to be considered diseases.

Bioethics began in the 1950s as an intellectual movement among a small group of physicians and theologians who started to examine the questions raised by the new medical technologies that were starting to emerge as the result of the heavy expenditure of public funds in medical research after World War II. They were soon joined by a number of philosophers who had become disillusioned with what they saw as the arid abstractions of much analytic philosophy at the time and by lawyers who sought to find principles in the law that would guide ethical decision making or, if such principles were not there, to develop them by case law and legislation or regulation. Although these four disciplines—medicine, theology, philosophy, and law—still dominate the field, today bioethics is an interdisciplinary effort, with political scientists, economists, sociologists, anthropologists, nurses, allied health professionals, policymakers, psychologists, and others contributing their special perspectives to the ongoing debates.

The issues discussed in this volume attest to the wide range of bioethical dilemmas, their complexity, and the passion they arouse. But if bioethics today is at the frontiers of scientific knowledge, it is also a field with ancient roots. It goes back to the most basic questions of human life: What is right? What is wrong? How should people act toward others? And why?

While the *bio* part of *bioethics* gives the field its urgency and immediacy, we should not forget that the root word is *ethics*.

Applying Ethics to Medical Dilemmas

To see where bioethics fits into the larger framework of academic inquiry, some definitions are in order. First, *morality* is the general term for an individual's or a society's standards of conduct, both actual and ideal, and of the character traits that determine whether people are considered "good" or "bad." The scientific study of morality is called *descriptive ethics;* a scientist—generally an anthropologist, sociologist, or historian—can describe in empirical terms what the moral beliefs, judgments, or actions of individuals or societies are and what reasons are given for the way they act or what they believe. The philosophical study of morality, however, approaches the subject of morality in one of two different ways: either as an analysis of the concepts, terms, and methods of reasoning (*metaethics*) or as an analysis of what those standards or moral judgments ought to be (*normative ethics*). Metaethics deals with meanings of moral terms and logic; normative ethics, with which the issues in this volume are concerned, reflects on the kinds of actions and principles that will promote moral behavior.

Because normative ethics accepts the idea that some acts and character traits are more moral than others (and that some are immoral), it rejects the rather popular idea that ethics is relative. Because different societies have different moral codes and values, ethical relativists have argued that there can be no universal moral judgments: What is right or wrong depends on who does it and where, and whether or not society approves. Although it is certainly true that moral values are embedded in a social, cultural, and political context, it is also true that certain moral judgments are universal. We think it is wrong, for example, to sell people into slavery—whether or not a certain society approved or even whether or not a person wanted to be a slave. People may not agree about what these universal moral values are or ought to be, but it is hard to deny that some such values exist.

The other relativistic view rejected by normative ethics is the notion that whatever feels good *is* good. In this view, ethics is a matter of personal preference, weightier than one's choice of which automobile to buy, but not much different in kind. Different people, having different feelings, can arrive at equally valid moral judgments, according to the relativistic view. Just as we should not disregard cultural factors, we should not overlook the role of emotion and personal experience in arriving at moral judgments. But to give emotion ultimate authority would be to consign reason and rationality—the bases of moral argument—to the ethical trash heap. At the very least, it would be impossible to develop a just policy concerning the care of vulnerable persons, like the mentally retarded or newborns, who depend solely on the vagaries of individual caretakers.

Thus, if normative ethics is one branch of philosophy, bioethics is one branch of normative ethics; it is normative ethics applied to the practice of medicine and science. There are other branches—business ethics, legal ethics, journalism ethics, and military ethics, for example. One common term for the entire grouping is *applied and professional ethics,* because these ethics deal with the ethical standards of the members of a particular profession and how they are applied in the professionals' dealings with each other and the rest of society. Bioethics is based on the belief that some solutions to the dilemmas that arise in medicine and science are more moral than others and that these solutions can be determined by moral reasoning and reflection.

Ethical Theories

If the practitioners of bioethics do not rely solely on cultural norms and emotions, what are their sources of determining what is right or wrong? The most comprehensive source is a theory of ethics—a broad set of moral principles (or perhaps just one overriding principle) that is used in measuring human conduct. Divine law is one such source, of course, but even in the Western religious traditions of bioethics (both the Jewish and Catholic religions have rich and comprehensive commentaries on ethical issues, and the Protestant religion has a less cohesive but still important tradition) the law of God is interpreted in terms of human moral principles. Recently, bioethicists have paid more attention to analyzing the teachings of other religious traditions, such as Islam, Buddhism, Confucianism, and other Eastern religions. A theory of ethics must be acceptable to many groups, not just the followers of one religious tradition. Most writers outside the religious traditions (and some within them) have looked to one of three major traditions in ethics: teleological theories, deontological theories, and natural law theories.

Teleological Theories

Teleological theories are based on the idea that the end or purpose (from the Greek *telos,* or end) of the action determines its rightness or wrongness. The most prominent teleological theory is *utilitarianism.* In its simplest formulation, an act is moral if it brings more good consequences than bad ones. Utilitarian theories are derived from the works of two English philosophers: Jeremy Bentham (1748–1832) and John Stuart Mill (1806–1873). Rejecting the absolutist religious morality of his time, Bentham proposed that "utility"—the greatest good for the greatest number—should guide the actions of human beings. Invoking the hedonistic philosophy of Epicurean Greeks, Bentham said that pleasure (*hedon* in Greek) is good and pain is bad. Therefore, actions are right if they promote more pleasure than pain and wrong if they promote more pain than pleasure. Mill found the highest utility in "happiness," rather than pleasure. (Mill's philosophy is echoed in the Declaration of Independence's espousal of "life, liberty, and the pursuit of happiness.") Other utilitarians have looked to a range of utilities, or goods (including friendship, love, devotion, and the like) that they believe ought to be weighed in the balance—the utilitarian calculus.

Utilitarianism has a pragmatic appeal. It is flexible, and it seems impartial. However, its critics point out that utilitarianism can be used to justify suppression of individual rights for the good of society ("the ends justify the means") and that it is difficult to quantify and compare "utilities," however they are defined.

Utilitarianism, in its many forms, has had a powerful influence on bioethical discussion, partly because it is the closest to the case-by-case risk/benefit ratio that physicians use in clinical decision making. Joseph Fletcher, a Protestant theologian who was one of the pioneers in bioethics in the 1950s, developed utilitarian theories that he called *situation ethics.* He argued that a true Christian morality does not blindly follow moral rules but acts from love and sensitivity to the particular situation and the needs of those involved. He has enthusiastically supported most modern technologies on the grounds that they lead to good ends.

Writers in this volume who use modified utilitarian theories to arrive at their moral judgments include Lawrence O. Gostin, who defends giving public health agencies sweeping powers in a bioterrorist threat, and Gregory E. Kaebnick, who supports synthetic biology experiments.

Deontological Theories

The second major type of ethical theory is *deontological* (from the Greek *deon*, or duty). The rightness or wrongness of an act, these theories hold, should be judged on whether or not it conforms to a moral principle or rule, not on whether it leads to good or bad consequences. The primary exponent of a deontological theory was Immanuel Kant (1724–1804), a German philosopher. Kant declared that there is an ultimate norm, or supreme duty, which he called the "Moral Law." He held that an act is moral only if it springs from a "good will," the only thing that is good without qualification.

We must do good things, said Kant, because we have a duty to do them, not because they result in good consequences or because they give us pleasure (although that can happen as well). Kant constructed a formal "Categorical Imperative," the ultimate test of morality: "I ought never to act except in such a way that I can also will that my maxim should become universal law." Recognizing that this formulation was far from clear, Kant said the same thing in three other ways. He explained that a moral rule must be one that can serve as a guide for everyone's conduct; it must be one that permits people to treat each other as ends in themselves, not solely as means to another's ends; and it must be one that each person can impose on himself or herself by his or her own will, not one that is solely imposed by the state, one's parents, or God. Kant's Categorical Imperative, in the simplest terms, says that all persons have equal moral worth and that no rule can be moral unless all people can apply it autonomously to all other human beings. Although on its own Kant's Categorical Imperative is merely a formal statement with no moral content at all, he gave some examples of what he meant: "Do not commit suicide," and "Help others in distress."

Kantian ethics is criticized by many who note that Kant gives little guidance on what to do when ethical principles conflict, as they often do. Moreover, they say, his emphasis on autonomous decision making and individual will neglects the social and communal context in which people live and make decisions. It leads to isolation and unreality. These criticisms notwithstanding, Kantian ethics has stimulated much current thinking in bioethics. In this volume, the idea that certain actions are in and of themselves right or wrong underlies, for example, Patrick Lee and Robert P. George's argument against abortion because it involves killing a human being, and Donald W. Herbe's defense of a pharmacist's right to refuse to fill some prescriptions on ground of conscience.

Two modern deontological theorists are philosophers John Rawls and Robert M. Veatch. In *A Theory of Justice* (1971), Rawls places the highest value on equitable distribution of society's resources. He believes that society has a fundamental obligation to correct the inequalities of historical circumstance and natural endowment of its least well-off members. According to this theory, some action is good only if it benefits the least well-off. (It can also benefit others, but that is secondary.) His social justice theory has influenced bioethical writings concerning the allocation of scarce resources.

Veatch has applied Rawlsian principles to medical ethics. In his book, *A Theory of Medical Ethics* (1981), he offers a model of social contract among professionals, patients, and society that emphasizes mutual respect and responsibilities. This contract model will, he hopes, avoid the narrowness of professional codes of ethics and the generalities and ambiguities of more broadly based ethical theories.

Natural Law Theory

The third strain of ethical theory that is prominent in bioethics is *natural law theory*, first developed by St. Thomas Aquinas (1223–1274). According to this theory, actions are morally right if they accord with our nature as human beings. The attribute that is distinctively human is the ability to reason and to exercise intelligence. Thus, argues this theory, we can know the good, which is objective and can be learned through reason. References to natural law theory are prominent in the works of Catholic theologians and writers; they see natural law as ultimately derived from God but knowable through the efforts of human beings. The influence of natural law theory can be seen in the issues on genetic enhancement and synthetic biology.

Theory of Virtue

The *theory of virtue,* another ethical theory with deep roots in the Aristotelian tradition, has recently been revived in bioethics. This theory stresses not the morality of any particular actions or rules but the disposition of individuals to act morally, to be virtuous. In its modern version, its primary exponent is Alasdair MacIntyre, whose book *After Virtue* (1980) urges a return to the Aristotelian model. Gregory E. Pence has applied the theory of virtue directly to medicine in *Ethical Options in Medicine* (1980); he lists temperance in personal life, compassion for the suffering patient, professional competence, justice, honesty, courage, and practical judgment as the virtues that are most desirable in physicians. Although this theory has not yet been as fully developed in bioethics as the utilitarian or deontological theories, it is likely to have particular appeal for physicians—many of whom have resisted formal ethics education on the grounds that moral character is the critical factor and that one can best learn to be a moral physician by emulating one's mentors. Although not explicit, assumptions about the qualities of a virtuous physician underlie the discussion in Issue 6 on physician-assisted suicide.

Although various authors, in this volume and elsewhere, appeal in rather direct ways to either utilitarian or deontological theories, often the various types are combined. One may argue both that a particular action is immoral in and of itself and that it will have bad consequences (some commentators say even Kant used this argument). In fact, probably no single ethical theory is adequate to deal with all the ramifications of the issues. In that case we can turn to a middle level of ethical discussion. Between the abstractions of ethical theories (Kant's Categorical Imperative) and the specifics of moral judgments (always obtain informed consent from a patient) is a range of concepts—ethical principles—that can be applied to particular cases.

Ethical Principles

In its 4 years of deliberation in the 1970s, the National Commission for the Protection of Human Subjects of Biomedical and Behavioral Research grappled with some of the most difficult issues facing researchers and society: When, if ever, is it ethical to do research on fetuses, on children, or on people in mental institutions? This commission—which was composed of people from various religious backgrounds, professions, and social strata—was finally able to agree on specific recommendations on these questions, but only after they had finished their work did the commissioners try to determine what ethical principles they had used in reaching a consensus. In their Belmont Report (1978), named after the conference center where they met to discuss this question, the commissioners outlined what they considered to be the three most important ethical principles (respect for persons, beneficence, and justice) that should govern the conduct of research with human beings. These three principles, they believed, are generally accepted in our cultural tradition and can serve as basic justifications for the many particular ethical prescriptions and evaluations of human action. Because of the principles' general acceptance and widespread applicability, they are at the basis of most bioethical discussions. Although philosophers argue about whether other principles—preventing harm to others or loyalty, for example—ought to be accorded equal weight with these three or should be included under another umbrella, they agree that these principles are fundamental.

Respect for Persons

Respect for persons incorporates at least two basic ethical convictions, according to the Belmont Report. Individuals should be treated as autonomous agents, and persons with diminished autonomy are entitled to protection. The derivation from Kant is clear. Because human beings have the capacity for rational action and moral choice, they have a value independent of anything that they can do or provide to others. Therefore, they should be treated in a way that respects their independent choices and judgments. Respecting autonomy means giving weight to autonomous persons' considered opinions and choices, and refraining from interfering with their choices unless those choices are clearly detrimental to others. However, since the capacity for autonomy varies with age, mental disability, or other circumstances, those people whose autonomy is diminished must be protected—but only in ways that serve their interests and do not interfere with the level of autonomy that they do possess. This subject is discussed in Issue 9 on adolescent life-and-death decision making.

Two important moral rules are derived from the ethical principle of respect for persons: informed consent and truth telling. Persons can exercise autonomy only when they have been fully informed about the range of options open to them, and the process of informed consent is generally considered to include the elements of information, comprehension, and voluntariness. Thus, a person can give informed consent to some medical procedure only if he or she has full information about the risks and benefits, understands them, and agrees voluntarily—that is, without being coerced or pressured into agreement. Although the principle of informed consent has become an accepted moral rule (and a legal one as well), it is difficult—some say impossible—to achieve in a real-world setting. It can easily be turned into a legalistic parody or avoided altogether. But as a moral ideal it serves to balance the unequal power of the physician and patient.

Another important moral ideal derived from the principle of respect for persons is truth telling. It held a high place in Kant's theory. In his essay "The Supposed Right to Tell Lies From Benevolent Motives," he wrote: "If, then, we define a lie merely as an intentionally false declaration towards another man, we need not add that it must injure another . . . ; for it always injures another; if not another individual, yet mankind generally. . . . To be truthful in all declarations is therefore a sacred and conditional command of reasons, and not to be limited by any other expediency." Truth telling is discussed in Issue 2.

Other important moral rules that are derived from the principle of respect for persons are confidentiality and privacy.

Beneficence

Most physicians would probably consider beneficence (from the Latin *bene,* or good) the most basic ethical principle. In the Hippocratic Oath it is used this way: "I will apply dietetic measures for the benefit of the sick according to my ability and judgment; I will keep them from harm and injustice." And further on, "Whatever houses I may visit, I will comfort and benefit the sick, remaining free of all intentional injustice." The phrase *Primum non nocere* (First, do no harm) is another well-known version of this idea, but it appears to be a much later, Latinized version—not from the Hippocratic period.

Philosopher William Frankena has outlined four elements included in the principle of beneficence: (1) One ought not to inflict evil or harm; (2) one ought to prevent evil or harm; (3) one ought to remove evil or harm; and (4) one ought to do or promote good. Frankena arranged these elements in hierarchical order, so that the first takes precedence over the second, and so on. In this scheme, it is more important to avoid doing evil or harm than to do good. But in the Belmont Report, beneficence is understood as an obligation—first, to do no harm, and second, to maximize possible benefits and minimize possible harms.

The principle of beneficence is at the basis of Marcia Angell's support of allowing physicians to assist some patients in suicide and of Angela Fagerlin and Carl E. Schneider's concerns that living wills fail to achieve the goal of good care for patients.

Justice

The third ethical principle that is generally accepted is justice, which means "what is fair" or "what is deserved." An injustice occurs when some benefit to which a person is entitled is denied without good reason or when some burden is imposed unduly, according to the Belmont Report. Another way of interpreting the principle is to say that equals should be treated equally. However, some distinctions—such as age, experience, competence, physical condition, and the like—can justify unequal treatment. Those who appeal to the principle of justice are most concerned about which distinctions can be made legitimately and which ones cannot (see Issue 20 on pharmacists' refusals on conscience grounds).

One important derivative of the principle of justice is the recent emphasis on "rights" in bioethics. Given the successes in the 1960s and 1970s of civil rights movements in the courts and political arena, it is easy to understand the appeal of "rights talk." An emphasis on individual rights is part of the American tradition, in a way that emphasis on the "common good" is not. The language of rights has been prominent in the abortion debate, for instance, where the "right to life" has been pitted against the "right to privacy" or the "right to control one's body." The "right to health care" is a potent rallying cry, though it is one that is difficult to enforce legally. Although claims to rights may be effective in marshaling political support and in emphasizing moral ideals, those rights may not be the most effective way to solve ethical dilemmas. Our society, as philosopher Ruth Macklin has pointed out, has not yet agreed on a theory of justice in health care that will determine who has what kinds of rights and—the other side of the coin—who has the obligation to fulfill them.

When Principles Conflict

These three fundamental ethical principles—respect for persons, beneficence, and justice—all carry weight in ethical decision making. But what happens when they conflict? That is what this book is all about.

On each side of the issues included in this volume are writers who appeal, explicitly or implicitly, to one or more of these principles. For example, in Issue 8, Jean Toal sees beneficence as paramount, and she would criminalize drug-using behavior by pregnant women in order to prevent harm to their fetuses. Lynn M. Paltrow finds such a policy unjust because it singles out certain risks and certain women for state intervention.

Some of the issues are concerned with how to interpret a particular principle: Whether, for example, it is more or less beneficent to allow a physician to assist in suicide, or whether society's interest in obtaining transplantable organs for those who need them and allowing hearts to be removed immediately after cardiac death.

Will it ever be possible to resolve such fundamental divisions—those that are not merely matters of procedure or interpretation but of fundamental differences in principle? Lest the situation seems hopeless, consider that some consensus does seem to have been reached on questions that seemed equally tangled a few decades ago. The idea that government should play a role in regulating human subjects research was hotly debated, but it is now generally accepted (at least if the research is medical, not social or behavioral in nature, and is federally funded). And the appropriateness of using the criterion of brain death for determining the death of a person (and the possibility of subsequent removal of their organs for transplantation) has largely been accepted and written into state laws, although there are continuing debates about terminology and public understanding. The idea that a hopelessly ill patient has the legal and moral right to refuse treatment that will only postpone dying is also well established (though it is often hard to exercise because hospitals and physicians continue to resist it). Finally, nearly everyone now agrees that health care is distributed unjustly in the United States—a radical idea only a few years ago. There is, of course, sharp disagreement about whose responsibility it is to rectify the situation—the government's or the private sector's.

In the 27 years since the first edition of this book was published, the dominance of principles as the foundation of bioethics has been challenged. Several philosophers have pointed out, as already noted, that the "mid-level" principles are not grounded in a unified moral theory. Other writers have described the philosophical mode of argument as too arid and abstract, and they have called for the inclusion of other forms of discourse, such as public policy, emotion-based reasoning, and narrative, or "storytelling."

Besides the virtue theory, already described, two other candidates have their defenders. The ethics of caring has been presented as an alternative to traditional bioethics reasoning. Women, it is claimed, embody an ethic of caring, which is itself a prime aim of healing relationships. An ethic of caring would focus on relationships rather than autonomy, on reconciliation rather than winning an argument, and on nurturing rather than imposing dominance. While the absence of caring relationships is clearly a problem in modern health care, this view has been severely criticized by many, including women, as failing to provide a sufficient basis for replacing ethical principles.

Another mode of analysis that is being revived is casuistry. Although associated with the Middle Ages and religious thinking, casuistry is simply a way of reaching consensus on principles by focusing on concrete cases—the clearest ones first, and then the harder ones. The casuist reaches principles from the bottom up, rather than deciding cases from the top (principles first) down.

A final form of analysis is clinical ethics. Its practitioners focus on the clinical realities of moral choices as they emerge in ordinary health care. It is not antithetical to principles but brings abstractions back to reality by measuring proposed solutions against the real world in which doctors and patients live and work.

Edmund Pellegrino, a distinguished physician and ethicist, has seen many changes in the more than 50 years he has been involved in medicine. Looking toward the future, he does not see the death of principles, but he does foresee some changes. "Physicians and other health workers must become familiar with shifts in contemporary moral philosophy," he says, "if they are to maintain a hand in restructuring the ethics of their profession." But clinicians, too, must change, to "provide a reality check on the nihilism and skepticism of contemporary philosophy. Medical ethics is too ancient and too essential . . . to be left entirely to the fortuitous currents of philosophical fashion or the unsupported assertion of clinicians."

Although there is consensus in some areas, in others there is only controversy. This book will introduce you to some of the ongoing debates. Whether or not we will be able to move beyond opposing views to a realm of moral consensus will depend on society's willingness to struggle with these issues and to make the hard choices that are required.

Internet References . . .

Agency for Healthcare Research and Quality (AHRQ)

The AHRQ Web site provides research-based information to increase the scientific knowledge needed to enhance consumer and clinical decision making, improve health care quality, and promote efficiency in the organization of public and private systems of health care delivery.

http://www.ahrq.gov

Bioethics Resources on the Web

Created by the National Institutes of Health Office of Science Policy, this is an excellent starting point and has links to other resources.

http://bioethics.od.nih.gov/

The National Reference Center for Bioethics Literature

Located at the Kennedy Institute of Ethics, Georgetown University, this site has extensive resources on physician–patient relationships and other topics and will perform data researches on request.

http://bioethics.georgetown.edu/

Bioethics: Web Resources

Professor Tom May at Southern Methodist University has created a comprehensive and detailed guide that lists resources by topic, as well as sections on theology and bioethics, institutional links, and journals and newsletters.

http://faculty.smu.edu/tmayo/bioweb.htm

The Hastings Center Bioethics Forum

Among the activities of this bioethics center is the Bioethics Forum, which has timely commentaries on controversial issues.

http://www.thehastingscenter.org/BioethicsForum/

Medical Decision Making

In earlier times medical decision making was of concern only to physicians. With their presumed greater knowledge and with patients' best interests at heart, they were entrusted with making life-and-death, as well as ordinary decisions. Ironically, although physicians had greater authority in those times than they do today, they also had less ability to treat. As medicine has grown more technologically and scientifically sophisticated, the range of people who have an interest in making decisions—and in some cases, a right to do so—among the medical options has grown. Law and ethics have reaffirmed the status of the patient as the primary decision maker. Nevertheless, many ambiguous and troubling situations remain in implementing patients' wishes. It is not even clear that patients have the moral right to make arbitrary decisions about aspects of their care, especially when their preferences impinge on the rights of others, such as family members, physicians, and other patients. Many cultural traditions find Western values, such as truth-telling, harmful to patients. Moreover, as marketplace values have entered medicine in dramatic ways, individuals are now seen more often as "consumers" rather than "patients." Prescription drug advertising that appeals directly to consumers raises questions about the balance between individual autonomy and physician beneficence. This section explores some of the issues that arise when making medical decisions.

- Is Informed Consent Still Central to Medical Ethics?
- Should Truth-Telling Depend on the Patient's Culture?
- Does Direct-to-Consumer Drug Advertising Enhance Patient Choice?

ISSUE 1

Is Informed Consent Still Central to Medical Ethics?

YES: Robert M. Arnold and Charles W. Lidz, from "Informed Consent: Clinical Aspects of Consent in Health Care," in Stephen G. Post, ed., *Encyclopedia of Bioethics,* vol. 3, 3rd ed. (Macmillan, 2003)

NO: Onora O'Neill, from *Autonomy and Trust in Bioethics* (Cambridge University Press, 2002)

ISSUE SUMMARY

YES: Physician Robert M. Arnold and professor of psychiatry and sociology Charles W. Lidz assert that informed consent in clinical care is an essential process that promotes good communication and patient autonomy despite the obstacles of implementation.

NO: Philosopher Onora O'Neill argues that the most evident change in medical practice in recent decades may be a loss of trust in physicians rather than any growth of patient autonomy. Informed consent in practice, she says, often amounts simply to a right to choose or refuse treatments, not a deeper and more meaningful expression of self-mastery.

Informed consent is undoubtedly one of the best-known and, arguably, one of the least-implemented concepts in modern medicine. Although much of modern medical ethics has ancient roots, the idea of informed consent is relatively recent. Until the mid-twentieth century most medical ethics were firmly based on the obligations of physicians to act for the benefit of their patients. Information was supposed to be managed carefully in order to protect patients from bad news and to keep them hopeful.

The first "Code of Medical Ethics" of the American Medical Association relied heavily on the work of Thomas Percival, a British physician whose book *Medical Ethics* (1803) played a crucial role in the field for more than a century. Percival believed that the patient's right to the truth was less important than the physician's obligation to benefit the patient. Deception, in the interest of doing good, was thus justified. The patient's consent to treatment, informed or otherwise, is not mentioned in early codes of medical ethics, although on a practical level doctors had to have a patient's permission to perform most procedures.

The modern concept of informed consent came to medical ethics through the courts. The earliest influential decision was *Schloendorff v. New York Hospital* (1914), in which the court ruled that a patient's right to "self-determination" obligated a physician to obtain consent. This case laid the basis for further litigation. The most influential series of decisions occurred in the 1950s and 1960s, when rulings went beyond the obligation to obtain consent to include an explicit duty to disclose information relevant to the patient who is making a decision about consent.

While the earlier cases had been based on the patient's right to be free from unwanted bodily intrusion (legally, "battery"), the court in *Natanson v. Kline* (1960) held that physicians who withheld information while obtaining consent were guilty of negligence. Imposing a legal duty on physicians to inform their patients of the risks, benefits, and alternatives to treatment exposed them to the risk of malpractice suits. Another factor that influenced the ascendance of informed consent in medical treatment were parallel discussions about the ethics of research involving human subjects. Voluntary consent to participate in research was a cornerstone of the Nuremberg Code of 1947, which was issued after the trials of Nazi physicians who had performed lethal experiments on nonconsenting prisoners.

Nevertheless, traditions die hard, and little change was seen in actual practice until the resurgence of interest in medical ethics in the 1970s. In 1972 the case of *Canterbury v. Spence* established a far-reaching patient-centered disclosure standard. The ruling stated, "The patient's right of self-decision can be effectively exercised only if the patient possesses enough information to enable an intelligent choice. . . . Social policy does not accept the paternalistic view that the physician may remain silent because divulgence might prompt the patient to forego needed therapy." In the 1980s and 1990s court cases have focused on individuals who lack the competence to provide informed consent, such as comatose patients, children, and mentally ill persons.

Although the physician's duty to obtain informed consent and the patient's right to information are now firmly established in law and grounded in the ethical principle of respect for persons, medical practice varies considerably. In Stephen G. Post, ed., *Encyclopedia of Bioethics* (2003), Tom L. Beauchamp and Ruth R. Faden, philosophers who have studied informed consent extensively, assert, "The overwhelming impression from the empirical literature and from reported clinical experience is that the actual process of soliciting informed consent often falls short of a serious show of respect for the decisional authority of patients."

The following selections illustrate two views of the future of informed consent. Robert M. Arnold and Charles W. Lidz reassert the importance of informed consent and offer ways in which the process can be improved in the clinical setting, despite the many obstacles. Onora O'Neill argues that informed consent has not enhanced patient autonomy but has had the opposite effect of lessening patient trust.

YES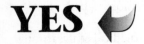

Robert M. Arnold and
Charles W. Lidz

Informed Consent: Clinical Aspects of Consent in Health Care

Clinical Aspects of Consent in Healthcare

Decision making is an everyday event in healthcare, not only for doctors and patients, but also for nurses, psychologists, social workers, emergency medical technicians, dentists, and other health professionals. Since the 1960s, however, the cultural ideal of how these decisions should be made has changed considerably. The concept that medical decision making should rely exclusively on the physician's expertise has been replaced by a model in which healthcare professionals share information and discuss alternatives with patients who then make the ultimate decisions about treatment.

The concept of informed consent gained its initial support as part of the general societal trend toward broadening access to decision making during the 1960s. Thus, the initial support for informed consent came from legal and philosophic circles rather than healthcare professionals. In the legal arena, informed consent has been used to develop minimal standards for doctor–patient interactions and clinical decision making (Berg et al.). Although there are some differences by jurisdiction, widely accepted legal standards require that healthcare professionals inform patients of the risks, benefits, and alternatives of all proposed treatments, and then allow the patient to choose among acceptable therapeutic alternatives.

In academia, informed consent has served as a cornerstone for the development of the discipline of bioethics. Based on the importance of autonomy in moral discourse, philosophers have argued that healthcare professionals are obligated to engage patients in discussions regarding the goals of therapy and the alternatives for reaching those goals, and that patients are the final decision makers regarding all therapeutic decisions.

While many physicians would express some support to the concept of shared decision making, this support is largely theoretical and does not seem to have made its way into routine medical practice. Physicians typically think of informed consent as a legal requirement for a signed piece of paper that is at best a waste of time, and at worst a bureaucratic, legalistic interference with their care for patients. Rather than seeing informed consent as a process that promotes good communication and patient autonomy, many healthcare

From *Encyclopedia of Bioethics* (5 volume set), vol. 3, rev. ed., 2003, pp. 1290–1296. Copyright © 2003 by Gale, a part of Cengage Learning, Inc. Reprinted by permission. www.cengage.com/permissions

professionals view it as a complex, legally prescribed recitation of risks and benefits that only frightens or confuses patients.

Objections to Informed Consent

There are various objections to informed consent that clinicians often make, and it will be useful to review those objections here.

Consent cannot be truly "informed" Many practicing clinicians report that their patients are unable to understand the complex medical information necessary for a fully rational weighing of alternative treatments. There is considerable research support for this view. A variety of studies document that patients recall only a small percentage of the information that professionals present to them (Meisel and Roth); that they are not as good decision makers when they are sick as at other times (Sherlock; Cassell, 2001); and that they often make decisions based on medically trivial factors. Informed consent thus appears either to promote uninformed—and thus suboptimal—decisions, or to encourage patients to blindly accept healthcare professionals' recommendations. In either case informed consent appears to be a charade, and a dangerous one at that.

However, the fact that patients often do have difficulty understanding important aspects of medical decisions does not mean that healthcare professionals are the best decision makers about the patient's treatment. Knowledge about medical facts is not enough. Wise house buyers will have a structural engineer check over an old house, but few would be willing to allow the engineer to choose their house for them. Just as structural engineers cannot decide which house a family should buy—because they lack knowledge about the family's pattern of living, personal tastes, and potential family growth—healthcare professionals cannot scientifically deduce the best treatment for a specific patient simply from the medical facts. What matters to individuals about their health depends on their lifestyles, past experiences, and values, so choosing the *optimal therapy* is not a purely objective matter (U.S. President's Commission). Thus, patients and healthcare professionals both contribute essential knowledge to the decision-making process: patients bring their knowledge of their personal situation, goals, and values; and healthcare professionals bring their expertise on the nature of the problem and the technology that may be used to meet the patient's goals (see Brock).

Informed-consent disclosures, even if they are well done, may not lead to what clinicians might consider optimal decisions. Most people make major life decisions, such as whom to marry and which occupation to take up, based on faulty or incomplete information. Patients' lack of understanding of medical information in choosing treatment is probably no worse than their lack of information in choosing a spouse, nor are medical decisions more important than spousal choice. Respecting patient autonomy means allowing individuals to make their own decisions, even if the healthcare professional disagrees with them. The informed-consent process can improve patient decisions, but it cannot be expected to lead to perfect decisions.

Moreover, although sick persons have defects in their rational abilities, so do healthcare professionals. In fact, some of the most famous research on the difficulties individuals have with the rational use of probabilistic data involves physicians (Dawson and Ackes). Health professionals must be careful not to be too pessimistic about patients' ability to become informed decision makers. Patients may not be able to become as technically well-informed as professionals, but they clearly can understand and make decisions based on relevant information. One study, for example, showed that patients' decisions regarding life-sustaining treatment changed when they were given accurate information about the therapy's chance of success and that patients, when given increased information about screening tests for prostate cancer, were less likely to have the test change their decision on having the test (Murphy et al.). Moreover, what seems to be an irrational decision may turn out to be, from the patient's point of view, rational. Thus, a patient may turn down a recommended treatment because of personal experience with surgery or because the long-term benefit is not seen as being worth the short-term risk.

Most important, the difficulty of educating sick persons does not justify unilateral decision making. Rather, it places a special obligation on healthcare professionals to communicate clearly with patients. Using technical jargon, trying to give all of the available information in one visit, and not asking what the patient wants to know is a recipe for confusing even the most intelligent patient. A growing literature deals with informational aides—ranging from question prompt-sheets to giving patients audiotapes of the interaction and formal decision aides—that can be used to promote patient understanding and shared decision-making. New technologies like interactive DVD offer patients the opportunity to participate more fully in shared decision making at their own rate. A limitation of many of these aides is that they are limited helping with specific decisions and need to be updated frequently (Barry). Healthcare professionals also need to become more familiar with different cultural patterns of communication in order to talk with patients from different cultural backgrounds. For example, although a simple, factual discussion of depression and its treatment may be acceptable to most middle-class Americans, it would be seen as inappropriate by a first-generation Vietnamese male, whose culture discourages viewing depression as a disease (Hahn). There is no reason, in principle, why a person who makes decisions at home and work cannot, with help, understand the medical data sufficiently to become involved in medical decisions. Healthcare professionals must learn how best to present that help and involve patients in the decision-making process.

Patients do not wish to be involved in decision making   Many healthcare professionals believe that it is unfair to force patients to make decisions regarding their medical care. After all, they argue, patients pay their healthcare professionals to make medical decisions. The empirical literature partially supports the view that patients want professionals to make treatment decisions for them (Steel et al.). For example, in a study of male patients' preferences about medical decision making regarding hypertension, only 53 percent wanted to participate at all in the decision-making process (Strull et al.). More recent data suggest that sicker patients are less interested in information about their disease and more willing to have doctors make decisions (Butow 1997; 2002).

There is no reason to force patients to be involved in decisions if they do not want to be. However, unless the health professional asks, he or she cannot know how involved a patient wants to be. Studies suggest that doctors' ability to predict their patients' interest in information, or their desire to be involved in decision making, is no better than flipping a coin (Butow 1997, 2002). In addition, roughly two-thirds of patients want to be involved in decision making, either by being the primary decision maker (the minority) or in shared decision making with the physician.

Patients may not always want to be involved in decision making, since many have been socialized into believing that "the doctor knows best." This is particularly true for poorer patients. Studies have shown that physicians wrongly assume that because patients with fewer socioeconomic resources ask fewer questions, they do not want as much information. These patients may in fact want just as much information, but they have been socialized into a different way of interacting with healthcare professionals (Waitzkin, 1984).

Patients may choose to allow someone else to make the decision for them. However, when a patient asks, "What would you do if you were me?" the underlying question may be, "As an expert in biomedicine, what alternative do you think will best maximize my values or interest?" If this is the case, the healthcare professional should respond by making a recommendation and justifying it in terms of the patient's values or interests. More frequently, the patient is asking, "If you had this disease, what therapy would you choose?" This question presumes that the professional and patient have the same values, needs, and problems, which is often not the case. Healthcare professionals should respond by pointing this out and emphasizing the importance of the patients' values in the decision-making process.

Although many patients do not want to be actively involved in decision making, they almost always want more information concerning their illness than the healthcare professional gives them. Healthcare professionals should not assume that just because patients do not wish to choose their therapy, they do not want information. Patients may desire information so as to increase compliance or make modifications in other areas of their lives, as well as to make medical decisions.

There are harmful effects of informing patients   Healthcare professionals often justify withholding information from patients because of their belief that informing patients would be psychologically damaging and therefore contrary to the principle of nonmaleficence. Many healthcare professionals, however, overestimate potential psychological harm and neglect the positive effects of full disclosure (Faden et al.). Some discussions that physicians assume are stressful, such as advance care-planning, have been shown to decrease patient anxiety and increase the patient's sense of control. Moreover, bad news can often be communicated in a way that ameliorates the psychological effects of the disclosure (Quill and Townsend). Truth-telling must be distinguished from "truth dumping." Explanation of the care that can be provided, and empathic attention to the patient's fears and uncertainties can often prevent or mitigate otherwise more painful news. Finally, sometimes the harm associated with bad news is unavoidable. It is normal to be sad after finding out that one has an incurable cancer, for example. That does not mean that one should not convey the information, only that it should be done in as sensitively and supportively as possible.

Informed consent takes too much time   Respecting autonomy and promoting patient well-being—the values served through informed consent—are fundamental to good medicine. However, adhering to the ideals of medical practice takes time—time to help patients understand their illness and work through their emotional reactions to stressful information, to discuss each party's preconceptions and to clarify the therapeutic goals, to decide on a treatment plan, and to elicit questions about diagnosis and treatment.

In U.S. healthcare, time is money. As many commentators have noted, physicians are less well reimbursed for talking to patients than for performing invasive tests. This may discourage doctors from spending enough time discussing treatment options with patients. This, along with the pressures of managed care has decreased the average outpatient encounter, allowing even less time for doctor–patient communication. The ultimate justification for spending time to facilitate patient decisions is the same as that for spending any time in medical care: that patients will be better cared for. Moreover, some of the new decision aides, such as question prompts, may in fact decrease the time spent in the patient visit, while simultaneously increasing patient understanding.

Clinical Approaches to Informed Consent

Many of the problems in implementing informed consent result, at least in part, from the way informed consent has been implemented in clinical practice. Informed consent has become synonymous with the *consent form,* a legal invention with a legitimate role in documenting that informed consent has taken place, but hardly a substitute for the discussion process leading to informed consent (Andrews).

A pro forma approach: an event model of informed consent   In many clinical settings, consent begins when *it is time to get consent,* typically just prior to the administration of treatment. The process of getting the patients' consent consists of the recitation by a physician or nurse of the list of material risks and benefits and a request that the patient sign for the proposed treatment. This "conversation" is a very limited one that emphasizes the transfer of information from the physician or nurse to the patient. While it does meet the minimal legal requirements for informed consent efficiently, it does not meet the higher ethical goal of informed consent, which is to empower patients by educating and involving them in their treatment plans. Instead, it imposes an almost empty ritual on an unchanged relationship between provider and patient (Katz).

The procedure just described assumes that care involves a series of dis-crete, circumscribed decisions. In fact, much of clinical medicine consists of a series of frequent, interwoven decisions that must be repeatedly reconsid-ered as more information becomes available. When "it is time to get con-sent," there may be nothing left to decide. Consider the operative consent form obtained the evening prior to an operation. After patients have discussed with their families whether to be admitted to the hospital, rearranged their work and child-care schedules, and undergone a long and painful diagnostic workup, the decision to have surgery seems preordained. The evening before the operation, patients do not seriously evaluate the operation's risks and ben-efits, so consent is pro forma. No wonder some healthcare professionals feel that *consent* is a waste of time and energy.

The event model for gathering informed consent falls far short of meeting the ethical goal of ensuring patient participation in the decision-making process. Rather than engaging the patient as an active participant in the decision-making process, the patient's role is to agree to or veto the health-care professionals' recommendations. Little attempt is made to elicit patient preferences and consider how treatment might address them.

A dialogical approach: the process model of informed consent   Fortu-ately, it is possible to fulfill legal requirements for informed consent while maximizing active patient participation in the clinical setting. An alternative to the event model described above, which sees informed consent as an aber-ration from clinical practice, the process model attempts to integrate informed consent into all aspects of clinical care (Berg et al). The process model of informed consent assumes that each party has something to contribute to the decision-making process. The physician brings technical knowledge and experience in treating patients with similar problems, while patients bring knowledge about their life circumstances and the ability to assess the effect that treatment may have on them. Open discussion makes it possible for the patient and the physician to examine critically their views and to determine what might be optimal treatment.

The process model also recognizes that medical care rarely involves only one decision made at a single point in time. Decisions about care frequently begin with the suspicion that something is wrong and that treatment may be necessary, and they end only when the patient leaves follow-up care. Deci-sions involve diagnostic as well as therapeutic interventions. Some decisions are made in one visit, while others occur over a prolonged period of time. Although some interactions between provider and patient involve explicit decisions, decisions are made at each interaction, even if the decision is only to continue treatment. The process model also recognizes that various health-care professionals may play a role in making sure that the patients' consent is informed. For example, a woman deciding on various breast cancer treatments may talk with an oncologist and a surgeon about the risks of various treat-ments, with a nurse about the side effects of medication, with a social worker about financial issues in treatment, and with a patient-support group about her husband's reaction to a possible mastectomy.

Ideally, then, informed consent involves shared decision making over a period of time; in a dialogue throughout the course of the patient's relationship with various healthcare professionals. Such a dialogue aims to facilitate patient participation and to strengthen the therapeutic alliance.

Tasks Involved in Informed Consent

Consent is a series of interrelated tasks. First, the patient and professional must agree on the problem that will be the focus of their work together (Eisenthal and Lazare). Most nonemergency consultations involve complex negotiations between healthcare professional and patient regarding the definition of the patient's problem. The patient may see the problem as a routine physical examination for a work release, the need for advice, or the investigation of a physical symptom. If professionals are to respond effectively to the patients' goals, they must find out the reason for the visit. Whereas physicians typically focus on biomedical information and its implications, patients typically view the problem in the context of their social situation (Fisher and Todd). The differences between the patient's perceptions of the problem and the professional's perceptions must be explicitly worked through, since agreement regarding the focus of the interactions will lead to increased patient satisfaction and compliance with further treatment plans (Meichenbaum and Turk).

Even when the professional and patient have agreed on what the problem is, substantial misunderstandings may arise regarding the treatment goals. Patients may expect the medically impossible, or they may expect outcomes based on knowledge of life circumstances about which the physician is unaware. Since assessing the risks and benefits of any treatment option depends on therapeutic goals, the professional and patient must agree on the goals the therapy aims to accomplish.

Finding out what the patient wants is more complicated than merely inquiring, "What do you want?" A patient typically does not come to the professional with well-developed preferences regarding medical therapy except "to get better," with little understanding of what this may involve (Cassell, 1985). As a patient's knowledge and perspective change over the course of an illness, so too may the patient's views regarding the therapeutic goals.

Because clinicians provide much of the medical information needed to ensure that the patient's preferences are grounded in medical possibility, healthcare professionals play a significant role in how a patient's preferences evolve. It is important that they understand that patients may reasonably hold different goals from those their practitioners hold. This is particularly true when they come from different economic strata. For example, a physician's emphasis on the most medically sophisticated care may pale in the light of the patient's financial problems. Therapeutic goals, like the definition of the problem, require ongoing clarification and negotiation.

After agreeing upon the problem and the therapeutic goals, the healthcare professional and the patient must choose the best way to achieve them. If patients have been involved in the prior two steps, the decision about a treatment plan will more likely reflect their values than if they are merely asked to assent to the clinician's strategy.

Healthcare professionals often ask how much information they must supply to ensure that the patient is an informed participant in the decision-making process (Mazur). There is, however, a more important question: Has the information been provided in a manner that the patient can understand? While the law only requires that healthcare professionals inform patients, morally valid consent requires that patients understand the information conveyed. Ensuring patient understanding requires attention to the quality as well as the quantity of information presented (Faden).

A great deal of empirical data has been collected concerning problems with consent forms. These forms have been criticized, for example, as being unintelligible because of their length and use of technical language (Berg et al.). Healthcare professionals thus need to be aware of, and facile in using, a variety of methods to increase patients' comprehension of information, including verbal techniques, written information, and interactive videodiscs (Stanley et al.).

Still, the question of how much information to present remains. The legal standards regarding information disclosure—what a reasonable patient would find essential to making a decision or what a reasonably prudent physician would disclose—are not particularly helpful. Howard Brody has suggested two important features: (1) the physician must disclose the basis on which the proposed treatment or the alternative possible treatments have been chosen; and (2) the patient must be encouraged to ask questions suggested by the physician's reasoning—and the questions need to be answered to the patient's satisfaction (Brody). Healthcare professionals must also inform patients when controversy exists about the various therapeutic options. Similarly, patients should also be told the degree to which the recommendation is based on established scientific evidence rather than personal experience or educated guesses.

Two other factors will influence the amount of information that should be given: the importance of the decision (given the patient's situation and goals) and the amount of consensus within the healthcare professions regarding the agreed-upon therapy. For example, a low-risk intervention, such as giving influenza vaccines to elderly patients, offers a clear-cut benefit with minimal risk. In this case, the professional should describe the intervention and recommend it because of its benefits. A detailed description of the infrequent risks is not needed unless the patient asks or is known to be skeptical of medical interventions. Interventions that present greater risks or a less clear-cut risk-benefit ratio require a longer description—for example, the decision to administer AZT to an HIV (human immunodeficiency virus)-positive, asymptomatic woman with a CD4 cell count of 350. In this situation, the data regarding starting medications are unclear and a patient's preference is critical. In this situation, one would need to talk about the major side effects of the medicines, the burden of taking medicines daily, the immunological benefit of anti-virals, etc. In neither case is a discussion of pathophysiology or biochemistry necessary. It must be emphasized that there is no formula for deciding how much a patient needs to be told or the length of time this will take. The amount of information necessary will depend on the patient's individual situation, values, and goals.

Finally, an adequate decision-making process requires continual updating of information, monitoring of expectations, and evaluation of the patient's progress in reaching the chosen or revised goals. Thus, the final step in informed consent is follow-up. This step is particularly important for patients with chronic diseases for which modifications of the treatment plan are often necessary.

The process model of informed consent has many advantages. Because it assumes many short conversations over time rather than one long interaction, it can be more easily integrated into the professional's ambulatory practice than the event model. It also allows patients to be much more involved in decision making and ensures that treatment is more consistent with their values. Furthermore, the continual monitoring of patients' understanding of their disease, the treatment, and its progress is likely to reduce misunderstandings and increase their investment in, and adherence to, the treatment plan. Thus, the process model of informed consent is likely to promote both patient autonomy and well-being.

Unfortunately, there are situations in which this approach is not very helpful. Some healthcare professionals, anesthesiologists, or emergency medical technicians, for example, are not likely to have ongoing relationships with patients. In emergencies, there is not time for a decision to develop through a series of short conversations. In these cases, informed consent may more closely approximate the event model. However, since most medical care is delivered by primary-care practitioners in an ambulatory setting, the process model of informed consent is more helpful.

Bibliography

Andrews, Lori B. 1984. "Informed Consent Status and the Decision-making Process." *Journal of Legal Medicine* 5(2): 163–217.

Barry, M. 2000. "Involving Patients in Medical Decisions: How Can Physicians Do Better?" *Journal of the American Medical Association* 282(24): 2356–2357.

Berg, Jessica; Appelbaum, Paul S.; Lidz, Charles W.; et al. 2001. *Informed Consent: Legal Theory and Clinical Practice,* 2nd edition. New York: Oxford University Press.

Brock, Dan W. 1991. "The Ideal of Shared Decision Making Between Physicians and Patients." *Kennedy Institute of Ethics Journal* 1(1): 28–47.

Braddock, C. H.; Fihn, S. D.; Levinson, W.; et al. 1997. "How Doctors and Patients Discuss Routine Clinical Decisions: Informed Decision Making in the Outpatient Setting." *Journal of General Internal Medicine* 12(6): 339–345.

Brody, Howard. 1989. "Transparency: Informed Consent in Primary Care." *Hastings Center Report* 19(5): 5–9.

Butow, P. N.; Dowsett, S.; Hagerty, R.; et al. 2002. "Communicating Prognosis to Patients with Metastatic Disease: What Do They Really Want to Know?" *Supportive Care in Cancer* 10(2): 161–168.

Butow, P. N.; Maclean, M.; Dunn, S. M.; et al. 1997. "The Dynamics of Change: Cancer Patients' Preferences for Information, Involvement, and Support." *Annals of Oncology* 8: 857–863.

Cassell, Eric J. 1985. *Talking with Patients.* 2 vols. Cambridge, MA: MIT Press.

Cassell, Eric J. 2001. "Preliminary Evidence of Impaired Thinking in Sick Patients." *Annals of Internal Medicine* 134(12): 1120–1123.

Dawson, Neal V., and Arkes, Hal R. 1987. "Systematic Errors in Medical Decision Making: Judgment Limitations." *Journal of General Internal Medicine* 2(3): 183–187.

Eisenthal, Sherman, and Lazare, Aaron. 1976. "Evaluation of the Initial Interview in a Walk-In Clinic." *Journal of Nervous and Mental Disease* 162(3): 169–176.

Faden, Ruth R. 1977. "Disclosure and Informed Consent: Does It Matter How We Tell It?" *Health Education Monographs* 5(3): 198–214.

Faden, Ruth R.; Beauchamp, Tom L.; and King, Nancy M. P. 1986. *A History and Theory of Informed Consent.* New York: Oxford University Press.

Fisher, Sue, and Todd, Alexandra D., eds. 1983. *The Social Organization of Doctor–Patient Communication.* Washington, D.C.: Center for Applied Linguistics.

Gadow, Sally. 1980. "Existential Advocacy: Philosophic Foundation of Nursing." In *Nursing: Images and Ideals: Opening Dialogue with the Humanities,* ed. Stuart F. Spicker and Sally Gadow. New York: Springer.

Hahn, Robert A. 1982. "Culture and Informed Consent: An Anthropological Perspective." In *Making Health Care Decisions: The Ethical and Legal Implications of Informed Consent in the Patient–Practitioner Relationship,* vol. 2. Washington, D.C.: U.S. President's Commission for the Study of Ethical Problems in Medicine and Biomedical and Behavioral Research.

Katz, Jay. 1984. *The Silent World of Doctor and Patient.* New York: Free Press.

Lidz, Charles W.; Meisel, Alan; Zerubavel, Eviatar; et al., eds. 1984. *Informed Consent: A study of Decision-Making in Psychiatry.* New York: Guilford.

Mazur, Dennis J. 1986. "What Should Patients Be Told Prior to a Medical Procedure? Ethical and Legal Perspectives on Medical Informed Consent." *American Journal of Medicine* 81(6): 1051–1054.

Meichenbaum, Donald, and Turk, Dennis. 1987. *Facilitating Treatment Adherence: A Practitioner's Guidebook.* New York: Plenum Press.

Meisel, Alan, and Roth, Loren H. 1981. "What We Do and Do Not Know About Informed Consent." *Journal of the American Medical Association* 246(21): 2473–2477.

Murphy, Donald J.; Burrows, David; Santilli, Sara; et al. 1994. "The Influence of the Probability of Survival on Patients' Preferences Regarding Cardiopulmonary Resuscitation." *New England Journal of Medicine* 330(8): 545–549.

Quill, Timothy E., and Townsend, Penelope. 1991. "Bad News: Delivery, Dialogue, and Dilemmas." *Archives of Internal Medicine* 151: 463–468.

Sherlock, Richard. 1986. "Reasonable Men and Sick Human Beings." *American Journal of Medicine* 80(1): 2–4.

Stanley, Barbara; Guido, Jeannine; Stanley, Michael; et al. 1984. "The Elderly Patient and Informed Consent: Empirical Findings." *Journal of the American Medical Association* 252(10): 1302–1306.

Steel, David J.; Blackwell, Barry; Gutmann, Mary C.; et al. 1987. "The Activated Patient: Dogma, Dream, or Desideratum." *Patient Education and Counseling* 10(1): 3–23.

Strull, William M.; Lo, Bernard; and Charles, Gerard. 1984. "Do Patients Want to Participate in Medical Decision-Making?" *Journal of the American Medical Association* 252(21): 2990–2994.

U.S. President's Commission for the Study of Ethical Problems in Medicine and Biomedical and Behavioral Research. 1982. *Making Health Care Decisions: A Report on the Ethical and Legal Implications of Informed Consent in the Patient–Practitioner Relationship.* Washington, D.C.: Author.

Waitzkin, Howard. 1984. "Doctor–Patient Communication: Clinical Implications of Social Scientific Research." *Journal of the American Medical Association* 252(17): 2441–2446.

Waitzkin, Howard. 1991. *The Politics of Medical Encounters: How Patients and Doctors Deal with Social Problems.* New Haven, CT: Yale University Press.

West, Candace. 1984. Routine Complications: *Troubles with Talk between Doctors and Patients.* Bloomington: Indiana University Press.

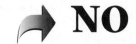

Gaining Autonomy and Losing Trust?

Contemporary Bioethics

Bioethics is not a discipline, nor even a new discipline; I doubt whether it will ever be a discipline. It has become a meeting ground for a number of disciplines, discourses and organisations concerned with ethical, legal and social questions raised by advances in medicine, science and biotechnology. The protagonists who debate and dispute on this ground include patients and environmentalists, scientists and journalists, politicians and campaigners and representatives of an array of civic and business interests, professions and academic disciplines. Much of the debate is new and contentious in content and flavour; some of it is alarming and some misleading.

The first occasion on which I can remember a discussion of bioethics—we did not then use the word, although it had been coined[1]—was in the mid-1970s at a meeting of philosophers, scientists and doctors in New York City. We were discussing genetically modified (GM) organisms: a topic of breathtaking novelty that was already hitting the headlines. Towards the end of the evening an elderly doctor remarked, with mild nostalgia, that when he had studied medical ethics as a student, things had been easier: the curriculum had covered referrals, confidentiality—and billing. Those simpler days are now very remote. . . .

During [recent] years no themes have become more central in large parts of bioethics, and especially in medical ethics, than the importance of respecting individual rights and individual autonomy. These are now the dominant ethical ideas in many discussions of topics ranging from genetic testing to geriatric medicine, from psychiatry to *in vitro* fertilisation, from beginning to end of life problems, from medical innovation to medical futility, from heroic medicine to hospices. In writing on these and many other topics, much time and effort has gone into articulating and advancing various conceptions of respect for persons, and hence for patients, that centre on ensuring that their rights and their autonomy are respected. Respect for autonomy and for rights are often closely identified with medical practice that seeks individuals' informed consent to all medical treatment, medical research or disclosure of personal information, and so with major changes in the acceptable relationships between professionals and patients. Medical practice has moved away from paternalistic traditions, in which professionals were seen as the proper judges of patients' best interests. Increased recognition and respect of patients' rights and insistence on the ethical importance of securing their consent are now viewed as standard and obligatory ways of securing respect for patients' autonomy.[2] . . .

We might expect the increasing attention paid to individual rights and to autonomy to have increased public trust in the ways in which medicine, science and biotechnology are practised and regulated. Greater rights and autonomy give individuals greater control over the ways they live and increase their capacities to resist others' demands and institutional pressures. Yet amid widespred and energetic efforts to respect persons and their autonomy and to improve regulatory structures, public trust in medicine, science and biotechnology has seemingly faltered. The loss of trust is a constant refrain in the claims of campaigning groups and in the press. . . .

Trust and Autonomy in Medical Ethics

[The] traditional model of the trusting doctor–patient relationship has been subject to multiple criticisms for many years. Traditional doctor–patient relationships, it has been said on countless occasions, have in fact nearly always been based on asymmetric knowledge and power. They institutionalise opportunities for abuse of trust. Doctor–patient relationships were viewed as relationships of trust only because a paternalistic view of medicine was assumed, in which the dependence of patients on professionals was generally accepted. The traditional doctor–patient relationship, so its critics claim, may have been one of trust, but not of reasonable trust. Rather, they claimed, patients who placed trust in their doctors were like children who initially must trust their parents blindly. Such trust was based largely on the lack of any alternative, and on inability to discriminate between well-placed and misplaced trust.

If there was one point of agreement about necessary change in the early years of contemporary medical ethics, it was that this traditional, paternalistic conception of the doctor–patient relationship was defective, and could not provide an adequate context for reasonable trust. A more adequate basis for trust required patients who were on a more equal footing with professionals, and this meant that they would have to be better informed and less dependent. The older assumption that relations of trust are in themselves enough to safeguard a weaker, dependent party was increasingly dismissed as naive. The only trust that is well placed is given by those who understand what is proposed, and who are in a position to refuse or choose in the light of that understanding. We can look at the same image with a less innocent eye, and see it as raising all these questions about the traditional doctor–patient relationship. In this second way of seeing the picture the doctor dominates: the white coat and intimidating office are symbols of her professional authority; the patient's anxious and discontented expression reveals how little this is a relationship of trust.

These considerations lie behind many discussions of supposedly better models of the doctor–patient relationship, in which patients are thought of as equal partners in their treatment, in which treatment is given only with the informed consent of patients, in which patient satisfaction is an important indicator of professional adequacy, in which patients are variously seen as consumers, as informed adults and are not infantilised or treated paternalistically and in which the power of doctors is curbed.[3] In this more sophisticated approach to trust, autonomy is seen as a precondition of genuine trust. Here, as one writer puts it, 'informed consent is the modern clinical ritual of trust',[4] a ritual of trust that embeds it in properly institutionalised respect for patient autonomy. So we can also read the image in the frontispiece in a third, more optimistic, way as combining patient autonomy with mutual trust in the new, recommended, respecting way. What we now see is a relationship between equals: the patient too is a professional, dressed in a suit and sitting like an equal at the desk; the patient has heard a full explanation and is being offered a consent form; he is deciding whether to give his fully informed consent. Trust is properly combined with patient autonomy.

This revised model of doctor–patient interaction demands more than a simple change of attitude on the part of doctors, or of patients. It also requires huge changes in the terms and conditions of medical practice and ways of ensuring that treatment is given only where patients have consented. Informed consent has not always been so central to doctor–patient relationships, which were traditionally grounded in doctors' duties not to harm and to benefit. Informed consent came to be seen as increasingly important in part because of legal developments, especially in the USA, and in part because of its significance for research on human subjects, and the dire abuse of research subjects by Nazi doctors. The first principle of the Nuremberg Doctors' Code of 1947 states emphatically that subjects' consent must be 'voluntary, competent, informed and comprehensive'.[5] Only later did the thought emerge clearly that consent was also central to clinical practice, and that patient autonomy or self-determination should not be subordinated to doctors' commitments to act for their patients' benefit or best interest. Yet despite the enormous stress laid on individual autonomy and patient rights in recent years, this heightened concern for patient autonomy does not extend throughout medicine: public health, and the treatment of those unable to consent are major domains of medical practice that cannot easily be subjected to requirements of respecting autonomy and securing informed consent.

From the patient's point of view, however, the most evident change in medical practice of recent decades may be loss of a context of trust rather than any growth of autonomy. He or she now faces not a known and trusted face, but teams of professionals who are neither names nor faces, but as the title of one book aptly put it, *strangers at the bedside*.[6] These strangers have access to large amounts of information that patients give them in confidence. Yet to their patients they remain strangers—powerful strangers. They are the functionaries of medical institutions whose structures are opaque to most patients, although supposedly designed to secure their best interest, to preserve confidentiality and to respect privacy. Seen 'from the patient's point of view every development in the post World War II period distanced the physician and the hospital from the patient, disrupting social connection and serving the bonds of trust'.[7]

From the practitioner's point of view, too, the situation has losses as well as gains. The simplicities of the Hippocratic oath and of other older professional codes have been replaced by far more complex professional codes, by more formal certification of competence to perform specific medical interventions, by enormous increases in requirements for keeping records and by many exacting forms of professional accountability.[8] In medicine, as in most other forms of professional life and public service, and 'audit society' has emerged.[9] The doctor now faces the patient knowing that he or she must comply with explicit standards and codes, that many aspects of medical practice are regulated, that compliance is monitored and that patients who are not properly treated may complain—or even sue.

These new relationships may live up to their billing by replacing traditional forms of trust with a new and better basis for trust. The new structures may provide reasons for patients to trust even if they do not know their doctors personally, and do not understand the details of the rules and codes that constrain doctors' action. Supposedly they can feel reassured that the power of doctors is now duly regulated and constrained, that doctors will act with due respect and that they can seek redress where doctors fail. Although traditional trust has vanished with the contexts in which it arose, a more acceptable basis for reasonable trust has been secured, which anchors it in professional respect for patients' rights. Supposedly the ideals of trust and autonomy have been reshaped and are now compatible. . . .

The Triumph of Informed Consent

Yet what does the supposed triumph of autonomy in medical ethics amount to? . . .

By insisting on the importance of informed consent we *make* it *possible* for individuals to choose autonomously, however that it is to be construed. But we in no way guarantee or require that they do so. Those who insist on the importance of informed consent in medical practice typically say nothing about individuality or character, about self-mastery, or reflective endorsement, or self-control, or rational reflection, or second-order desires, or about any of the other specific ways in which autonomous choices supposedly are to be distinguished from other, mere choices.

In short, the focus of bioethical discussions of autonomy is not on patient autonomy or individual autonomy of any distinctive sort. What is rather grandly called 'patient autonomy' often amounts simply to a right to choose or refuse treatments on offer, and the corresponding obligations of practitioners not to proceed without patients' consent. Of course, some patients may use this liberty to accept or refuse treatment with a high degree of reflection and individuality, hence (on some accounts) with a high degree of individual or personal autonomy. But this need not generally be the case. Requirements for informed consent are relevant to specifically autonomous choice only because they are relevant to choice of all sorts. What passes for patient autonomy in medical practice is operationalised by practices of informed consent: the much-discussed triumph of autonomy is mostly a triumph of informed consent requirements.

This minimalist interpretation of individual or personal autonomy in medical ethics in fact fits rather well with medical practice. When we are ill or injured we often find it hard to achieve any demanding version of individual autonomy. We are all too aware of our need and ignorance, and specifically that we need help from others whose expertise, control of resources and willingness to assist is not guaranteed. A person who is ill or injured is highly vulnerable to others, and highly dependent on their action and competence. Robust conceptions of autonomy may seem a burden and even unachievable for patients; mere choosing may be hard enough. And, in fact, the choices that patients are required to make typically quite limited. It is not as if doctors offer patients a smorgasbord of possible treatments and interventions, a variegated menu of care and cure. Typically a diagnosis is followed with an indication of prognosis and suggestions for treatment to be undertaken. Patients are typically asked to choose from a smallish menu—often a menu of one item—that others have composed and described in simplified terms. This may suit us well when ill, but it is a far cry from any demanding exercise of individual autonomy.

It is probably a considerable relief to many patients that they are not asked to muster much in the way of individual autonomy. When we are ill or injured we often lack the skills or energy for demanding cognitive tasks. Our highest priority is to get help from others and in particular from others with relevant skills and knowledge. The traditional construction of doctor–patient relations as relations of trust, as quasi-personal, as guided by professional concern for the patient's best interests makes sense to many patients because (if achievable) it would secure what they most need. The point and the context of the older, trust-centred model of doctor–patient relationships are not at all obscure.

However, at a time at which the real relations between doctors and patients are no longer personal relationships, nor even one-to-one relationships, but rather relationships between patients and complex organisations staffed by many professionals, the older personal, trust-based model of doctor–patient relationships seems increasingly obsolete. Contemporary relations between professionals and patients are constrained, formalised and regulated in many ways, and may erode patients' reasons for trusting. The very requirements to record and file medical information, for example, while intended to control information and protect patients, can inhibit doctors' abilities to communicate freely. Doctors, like many other professionals, find themselves pressed to be accountable rather than to be communicative, to conform to regulations rather than to enter relations of trust. As layers of regulation and control are added with the aim of protecting dependent, ignorant and vulnerable patients, as professionals are disciplined by multiple systems of accountability backed by threats of litigation on grounds of professional negligence in case of failure to meet these requirements, relations between patients and professionals are inevitably reshaped. Much is demanded of informed consent requirements if they are to substitute for forms of trust that are no longer achievable (or perhaps were never widely achieved, and still less widely warranted), and safeguard the interests of patients who find strangers at their bedsides. . . .

Notes

1. The Kennedy Institute in Washington DC was founded in 1971 with the full name 'The Joseph and Rose Kennedy Institute for the Study of Human Reproduction and Bioethics'. See W.T. Reich, 'The Word 'Bioethics': Its Birth and the Legacies of Those Who 'Shaped It', *Kennedy Institute of Ethics Journal,* 4, 1994, 319–35.

2. For a highly informative account of these changes, . . . see Ruth Faden and Tom Beauchamp, *A History and Theory of Informed Consent,* Oxford University Press, 1986; for a sociological perspective see Paul Root Wolpe, 'The Triumph of Autonomy in American Bioethics: A Sociological View', in Raymond DeVries and Janardan Subedi, eds., *Bioethics and Society: Constructing the Ethical Enterprise,* Prentice-Hall, 1998, 38–59.

3. R.A. Hope and K.W.M. Fulford, 'Medical Education: Patients, Principles, Practice Skills', in R. Gillon, ed., *Principles of Health Care Ethics,* John Wiley & Sons, 1993.

4. Wolpe, 'The Triumph of Autonomy', 48.

5. See Faden and Beauchamp, *A History and Theory of Informed Consent;* Ulrich Tröhler and Stella Reiter-Theil, *Ethics Codes in Medicine: Foundations and Achievements of Codification Since 1947,* Ashgate; Lori B. Andrews, 'Informed Consent Statutes and the Decision-Making Process', *Journal of Legal Medicine,* 30, 163–217; World Medical Association, Declaration of Helsinki, 2000; see institutional bibliography.

6. David J. Rothman, *Strangers at the Bedside: A History of How Law and Ethics Transformed Medical Decision-Making,* Basic Books, 1991. Rosamond Rhodes and James J. Strain, 'Trust and Transforming Healthcare Institutions', *Cambridge Journal of Healthcare Ethics,* 9, 2000, 205–17.

7. Rothman, *Strangers at the Bedside.*

8. Nigel G.E. Harris, 'Professional Codes and Kantian Duties', in Ruth Chadwick, ed., *Ethics and the Professions,* Amesbury, 1994, 104–15.

9. Michael Power, *The Audit Explosion,* Demos, 1994 and *The Audit Society: Rituals of Verification,* Oxford University Press, 1994.

POSTSCRIPT

Is Informed Consent Still Central to Medical Ethics?

In October 2008, California governor Arnold Schwarzenegger signed a bill requiring physicians to provide patients diagnosed with a terminal illness information about all legal end-of-life treatment options, including hospice and palliative care. Patients have to request this information, and physicians are not obligated to provide any treatment with which they disagree. Opponents claimed that the bill was unnecessary since state laws already require informed consent and that the bill was a step toward physician-assisted suicide. See Issue 6, *Should Physicians Be Allowed to Assist in Patient Suicide?*

In the 1993 case of *Arato v. Avedon,* the California Supreme Court supported information sharing and patient-centered decision making but ruled that doctors need not supply explicit statistical information about life expectancy to patients. See George J. Annas, "Informed Consent, Cancer, and Truth in Prognosis," *The New England Journal of Medicine* (January 20, 1994).

Nonetheless, the concept of informed consent, from Western political and ethical theories that place a high value on individual self-determination, remains a central principle in the United States. Cultural groups who have different traditions may not share this value. Two articles in the *Journal of the American Medical Association* (September 13, 1995)—"Western Bioethics on the Navajo Reservation," by Joseph A. Carrese and Lorna A. Rhodes, and "Ethnicity and Attitudes Toward Patient Autonomy," by Leslie J. Blackhall—suggest that disclosing negative information and involving patients in decision making may be contrary to the beliefs of certain ethnic populations. For more on this subject, see Issue 2, *Should Truth-Telling Depend on the Patient's Culture?*

The most comprehensive account of informed consent is *A History and Theory of Informed Consent* by Ruth L. Faden, Tom L. Beauchamp, and Nancy M. P. King (Oxford University Press, 1986). Another useful volume, particularly in terms of psychiatric treatment, is *Informed Consent: Legal Theory and Clinical Practice* by Paul S. Appelbaum, Charles W. Lidz, and Alan Meisel (Oxford University Press, 1987). Jay Katz's *The Silent World of Doctor and Patient* (Free Press, 1984; paper edition 2002, Johns Hopkins University Press) is an insightful discussion of the reasons physicians may be reluctant to disclose information to their patients. See also, Jessica W. Berg, Paul S. Appelbaum, Charles W. Lidz, and Lisa S. Parker, *Informed Consent: Legal Theory and Clinical Practice,* 2d ed. (Oxford University Press, 2001), and Terrance C. McConnell, *Inalienable Rights: The Limits of Consent in Medicine and the Law* (Oxford University Press, 2000).

For further elaboration of Onora O'Neill's critique of informed consent, see Neil C. Manson and Onora O'Neill, *Rethinking Informed Consent in Bioethics* (Cambridge University Press, 2007). *The Ethics of Consent: Theory and Practice,* edited by Franklin Miller and Alan Wertheimer, brings together expert views on informed consent in many fields beyond bioethics (Oxford University Press, 2009).

ISSUE 2

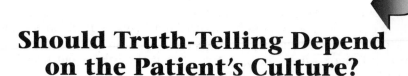

Should Truth-Telling Depend on the Patient's Culture?

YES: Leslie J. Blackhall, Gelya Frank, Sheila Murphy, and Vicki Michel, from "Bioethics in a Different Tongue: The Case of Truth-Telling," *Journal of Urban Health* (March 2001)

NO: Mark Kuczewski and Patrick J. McCruden, from "Informed Consent: Does It Take a Village? The Problem of Culture and Truth Telling," *Cambridge Quarterly of Healthcare Ethics* (2001)

ISSUE SUMMARY

YES: Leslie J. Blackhall, Gelya Frank, and Sheila Murphy, from the University of Southern California, and Vicki Michel, from the Loyola Law School, advise clinical and bioethics professionals facing truth-telling dilemmas to make room for the diverse ethical views of the populations they serve.

NO: Philosopher Mark Kuczewski and bioethicist Patrick J. McCruden argue that by insisting on informed consent or an appropriate waiver process, the health care system respects cultural differences rather than stereotyping them.

In his powerful short story "The Death of Ivan Ilych," Leo Tolstoy graphically portrays the physical agony and the social isolation of a dying man. However, "What tormented Ivan Ilych most was the deception, the lie, which for some reason they all accepted, that he was not dying but was simply ill, and that he only need keep quiet and undergo a treatment and then something very good would result." Instrumental in setting up the deception is Ivan's doctor, who reassures him to the very end that all will be well. Hearing the banal news from his doctor once again, "Ivan Ilych looks at him as much as to say: 'Are you really never ashamed of lying?' But the doctor does not wish to understand this question."

Unlike many of the ethical issues discussed in this volume, which have arisen as a result of modern scientific knowledge and technology, the question of whether or not to tell dying patients the truth is an old and persistent one. But this debate has been given a new urgency in two ways. First, medical practices today are so complex that it is often difficult to know just what the "truth" really is. A dying patient's life can often be prolonged, although at great financial and personal cost, and many people differ even over the definition of a terminal illness. Second, the American population now includes many people from different cultures whose beliefs about truth-telling differ from those of conventional Western medicine.

At a basic level what must be balanced in this decision are two significant principles of ethical conduct: the obligation to tell the truth and the obligation not to harm others, in this case, not just the patient but the patient's family members who seek to withhold the truth from their dying relative. Moral philosophers, beginning with Aristotle, have regarded truth as an absolute value or one that, at the very least, is preferable to deception. The great nineteenth-century German philosopher Immanuel Kant argued that there is no justification for lying (although some later commentators feel that his absolutist position has been overstated). Other philosophers have argued that deception is sometimes justified. For example, Henry Sidgwick, an early-twentieth-century British philosopher, believed that it was entirely acceptable to lie to invalids and children to protect them from the shock of the truth. Although the question has been debated for centuries, no clear-cut answer has been reached. In fact, the case of a benevolent lie to a dying patient is often given as the prime example of an excusable deception.

While the philosophical debate continued, American medical practice underwent a pronounced shift beginning in the 1960s. Influenced by the growing attention to the principle of patient autonomy, doctors began involving patients in their health care decisions and telling them the facts of their diagnosis and prognosis. In recent years, however, greater attention to cultural sensitivity has led to a new debate: whether or not to withhold the truth from dying patients because family members demand it in the name of their cultural belief that truth-telling would harm the patient.

In the following selections, Leslie J. Blackhall and her colleagues present data from their study of cultural beliefs about truth-telling to argue that it is important to respect the ways in which people differ as to how the truth should be told. They question even what "truth" and "telling" really mean. Mark Kuczewski and Patrick J. McCruden rebut this emphasis on cultural relativism and reinforce the significance of informed consent.

YES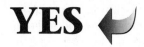

Leslie J. Blackhall et al.

Bioethics in a Different Tongue: The Case of Truth-Telling

Introduction

The study discussed in this [selection] began with the concern that much of bioethics was a top-down affair. The ethical problems surrounding end-of-life care and the solutions to these problems have been defined by professionals (like the authors) who are mainly white, middle-class people with advanced educational degrees and good (or at least decent) health insurance. When we looked at care at the end of life, we were concerned about excessive, burdensome, and futile medical technology and with the right to choose and, especially, to refuse treatments. Advance care directives were invented to address these problems, to ensure that patients' rights to refuse excessive care were preserved when they were so demented or comatose that they were unable to communicate, or even know, what those wishes were. Having decided what the problem was (too much futile care at the end of life) and the solution (advance care directives), much space then was devoted in the literature on bioethics to promoting these documents. However, most studies that look at the use of advance directives, even those studies with interventions designed to increase accessibility, show that relatively few people actually have completed a directive.[1-6]

The reasons why people do not complete advance directives are many and complex, but one reason may be that the concerns of bioethics professionals about care at the end of life are not necessarily those most important to all segments of the population. For example, it is questionable whether patients, many of whom have no health insurance, who receive care at major urban hospitals are worried about getting too much medical care at the end of life. At these hospitals, their experience is more likely to be a fight for every bit of medical attention they receive, not fending off excessive care. Also, in the clinical experience of one of us (L.J.B.), it is not uncommon for patients and their families, particularly recent immigrants, to seem puzzled by, if not downright hostile to, attempts to involve them in end-of-life decisions.

Observations and reflections such as these led us to undertake a study to look at attitudes concerning end-of-life care among elderly people of different ethnicities. The purpose of this study was to examine and compare the attitudes and life experiences of people from African-American, European-American,

Korean-American, and Mexican-American ethnic groups with respect to topics such as truth-telling, patient autonomy, advance care directives, and forgoing life support. This [selection] presents qualitative data from the portion of the study that dealt with the issue of truth-telling. . . .

Results

The data from this survey have been published elsewhere[7]; they are reviewed only briefly here. Almost all of the African-American and European-American subjects in our study believed that patients should be told the truth about a diagnosis of cancer (87% and 89%, respectively). Only 47% of Korean-Americans and 65% of Mexican-Americans believed in telling the truth about the diagnosis. With respect to telling the truth about a terminal prognosis, again the European-American and African-American respondents were much more likely to believe in open disclosure, with 63% of African-American and 69% of European-American subjects agreeing that a patient should be told. Only 33% of the Korean-American and 48% of the Mexican-American subjects agreed with telling a terminally ill patient about the patient's prognosis. Among the Mexican-American and Korean-American respondents, more years of education, higher income, younger age, and the ability to speak and read English predicted a positive attitude toward truth-telling.* Statistical analysis of the data, controlling for variables such as income, education, and access to care, revealed that ethnicity was the most important factor contributing to attitudes toward truth-telling.

Although large differences among the attitudes of our groups with respect to truth-telling are apparent from the survey data, the reasons for these differences cannot be determined from the survey responses alone. For this reason, in the ethnographic interviews, we repeated the case and asked not only whether should the patient be told, but also why. Why is it okay or not okay to tell? If it generally is not okay to tell, does that include you? Would you want to be kept in the dark? Have you ever had the experience of telling or not telling the truth to a relative or friend? The remainder of this article presents the results of our analysis of these ethnographic interviews; these results have not been published previously. The themes that emerged from the interviews are presented below; quotations from subjects are included to illustrate each point. In the sections that follow, subjects are identified by RP (research participant) number and ethnicity (EA, European-American; AA, African-American; MA, Mexican-American; KA, Korean-American).

---

*This was particularly important in the Mexican-American group, which was divided into two groups, one that spoke and read English and got their news from English-language media. The group generally had a higher socioeconomic status. The attitudes of those in this group on the survey tended to look more like those of the European-American group. The second group of Mexican-Americans spoke, read, and thought in Spanish; had a generally lower socioeconomic status; and had attitudes that were more negative toward truth-telling. The Korean-American group was much less diverse. In general, this group had immigrated to Los Angeles from Korea more recently, and few of them spoke English.

Themes

Patient autonomy: "Because it's me." Among the European-American and African-American subjects, the theme that emerged most frequently was that patients in general and the subjects themselves should know the truth because, as RP 001 (EA) put it, "I'd want to know the worst because it's me; I would have to face it." For the participants holding this belief, information about their bodies is theirs to know, good or bad, simply because it is their body.

Although the knowledge of a terminal prognosis may be distressing, if you are not told, someone else is making decisions that are properly yours, and this lack of control is even more distressing than the bad news. As RP 008 (EA) said, "If there's anything wrong with me, tell me; it's my decision what to do. . . . I happen to be a person that wants to control my destiny as much as I can." Even if there is nothing that can be done to cure the disease, the knowledge itself is a form of power. To be the owner of your own body and life, you need to know about yourself. RP 259 (AA) stated this succinctly: "I want to know everything about me." It is a patient's right to know this information and the doctor's duty to tell it since "the person was intelligent enough to go to the doctor because he knew something was wrong, and he wanted to know what was wrong with him" (RP 263, AA). This complex of ideas, which is consistent with the patient autonomy model of bioethics, was mentioned by almost every African-American and European-American respondent interviewed. Many qualified their support for truth-telling with the idea that some people were not able to handle such information: "Some people, it would frighten them very much" (RP 022, EA). However, even those who worried that some were too fragile to hear the truth seemed to feel that most people could and should be told their diagnosis and prognosis, and that doctors should err on the side of truth-telling. The Korean-American and Mexican-American subjects, as we show below, were more likely to see truth-telling as cruel and potentially harmful rather than empowering, and they rarely mentioned the idea of a "right" to the truth.

You know anyway. Related to the idea of truth as a right of the patient is the idea that patients will know, intuitively, that they are very sick or even dying, so there is no harm in telling them. RP 133 (EA) put it this way: "I think we have a sense of our bodies, and you know something's wrong, and it's better . . . to know exactly what." RP 108 (EA) said, "The person has a right to know, and I think internally a person has a feeling as to what the prognosis might be." The right to know is connected to the ability to know for these subjects. "It's my life, and I ought to know, cause you got a feeling anyway. You know" (RP 301, AA). Ownership of your body gives you a right to truthful information; it also gives you the ability to sense this information before it is told. In comparison, some of the Korean-American and Mexican-American subjects agreed that the patient will know, but for these participants, this was a reason not to tell the patient the truth. "You don't have to tell the person about such a thing because, unless the person is a dummy, he or she will figure it out" (RP 451, KA).

Getting your things in order.   One of the most common reasons given by our European-American respondents for wanting to know the truth about a terminal prognosis was so they could get their "things" in order. This rationale was much less common in our other groups. As RP 008 (EA) put it, doctors should tell the truth because "so many people don't have wills or anything else." "We feel that you need to take care of your business . . . make provisions for those who need to have provisions made for them. To me that's simply manly" (RP 22, EA). By getting your things in order, you can ensure that your family is cared for or, at the very least, prevent them from being burdened with complex financial matters after your death:

> You settle your affairs. You've got to have a trust or a will . . . and let your wife know where everything is, and go over the things with your kids and your family so you know that by the time I'm gone this is what's here and you do this and you do that. (RP 171, EA)

A subtext here is the desire to exert control in the face of an uncontrollable process, death. In this way, one could almost link the desire to complete a will prior to death with the desire to complete a living will prior to becoming incompetent. Both are attempts to extend the reach of one's control into situations in which, by definition, one otherwise is unable to exert any control. This interpretation is supported by the fact that, when our respondents were asked about living wills or durable power of attorney for health care, they frequently discussed the concepts of living trust and durable power of attorney for financial matters. At first, it seemed that our respondents were confusing the two concepts, but when pushed by our interviewers, it became clear that these two concepts simply were linked very tightly in their minds. Both types of document usually were completed in the same place (an attorney's office), often at the same time, and were saturated with complex meanings that revolved around the themes of mortality, burdensomeness, and control.

Get it right with God.   When asked about truth-telling, some of our subjects discussed the issue as one having religious or spiritual significance. According to this idea, you should know the truth so that you can get it right with God. This theme was mentioned most frequently by our African-American respondents. If you know the truth, you have time to "get right with the good Lord . . . so when you die, your soul is saved" (RP 347, AA). "There are too many things a person has to do with his life at that point, to be in ignorance of his death . . . he has to go to his minister and . . . make whatever peace you have to make with your minister" (RP 252, AA). Even in the face of this knowledge, "When the Lord is with you, the devil can't do you no harm" (RP 289, AA).

Getting it right with God does not necessarily mean simply preparing your soul for death. If your doctor tells you that you have cancer, you have an opportunity to bring the problem to God, whose healing powers are greater than a doctor's. "I got another doctor, that's Doctor Jesus" (RP 201, AA). "[I would want him to tell me] because . . . I got another doctor I would go to that's the master of the universe, and let him tell me what to think about it" (RP 208, AA). If you know the truth, "you can prepare for it . . . ask your God [if you can live a longer life]" (RP 280, AA). "I want to know, can he help me; if he can't, tell me. If he can't help me, I go to the next person; that's the man above" (RP 364, AA). These answers reflect the belief that doctors are fallible and frequently cannot know whether a patient will live or die. Only God is capable of having that kind of knowledge. As RP 289 (AA) said, "I wouldn't care if he told me because it wouldn't make it true. . . . I believe in the Lord just because he [the doctor] said you're going to die next week, I never will believe nothing like that." "Some [doctors] they say that, and they come out of it" (RP 280, AA). Doctors have one kind of knowledge and power; God another. "The doctors say what . . . the afflictions of the righteous is, but God delivers them out of it all" (RP 201, AA).

Interestingly, this theme of needing to know the truth so that one could become closer to God either for healing or for absolution simply was not mentioned by any of the subjects in the European-American group. This was a religiously diverse group that included (in roughly equal numbers) Protestants, Catholics, and Jews. Only one of our Korean-American subjects, a deeply religious convert to Christianity, mentioned this rationale: "Yes, I would [want to know the truth]. Then, I could repent for my sins before God" (RP 409, KA). Several of the Mexican-American subjects made similar comments: "I would not want to be deceived. . . . I would put myself in God's hands; I would repent for all my sins and for the bad things I have done" (RP 607, MA).

It is cruel to tell.   In contrast to the European-American and African-American subjects, most of our Korean-American and Mexican-American subjects did not perceive the truth (especially the truth about a fatal prognosis) as empowering. Rather than envisioning the patient as an autonomous agent who needs information to make decisions and maintain control and dignity, the Mexican-American and Korean-American respondents viewed the patient as sick, weak, and in need of protection by the doctor and the family. Telling the truth in this context was seen as cruel. "Tell him [the patient] that he is getting better . . . because we should not be so cruel as to tell him, 'You are going to die, and it will be on such and such a day'" (RP 607, MA). Instead, it is kinder to "give him hope, console him . . . [so he can] always have hope that he will get better" (RP 607, MA).

> Anyway, the patient will die, so what is the use of saying you are going to die of cancer, right? The doctor should say, "You are okay; you will be fine. . . . Just take the medicine which will get you better." He shouldn't say that you have cancer so that you will die in a few months. Isn't that common sense? (RP 414, KA)

When one of our anthropologists commented to a Korean-American subject that, in America, most people were informed of their diagnosis and prognosis, the subject replied, "Yes, they are, because this allows patients to be prepared for death, but it must be very painful for those patients" (RP 447, KA).

The benefit of "being prepared" here is seen as insufficient to outweigh the pain caused by knowledge of the truth. Of a son dying with liver cancer, one Korean-American respondent stated, "We just couldn't tell him because it was cruel" (RP 451, KA). She went on to illustrate this by telling how her son had guessed that he had cancer and had been very distressed:

> Holding on to me, he cried very, very sadly, saying, "Mother, I do not remember that I have done anything bad to others in my whole life. I do not know how I got stricken with this bad disease." . . . So, both he and I cried to the last drop of our tears.

This mother felt guilty that she had not been able to protect her son from the truth and did her best to make up for it: "After that, I comforted him so that he would not give up hope on himself."

Most of these subjects agreed not only that the truth should be withheld in general, but also that they would not want to know it themselves: "If they tell me . . . I have the terminal cancer, I will become more depressed because my life is coming to an end" (RP 605, MA). "I wouldn't [want to know]. . . . I would be afraid of dying" (RP 640, MA). One of our Korean-American subjects told us that, for many years, her children had hidden from her the knowledge that a surgical procedure was for cancer, and she stated, "My children did a good thing for me, not a bad thing. If I had researched what it was, then it would be bad for everyone" (RP 480, KA, after a cone biopsy).

Many of the respondents, especially the Korean-American respondents, were aware that patients often come to know the truth even if they are not told directly. As one subject put it, "The patient in critical condition could get an idea of what she or he has by the doctor's attitude. However, there is a difference in knowing about one's disease from guessing and from confirmation by others. I feel I don't want to know about my impending death . . . without hope, one cannot live. . . . So anyone who says that she or he wants to know about having a disease is out of their minds because the knowing itself is painful. If the patients have more stress, their lives are shortened" (RP 414, KA). This is discussed in more detail below; here, we just note that knowing, or rather guessing, is better than being told directly because it allows for some ambiguity and for the possibility of hope.

If you know you die faster.   The truth not only is distressing according to these respondents, but also it potentially is harmful, even fatal. "It's not good to tell people what's wrong with them because they die sooner. . . . I told the doctor not to tell him" (RP 605, MA). "If the spreading cancer didn't kill her, the fear would" (RP 640, MA). One respondent told us the story of his brother, who died of cancer in rural Mexico. The truth had been kept carefully from him until almost the end of his life, when he happened to come by a mirror and see himself. Seeing how wasted he looked, he realized his condition. After that, according to his brother, "He never recuperated. . . . That is when he gave up. I think that [noticing how grave the illness is] is very bad for a deathly ill patient. If he has something to pick him up, his life is prolonged"

(RP 666, MA). One of our Korean-American subjects brought his wife from Seoul, Korea, to Sacramento, California, for treatment without informing her of her condition: "We kept it a tight secret. . . . If she knew, she would not be able to live longer because of the fear" (RP 447, KA).

Some people can't take it. These themes, that the truth is cruel and harmful to patients, could be found in the transcripts of European-American and African-American subjects as well. Here, it almost always took the form of a statement that the truth is harmful for *some* people: "Some people just are not able, for whatever reason, to deal with unpleasant facts" (RP 007, EA). This almost always was qualified: "But, in general, I think you've got to level with people." (This statement was made by a man who felt that he could take it, but was not sure about his wife.) In this view, some people will not be able to cope after they receive such bad news; for these few, the truth is not empowering, but disabling. "Some people fall apart over nothing. And if the doctor knows the patient at all, he should be able to determine whether this person could handle it or not" (RP 259, AA). Some even admitted that they were one of the ones who couldn't take it: "I think it depends on the person. Some people can take the news better than others. . . . I'm a worry-wart, and they tell me that; all positive things I would throw out of my mind" (RP 258, AA).

Not the truth, but hope. Although superficially the attitudes of our Korean-American and Mexican-American subjects toward the truth seemed identical, there were differences between them. As we reviewed the data from our Mexican-American subjects, we were confused initially by what seemed to be a contradictory and ambiguous attitude toward the truth in many of the transcripts. For example, one of our Mexican-American subjects told us that, "It is my opinion that the truth must always be told [to everyone]. . . . I would want the doctor to tell me directly" (RP 658, MA). However, speaking of a cousin with cancer, she told this story:

> She suffered a lot . . . and always asked me, "Isn't it true that I have cancer?" I told her, "C'mon, what cancer? It's not cancer." . . . It would have been more suffering if she had known what she had. (RP 658, MA)

A respondent (RP 666, MA) (mentioned above), said, "I think that [noticing how grave the illness is] is very bad for a deathly ill patient," about his brother, who died after looking in a mirror. Further in that same transcript, this respondent said that, "Knowing the truth helps to make you feel better because you can look for a way to cheer up and not get to the end of the road like the doctors thought" (RP 666, MA). When asked by our anthropologist how a doctor should tell a patient the truth, he replied:

> He would tell you gently [saying], "Now, we are going to do everything in our hands so you feel better; however, we will not stop you from dying, but the 2 or 3 days you have left should be happy, and don't think about leaving because maybe it won't happen." (RP 666, MA)

That is, the doctor should tell the patient that the patient will die in 2 or 3 days, but at the same time tell the patient that maybe they aren't going to die at all.

Another subject (RP 730) answered an emphatic "Yes" to the truth-telling question and at first denied that people die faster when they are told ("Those are just rumors"), but later told us that the patient should not be told about the prognosis: "It's better not to tell them that part to encourage her so that she thinks she's going to live more than she will actually live" (RP 730, MA).

Some of these seeming contradictions simply may be an expression of the complexity of the subject. However, the perceived contradictory nature of these answers actually may be another variant of the top-down problem mentioned above. At the start of this study, the authors identified an ethical problem: truthtelling. The issue for us was whether the doctor should tell the truth. But, for these subjects, it appears that the more appropriate ethical category is "hope," and the issue is whether the doctor and family take away hope. Taking away hope is prohibited because it is cruel and because it makes the patient die faster. The truth is not the main issue; the truth can be told as long as it is told in such a way as not to remove hope. You can tell the patient that he or she is going to die as long as you tell the patient that he or she might not die. This is why telling the prognosis is so much worse than telling the diagnosis. As long as you tell the patient that the cancer can be cured, it is not so bad to tell the patient that they have cancer.

This interpretation is supported by two respondents in the Mexican-American group who actually had cancer. One of them had lung cancer. He agreed that people should be told the truth about their diagnosis, as he was. However, he admitted that he wouldn't want to know about a terminal prognosis: "No [don't tell me]. . . . It would torment me" (RP 615, MA). As far as could be determined from his description, he had only palliative (not curative) treatment (draining pleural effusions), but was convinced he was cured, or as he put it, "The tumor is dry" (RP 615, MA). . . . The patient was told the truth about his diagnosis, but given hope.

Another respondent, with head and neck cancer, had a similar story. When asked if it was appropriate to tell the truth, he stated, "Oh, yes, because then [they could] connect me to a machine instead of having surgery and giving me therapy and X-rays. . . . He [the doctor] told me that it was going to get better with the machines" (RP 754, MA). Later, when asked about being told the prognosis, he said it was okay "for the doctor to tell me, but so that I won't become discouraged, to tell me that I am [going to live longer] even though I am not." Tell me the truth about my dying, but tell it in such a way that I do not have to face it without hope that I will live. . . .

Conclusion

This study of 800 elderly subjects showed that major differences exist in the way people of different ethnicities view the issue of truth-telling. One of the core differences, around which many of the themes circled, is the question of how the truth affects the terminally ill patient. On one hand, the truth can be seen as an essential tool that allows the patient to maintain a sense of personal agency and control. Seen in this light, telling the truth, however painful, is empowering. On the other hand, the truth can be seen as traumatic and demoralizing, sapping the patient of hope and the will to live. For those who hold this view, truth-telling is an act of cruelty.

In fact, many, if not most, of our subjects held both views. They differed in the relative weight given to each view. In weighing the positive benefits of the truth versus its potential to harm, the deciding factor seems to be the way the self is understood. Are we mainly autonomous agents whose dignity and worth come from the individual choices we make with our lives, or is our most important characteristic the web of social relations in which we exist? If we hold the former view (as most of our African-American and European-American respondents did), then lack of access to the truth is almost dehumanizing since it strips us of our ability to make choices, without which we are something less than fully human. If, however, we tend to see ourselves not as individuals, but as a part of a larger social network (as was more common in the Mexican-American and Korean-American groups), then the notion of personal choice loses something of its force, and we may expect that those close to us will act on our behalf to protect and nurture us in our time of need.

The second meta-theme that emerged from these data has to do with the many meanings of telling. When we began this study, we assumed that there were two possibilities: The truth could be told to or withheld from the patient. This is how the survey instrument was designed; respondents had to answer yes or no to questions about telling the diagnosis and prognosis to a patient with terminal cancer. However, many of our subjects, particularly in the Mexican-American and Korean-American groups, had a view with more nuances of how the patient could be told, or could come to know, the truth. According to these respondents, the truth could be told vaguely, partially; could be understood without telling, by context and hints; or could be known by nunchi. These types of telling allow for ambiguity and therefore for hope. This adds another layer of complexity to the issue of truth-telling and calls into question not only whether, but also how, we should tell the truth and even what telling and the truth mean.

References

1. Hare J, Nelson C. Will outpatients complete living wills? A comparison of two interventions. *J Gen Intern Med.* 1991;6:41–46.

2. Sachs GA, Stocking CB, Miles SH. Empowering the older patient? A randomized controlled trial to increase discussion and use of advance directives. *J Am Geriatric Soc.* 1992;40:269–273.

3. Caralis PV, Davis B, Wright K, Marcial E. The Influence of ethnicity and race on attitudes toward advance directives, life-prolonging treatments and euthanasia. *J Clin Ethics.* 1993;4:155–166.

4. Teno JM, Fleishman J, Brock DW, Mor V. The use of Formal Prior Directives among patients with HIV-related diseases. *J Gen Intern Med.* 1990;5:490–494.

5. Sugarman J, Weinberger M, Samsa G. Factors associated with veterans' decisions about living wills. *Arch Intern Med.* 1992;152:343–347.

6. Murphy ST, Palmer JM, Azen S, Frank G, Michel V, Blackhall LJ. Ethnicity and advance care directives. *J Law Med Ethics.* 1996;24:108–117.

7. Blackhall LJ, Murphy S, Frank G, Michel V, Azen S. Ethnicity and attitudes toward patient autonomy. *JAMA.* 1995;274:820–825.

**Mark Kuczewski and
Patrick J. McCruden**

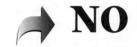 **NO**

Informed Consent: Does It Take a Village? The Problem of Culture and Truth Telling

Bioethicists have become very interested in the importance of social groups. This interest has spawned a growing literature on the role of the family[1] and the place of culture[2] in medical decisionmaking. These ethicists often argue that much of medical ethics suffers from the individualistic bias of the dominant culture and political tradition of the United States. As a result, the doctrine of informed consent has come under some scrutiny. It is believed that therein lies the source of the problem because the doctrine incorporates the assumptions of the larger society. Thus, informed consent has been reexamined, reinterpreted,[3] and even abandoned as unworkable.[4]

Our society embraces certain liberal democratic ideals such as the right of individuals to the maximum amount of freedom; that is, to do what they want, as long as they don't hurt anybody.[5] Of course, we also look for society to provide a certain equality of opportunity.[6] Otherwise one's freedom wouldn't mean much. These principles, liberty and equality, provide the foundation for the individual's pursuit of his or her particular vision of the good life. The state should remain neutral toward competing visions of the good life as long as these visions do not infringe on the rights of others. As a result, the state does not advocate a substantive morality but embraces a procedural ethic that allows each to play out his or her own life without interference from the value judgments of others.

Bioethicists have recently called our attention to the fact that this kind of ethic often works better in theory than in practice. Boundaries among individuals are sometimes not clearly demarcated. Although it is fine to speak about the rights of the individual, respecting patient autonomy usually requires a process of collaborative decisionmaking. This process involves not only the patient and physician but those who are close to the patient. Patient autonomy becomes a reality when treatment decisions are made in the way that patients typically make their other significant decisions. This often creates a legitimate role for the family in the decisionmaking schema.[7]

Similarly, some have noted that it is not only the significant interpersonal relationships that challenge medical ethics' conception of patient autonomy

From *Cambridge Quarterly of Healthcare Ethics,* by Mark Kuczewski and Patrick J. McCruden, vol. 10, no. 1, 2001, pp. 34–35, 37–41, 45–46. Copyright © 2001 by Cambridge University Press. Reprinted by permission.

but also the patient's culture.[8] The very concept of patient autonomy is a product of our Western culture, which values individual freedom and self-determination. Insofar as these cultural assumptions are shared by the parties in the clinical encounter, medical ethics is equipped to handle the situation. However, when the patient and the patient's family are from a culture whose values are quite different, our ethic may be invalidated. If so, it is not clear how the clinician should proceed. It could follow from these premises that medical ethics is relative to culture and physician behavior would best be guided by the norms of the patient's community. In short, one could argue for a culturally relative medical ethics.[9, 10]

We believe that the concerns about the individualistic nature of medical ethics are important. The rhetoric of informed consent still emphasizes self-determination despite the fact that good scholarship has expanded what bioethicists mean by that term. This scholarly trend toward a less individualistic, more process-oriented notion of informed consent and its resulting role for close others is salutary. However, it is not exactly clear what many of these critics of informed consent are seeking. Typically, compromises are called for because the "dominant Western bioethical concepts and principles are problematic" and "routine application of these concepts and principles may pose difficulties."[11] Although cautious, some argue that informed consent can be compromised. For instance, "[d]eviation from the usual formal standards of informed consent would be justified only by reference to patient-centered values."[12] And, of course, others have astutely observed that, in practice, informed consent is often compromised and truth withheld in the attempt to be culturally sensitive.[13]

Although cultural sensitivity is important, we shall argue that any suggestion that we should step outside our ethical framework entirely in favor of the ethic of the patient's culture is mistaken.[14] Such suggestions should not guide clinical behavior. We will justify this claim in two ways: (1) by reiterating the reasons our culture holds informed consent so dear and building on this foundation, and (2) by rebutting the epistemological assumptions of a culturally relative medical ethics. Furthermore, our skepticism regarding the use of culture in clinical decisionmaking might suggest that the study of culture is of no use to the clinician. We offer some preliminary speculations regarding why we believe that conclusion is overstated. . . .

The Cultural Challenge to Informed Consent

The doctrine of informed consent has certain basic features. The patient must be given information. In other words, disclosure of the diagnosis and prognosis must be made, treatment proposed, the risks and benefits of the treatment outlined, alternative options highlighted. The patient must, to some extent, grasp the information and then make a choice to accept or refuse the treatment. Certain conditions must also obtained. That is, the patient must be free from undue influence or coercion and the patient must have the cognitive and affective capacity to make the decision (i.e., the patient must be competent). Competence provides a road into the consent process for social groups.

When informed consent is a relatively straightforward onetime event, such as might occur immediately before a lifesaving emergency appendectomy, the patient may have little need of close others to provide a valid consent. However, many long-term chronic illnesses create an ongoing process of informed consent in which the patient's knowledge of treatment options and their attendant effects grows through experience. Through this experience, the patient gains insight into her illness and develops certain evaluations of the treatment options. The physician also goes through a process of refining the diagnosis and prognosis and continues to reassess her evaluations of the treatment options. The physician and patient mutually monitor each other to ascertain how their respective understandings and evaluations are proceeding.[15]

For the patient to make competent treatment choices, his or her values must be relatively stable. When consent is an event, the patient issues competent choices from existing values. But when illness demands that the patient reinterpret or develop new values to cope with the situation, close others will be needed to aid the patient in this process of reality testing and personal growth. The communitarian understanding of the interpersonal development of values through mutual self-discovery will clearly come into play. For instance, values or interpretations of values may become stable for the patient through the support of family and friends or, conversely, by standing up to the objections of these persons. Thus, the decisionmaking capacity of the patient is partially a group function. But, exactly to what degree is the person constituted by the group? Consider the following case.

Case 1

Oscar Ramirez, a 55-year-old patient of Mexican descent, presented with a large growth in his throat. He was told that the growth was cancerous. Mr. Ramirez was also told that he would need to have the tumor removed and start an aggressive round of chemotherapy. Mr. Ramirez agreed to the proposed treatment. However, Ramirez's wife and children told the oncologist that complete truthfulness would devastate him and that it was their duty to protect him. They supported this claim by saying that their background required that "la familia" take this protective role. They added that their culture does not place the same value on the individual's control of his own life that most Americans do. Thus, when the tumor could not be completely removed, Mr. Ramirez was merely told that his recovery would be lengthy and that much treatment would be needed to keep the cancer from recurring. Because of great skill in deception and a tightly orchestrated effort to conceal the truth, Oscar Ramirez died without ever being told of his terminal illness.

Let us tease out some moral intuitions regarding this case. Case-based reasoning, also known as casuistic method, will be of help. Casuistry suggests that we should not plunge directly into a case in which our intuitions are unclear. We should look at similar cases in which the right action readily suggests itself. Then, by analogy to these paradigms, we can illuminate our path in this problematic case.

A good casuist would tell us to pursue two different paradigms; one in which it seemed correct to withhold the truth from Mr. Ramirez and one in which it was clearly wrong. We can try out a number of different scenarios in search of these paradigms, but this does not seem to be a difficult exercise. One clear paradigm case in which it would be correct to withhold the truth is one in which Mr. Ramirez would be devastated by the bad news. After hearing of the difficulties in removing the tumor, Mr. Ramirez would slip into a deep, permanent depression and lose any possible enjoyment of the remainder of his life. Similarly, we would also have a similar paradigm case in one in which Mr. Ramirez wanted the truth withheld. For a variety of reasons, he may prefer this course of action. Such reasons might include that he simply does not like negative medical news, that bad news would drain off psychological energy that could be used to fight the disease, that he wishes this situation to be managed in accord with the traditional familial roles his family outlined, and so on. But the reason seems somewhat inconsequential to the choice of the correct action. If Mr. Ramirez clearly does not want to know his diagnosis, we are obligated to withhold it. On the other hand, when we look for a paradigm of truth telling in this instance, it would usually involve a desire by Mr. Ramirez to want to know his diagnosis. Perhaps he wishes to know for any of a variety of the usual reasons, including setting his affairs in order, finishing the "unfinished business" of life, and simply managing his end-of-life decisions.

As we compare these paradigms of information withholding and truth telling, we realize that we do not consider them to be equal. We favor those paradigms that contain some direct expression of patient autonomy, either by waiver of his informed consent rights or by providing full disclosure to be more applicable. Is this merely because we are members of a liberal democratic society? Probably not. Not so long ago we thought that persons who were given bad news routinely became irreversibly depressed. Then, we became familiar with the idea that the adverse reactions patients endured were transient and that they usually reacted better in the long run if allowed to remain in control of their life and destiny. Even so, the practices of clinicians continued (and might still continue) to be less than completely truthful.[16] Nevertheless, we realize that there is no need for a paradigm to justify telling the truth. We are in need of paradigms that can justify withholding information.

It is undoubtedly true that, in the short run, Mr. Ramirez does not want bad information. But the traditional doctrine of informed consent is founded on his right to have that information, even when it's bad, and the empirical postulate that he will be better off in the long run for it. Through the normal social and psychological processes of living, Mr. Ramirez will adapt to the harsh realities and do well. In this belief, communitarian and liberal theorists agree. However, the communitarian has a deeper appreciation for the fact that such processes might be culturally relative and without a community that values taking control of one's affairs, such processes might not proceed according to the paradigm.

So the disagreement between a communitarian perspective and a liberal theorist about how to proceed in a clinical case of this type may come down to a different rebuttable presumption. The liberal rights-oriented theorist requires some direct expression of autonomy even if it be via a waiver of informed consent. A more communitarian perspective argues that this delegation of authority can also be implicit. Edmund Pellegrino writes:

> . . . among many ethnic groups in the United States . . . this delega-
> tion of authority is culturally implicit. . . . Withholding the truth from
> a patient demands, of course, the utmost care in responding to any
> occasion when the patient wishes to exert more control.[17]

If we wish to be true to the process notion of informed consent and retain its communitarian concept of the person, must this conclusion follow? If the patient is from one of the requisite cultures that do not value autonomy, should we accept the family's statement that such news would "kill him"? We think not.

Justifying the Hegemony of Informed Consent

Communitarianism and cultural sensitivity are complex phenomena. It is all too easy to fall prey to simple-minded solutions. In general, we believe that the communitarian view sketched above suffers from (1) a simple-minded episte-mology and (2) a focus that excludes the culture and community of the health-care professions. Once community membership is seen as the complex matter it is and cultural sensitivity is also extended to the culture of the clinic, we believe that it will be clear that patients must waive their right to information to justify physicians withholding it.

The epistemology of this radical communitarian position posits cultures as opaque to those outside of them. We supposedly cannot appreciate the way that a different culture sees the respective roles of the persons involved. This assumes a sharp distinction between the "inside" and "outside" of a culture. Only those on the inside can understand its working whereas those on the outside must simply accept what the insiders tell us about it. The rationality of a culture is an internal one and cannot be evaluated externally.[18] As a result, we are at the mercy of the reports Mr. Ramirez's children supply about their culture and any survey data about that culture that can confirm a dissimilarity between his culture and those of the clinicians. The opacity of the culture has been substituted for the opacity of the individual of Western liberal theory.

The main problem with this epistemology is that we have little reason to believe that cultures are, in fact, so opaque and able to enforce rigid bound-aries between insiders and outsiders. Mr. Ramirez's case causes us a problem on the gut level because we have a cultural situation explained to us but are not sure how this patient relates to his own culture. Many people who seem to be clearly ensconced in a culture still pick and choose from its beliefs on many points. Mr. Ramirez does not live in one culture but in at least two. Otherwise he would not be in this particular hospital. How he relates to the beliefs of each is currently opaque. But, it need not remain so. We can simply ask him.

This would allow him to request information or to provide an explicit waiver of consent.

Second, and perhaps as important, is the fact that we have been speaking as if patients and their families come from cultures but the healthcare providers have none or one that is not authentic. This radical communitarian view caricatures them as value-free and adaptable to any culture. They normally live and die by the doctrine of informed consent because they usually encounter people from the Western liberal tradition that values freedom and individualism. Or, healthcare providers are themselves part of a culture that is value-free in valuing the autonomy of individuals. As a result, the communitarian counsels suggest that they must rein that tendency in when dealing with the contentladen value systems of other cultures. Surely, such a view is mistaken.

The clinic has its own culture and values. Typically, these are health-related values that favor treatment of illness and prolongation of life over pleasure and most other personal lifestyle choices. Clinicians, especially those engaged in clinical research or graduate medical education, also place a strong emphasis on the advancement of knowledge. Similarly, clinical practice is often thought to have an implicit ethos that varies among medical specialties or particular healthcare professions, their "standard of care." And, because healthcare professionals are highly educated and respected, they are probably likely to assume that others share these values or to overvalue the worth of their treatments. The doctrine of informed consent evolved to safeguard us from the imposition of this clinical culture on patients.

As we noted at the outset, the doctrine of informed consent requires that the physician disclose all of the pertinent facts about the diagnosis and treatment options so that the patient may decide if he or she values them to the same degree as the physician. We also saw that this required a certain process, given that it is not always obvious to the patient exactly how he or she values the proposed course of action. This process involved the relaxing of boundaries among persons as values were formed or interpreted. And, this situation can raise concerns regarding the occasional need for the healthcare provider to act as the patient's advocate in dealing with domineering family members and similar situations that may involve undue influence.[19] Clinical judgment is often strained at such moments and there are few objective signposts to guide the clinician. In these situations, some solace is found in the fact that the informed consent process is teleological in nature. That is, patient autonomy is considered the goal or outcome of the consent process. At some point, when the patient's values and preferences toward a treatment choice clearly become stable, the physician is clearly again the patient's advocate. Then, communitarian formulations recede as the patient again has an individual identity.

This teleological element is the ultimate safeguard in process models of informed consent. Concerns about the imposition of the values of family members and healthcare professionals on a vulnerable patient are assuaged by knowing that at some point, the end point, the patient will make an autonomous decision. A culturally relative medical ethics requires that we suspend this teleological element. In Mr. Ramirez's case, there was no point at which patient autonomy clearly emerged. Thus, the only safeguard against the tyranny of the culture of the clinic, a tyranny that never sought the patient's input on the level of aggressiveness of treatment, was suspended. One might attempt to argue that the clinicians and family were merely trying to respect the patient's implicit expression of autonomy, but we have absolutely no way to know whether this was more than wishful thinking. . . .

The Use of Culture in the Clinic

We are arguing for a position that recognizes the limits of healthcare professionals to step outside of their own cultural worldview and norms. We believe that it is epistemologically naïve to think otherwise as well as condescending to persons of other cultures to believe that they have no ability to engage in dialogue that stretches their limitations as well. By insisting on the doctrine of informed consent or an appropriate waiver process, we think that our healthcare system respects cultural differences rather than condescends to them. We propose that we accept these limitations and advocate the continued use of the safeguards afforded by the doctrine of informed consent and the possibilities available through explicit waivers by individuals.

If the ethics of healthcare practice are not culturally relative, then why should clinicians be concerned with culture at all? This is an interesting question. Informed consent is a conversational process and hearing what patients have to say requires some knowledge of cultures. Conversational norms are often cultural and colored by a variety of other factors such as gender. We will do well to know what norms we are likely to encounter in the clinic. But, we must never assume that a cultural generalization tells us the whole story. We should not try to get beyond our own cultural norm of informed consent that requires we ask patients what they mean.

It is also true that cultural sensitivity and understanding is worthwhile to clinicians even if it does not translate directly in behavioral change in the way things are done in the clinic. It is obvious that the encounter of other cultures increases the clinician's awareness of the culture of his or her setting. The clinician not only learns something about patients in understanding their cultures but also comes to understand himself. This reward of the practice of medicine and the healthcare specialties should not be dismissed lightly. Informed consent is, ideally, not just a process of discovery by the patient; it also holds the promise of being one of mutual self-discovery.

Notes

1. Nelson HL, Nelson JL. *The Patient in the Family: An Ethics of Medicine and Families.* New York: Routledge, 1995.

2. Pellegrino ED, Mazzarella P, Corsi P, eds. *Transcultural Dimensions in Medical Ethics.* Frederick, Md.: University Publishing Group, 1992.

3. Lidz CW, Appelbaum PS, Meisel A. Two models of implementing informed consent. *Archives of Internal Medicine* 1988;148:1385–9.

4. Veatch RM. Abandoning informed consent. *Hastings Center Report* 1995; 25(2):5–12.

5. Rawls J. *A Theory of Justice.* Cambridge, Mass.: Harvard University Press, 1971.

6. Daniels N. *Just Health Care.* New York: Cambridge University Press, 1985.

7. Kuczewski MG. Reconceiving the family: the process of consent in medical decisionmaking. *Hastings Center Report* 1996;26(2):30–7.

8. Blackhall LJ, Murphy ST, Frank G, Michel V, Azen S. Ethnicity and attitudes toward patient autonomy. *JAMA* 1995;274(10):820–5.

9. Carrese J, Rhodes L. Western bioethics on the Navajo reservation. *JAMA* 1995;274(10):826–9 at 826.

10. Pellegrino, ED. Is truth telling to the patient a cultural artifact? *JAMA* 1992; 268(13):1734–5.

11. See note 9, Carrese and Rhodes 1995:829.

12. Gostin LO. Informed consent, cultural sensitivity and respect for persons. *JAMA* 1995;274(10):844–5 at 845.

13. Freedman B. Offering truth: one ethical approach to the uninformed cancer patient. *Archives of Internal Medicine* 1993;153(5):572–6.

14. Gordon E. Decisionmaking: the notion of informed waiver. *Fordham Urban Law Journal* 1996;23(4):1321–62 at 1344.

15. See note 3, Lidz, Appelbaum, Meisel 1988:1386.

16. Novack D, Detering B, Arnold R, Forrow L, Ladinsky M, Pezzullo J. Physicians' attitudes toward using deception to resolve difficult ethical problems. *JAMA* 1989;261(20):2980–5.

17. See note 10, Pellegrino 1992:1735.

18. This position is also known as "whole tradition communitarianism." . . .

19. See note 7, Kuczewski 1996:35.

POSTSCRIPT

Should Truth-Telling Depend on the Patient's Culture?

The classic book on truth-telling is Sissela Bok's *Lying: Moral Choice in Public and Private Life* (Pantheon Books, 1978). Written at a time when many American physicians were reluctant to tell patients the truth, she challenged that view by arguing that the harm resulting from disclosure is less than believed and is outweighed by the benefits, including the important one of giving the patient the right to choose among treatments.

Much of the literature on withholding the truth from patients concerns cancer. Mary R. Anderlik, Rebecca D. Pentz, and Kenneth R. Hess, in "Revisiting the Truth-Telling Debate: A Study of Disclosure Practices at a Major Cancer Center," *The Journal of Clinical Ethics* (Fall 2000), found that in the previous year a majority of physicians had encountered a family's request to withhold information about a prognosis or diagnosis. The majority of physicians combined a general commitment to disclosure with a willingness to be flexible in some cases, more often in prognosis than in diagnosis.

Physicians Margaret A. Drickamer and Mark S. Lachs address a different disease in their essay, "Should Patients with Alzheimer's Disease Be Told Their Diagnosis?" *The New England Journal of Medicine* (April 2, 1992). Although they favor truth-telling, they present the case for not telling, including such factors as the difficulty of conclusive diagnosis, the impaired decision-making capacity and competence of patients with Alzheimer's, and the limited therapeutic options.

An often-cited article that offers a compromise position is Benjamin Freedman's "Offering Truth: One Ethical Approach to the Uninformed Cancer Patient," *Annals of Internal Medicine* (March 8, 1993). Another article by the Blackhall team, this one with Gelya Frank as the lead author, is "Ambiguity and Hope: Disclosure Preferences of Less Acculturated Elderly Mexican Americans Concerning Terminal Cancer—A Case Story," *Cambridge Quarterly of Healthcare Ethics* (vol. 11, 2002). Heather J. Gert offers an alternative to complete disclosure: giving patients enough information that they will not be surprised by whatever happens—unless the physician is also surprised ("Avoiding Surprises: A Model for Informing Patients," *Hastings Center Report,* September–October 2002).

See also J. S. Barclay, L. J. Blackhall, and J. A. Tulsky, "Communication Strategies and Cultural Issues in the Delivery of Bad News" (*Journal of Palliative Medicine,* August 2007).

ISSUE 3

Does Direct-to-Consumer Drug Advertising Enhance Patient Choice?

YES: Paul Antony, from "Testimony Before the Senate Special Committee on Aging, United States Senate" (September 29, 2005)

NO: David A. Kessler and Douglas A. Levy, from "Direct-to-Consumer Advertising: Is It Too Late to Manage the Risks?" *Annals of Family Medicine* (January/February 2007)

ISSUE SUMMARY

YES: Paul Antony, Chief Medical Officer of Pharmaceutical Research and Manufacturers of America (PhRMA), asserts that direct-to-consumer advertising can be a powerful tool in educating millions of people and improving their health through better communication with physicians, better adherence to medication regimens, and more active involvement in their own health care.

NO: Physicians David A. Kessler and Douglas A. Levy contend that as a result of direct-to-consumer advertising, consumers ultimately take medicines they may not need, spend money on brand medicines that may be no better than alternatives, or avoid healthy behaviors.

Most uses of the term *ethical* describe a person, an action, a policy, a belief, or a theory, not a product. Yet in 1976, the Subcommittee on Health and the Environment of the U.S. House of Representatives in its "Discursive Dictionary of Health Care" defined *ethical drug* as "a *drug* which is advertised only to physicians and other *prescribing* health *professionals*. Drug manufacturers which make only or primarily such drugs are referred to as the ethical drug industry. Synonymous with *prescription drug*" (italics in original).

Less than a decade later, pharmaceutical companies began advertising directly to consumers, and now one seldom hears the term *ethical drug*. Manufacturers still advertise to physicians, and physicians must still prescribe the drugs, but consumers are now a prime marketing target, especially through television. In 1983, the Food and Drug Administration (FDA), which regulates the approval and marketing of medications, imposed a moratorium on this type of marketing but lifted it two years later. In 1997, the agency changed its guidelines to allow more flexibility in television advertising in describing medication risks.

As any television viewer or magazine reader knows, the amount and intensity of drug advertising has been escalating ever since. In its November 2006 report, "Prescription Drugs: Improvements Needed in FDA's Oversight of Direct-to-Consumer Advertising," the General Accounting Office (GAO) of the U.S. House of Representatives reported that drug company spending on prescription drugs increased twice as fast from 1997 through 2005 as spending on promotion to physicians or on research and development. The FDA reviews only a small portion of the direct-to-consumer material it receives, is issuing fewer regulatory letters than it did in a 2002 GAO study, and is taking longer to issue them. The GAO concluded that the agency "cannot ensure that it is identifying or reviewing those materials that it would consider to be of the highest priority."

According to a content analysis of drug advertising in magazines from 1989 through 1998, conducted by Michael Wilkes and his colleagues at the University of California at Los Angeles, the most common medical conditions in these ads were allergies, obstetrical/gynecological, dermatological, cardiovascular, HIV/AIDS, and tobacco addiction. Women were more likely to be targeted than men.

The ads worked. The GAO report found that between 1999 and 2000 the number of prescriptions dispensed for the most heavily advertised drugs rose 25 percent but increased only 4 percent for not-so-visibly promoted drugs. Nicotine patches for tobacco addiction became an $800 million business as a result of advertising. Aggressive marketing of Claritin, produced by Schering-Plough, resulted in this drug accounting for more than half of the $1.8 billion spent in its marketing category. (In November 2002, the FDA took Claritin off the prescription drug list so that it is now available over the counter.)

A national survey conducted by *Prevention Magazine* in 1998 found that more than 53 million consumers talked to their physicians about an advertised medication, and another 49 million looked for information from another source, such as an Internet site. The GAO report estimates that about 8.5 million consumers (5 percent of the total) have both requested and received a prescription for a particular drug as a result of seeing a direct-to-consumer ad.

Although studies have found that consumers remember drug advertising, the consumers have misconceptions about a government's role in regulating this practice. Half of the respondents in a Sacramento County survey conducted by Wilkes and his UCLA colleagues believed that drug ads had to be submitted to the government for prior approval, which is not the case. Nor is it true, as 43 percent believed, that only completely safe drugs can be advertised or that drugs with serious side effects cannot be advertised, as 22 percent believed. Drug manufacturers are only required to truthfully present a fair balance of risks and effectiveness.

On balance, is direct-to-consumer advertising ethically justified or not? Does it enhance patient autonomy by giving information that in earlier decades was available only to physicians? The following selections provide two views of the debate. From an industry standpoint, Paul Antony finds benefits to individual health from alerting consumers to treatable conditions and encouraging them to take their medicines as prescribed. From their perspectives as physicians, David A. Kessler and Douglas A. Levy question whether industry spending on direct-to-consumer advertising is for patient benefit and may in fact lead to unnecessary and risky choices.

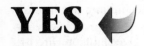

YES

Paul Antony

Testimony Before the Senate Special Committee on Aging

Mr. Chairman, Ranking Member Kohl and Members of the Committee, on behalf of the Pharmaceutical Research and Manufacturers of America (PhRMA), I am pleased to appear at this hearing today on direct-to-consumer (DTC) advertising. I am Paul Antony, M.D., Chief Medical Officer at PhRMA.

DTC advertising has been proven to be beneficial to American patients. And, continuing regulatory oversight by the FDA helps ensure that the content of DTC advertising informs and educates consumers about medical conditions and treatment options. PhRMA and its member companies have a responsibility to ensure that ads comply with FDA regulations. We take that job seriously. We want to continue to be a valuable contributor to improving public health.

DTC advertising can be a powerful tool in educating millions of people and improving health. Because of DTC advertising, large numbers of Americans are prompted to discuss illnesses with their doctors for the first time. Because of DTC advertising, patients become more involved in their own health care decisions, and are proactive in their patient–doctor dialogue. Because of DTC advertising, patients are more likely to take their prescribed medicines.

PhRMA's Guiding Principles on Direct-to-Consumer Advertisements about Prescription Medicines

PhRMA and its member companies have long understood the special relationship we have with the patients that use our innovative medicines. Despite the very positive role DTC advertising plays in educating patients about health issues and options, over the years, we have heard the concerns expressed about DTC advertising—that some ads may oversell benefits and undersell risks; that some ads may lead to inappropriate prescribing; that some patients may not be able to afford the advertised medicines; and that some ads may not be appropriate for some audiences. Some doctors have also complained that drug companies launch advertising campaigns without helping to educate doctors in advance. Although actual practice and data on the effects of DTC advertising differ from these concerns, PhRMA recognized our obligation to act. On July 29,

2005, PhRMA's Board of Directors unanimously approved Guiding Principles on Direct-to-Consumer Advertisements About Prescription Medicine. These principles help ensure that DTC advertising remains an important and powerful tool to educate patients while at the same time addressing many of the concerns expressed about DTC advertising over the past few years.

First, PhRMA member companies take their responsibility to fully comply with FDA advertising regulations very seriously. Our advertising is already required to be accurate and not misleading; it can only make claims supported by substantial evidence; it must reflect the balance between risks and benefits; and it must be consistent with FDA-approved labeling. However, patients, health care providers and the general public expect us to do more than just meet our exacting legal obligations, and our Guiding Principles do go further.

Our principles recognize that at the heart of our companies' DTC communications efforts is patient education. This means that DTC communications designed to market a medicine should responsibly educate patients about a medicine, including the conditions for which it may be prescribed. DTC advertising should also foster responsible communications between patients and health care professionals to help the patient achieve better health and a better appreciation of a medicine's known benefits and risks. Specifically, the Principles state that risk and safety information should be designed to achieve a balanced presentation of both risks and benefits associated with the advertised medicines.

Our Guiding Principles recognize that companies should spend appropriate time educating health care professionals about a new medicine before it is advertised to patients. That way, providers will be prepared to discuss the appropriateness of a given medication with a patient.

Current law provides that companies must submit their DTC television advertisements to FDA upon first use for FDA's review at its discretion. Companies that sign onto these Guiding Principles agree to submit all new DTC television ads to the FDA before releasing these ads for broadcast, giving the agency an opportunity to review consistent with its priorities and resources. Companies also commit to informing FDA of the earliest date the advertisement is set to air. Should new information concerning a previously unknown safety risk be discovered, companies commit to work with FDA to "responsibly alter or discontinue a DTC advertising campaign."

In addition, the Principles encourage companies to include, where feasible, information about help for the uninsured and underinsured in their DTC communications. Our member companies offer a host of programs that can assist needy patients with their medicines.

The Principles also recognize that ads should respect the seriousness of the health condition and medicine being advertised and that ads employing humor or entertainment may not be appropriate in all instances.

As a result of concerns that certain prescription drug ads may not be suitable for all viewing audiences, the Guiding Principles state that, "DTC television and print advertisements should be targeted to avoid audiences that are not age appropriate for the messages involved."

Signatory companies are committed to establishing their own internal processes to ensure compliance with the Guiding Principles and to broadly disseminate them internally and to advertisers. In addition, PhRMA's Board unanimously approved the creation of an office of accountability to ensure the public has an opportunity to comment on companies' compliance with these Principles. The office of accountability will be responsible for receiving comments from the general public and from health care professionals regarding DTC ads by any company that publicly states it will follow the principles. The PhRMA office of accountability will provide to these companies any comment that is reasonably related to compliance with the Principles. Periodic reports will be issued by the PhRMA office of accountability to the public regarding the nature of the comments. Each report will also be submitted to the FDA.

PhRMA's Board also agreed to select an independent panel of outside experts and individuals to review reports from the office of accountability after one year and evaluate overall trends in the industry as they relate to the Principles. The panel will be empowered to make recommendations in accordance with the Principles. The Principles will go into effect in January 2006.

We believe these Principles will help patients and health care professionals get the information they need to make informed health care decisions.

The Value of DTC Advertising

Informing and Empowering Consumers

Surveys indicate that DTC advertising makes consumers aware of new drugs and their benefits, as well as risks and side effects with the drugs advertised. They help consumers recognize symptoms and seek appropriate care. According to an article in *The New England Journal of Medicine,* DTC advertising is concentrated among a few therapeutic categories. These are therapeutic categories in which consumers can recognize their own symptoms, such as arthritis, seasonal allergies, and obesity; or for pharmaceuticals that treat chronic diseases with many undiagnosed sufferers, such as high cholesterol, osteoporosis, and depression.

DTC advertising gets patients talking to their doctors about conditions that may otherwise have gone undiagnosed or undertreated. For example, a study conducted by RAND Health and published in *The New England Journal of Medicine* found that nearly half of all adults in the United States fail to receive recommended health care. According to researchers on the RAND study, "the deficiencies in care . . . pose serious threats to the health of the American public that could contribute to thousands of preventable deaths in the United States each year." The study found underuse of prescription medications in seven of the nine conditions for which prescription medicines were the recommended treatment. Conditions for which underuse was found include asthma, cerebrovascular disease, congestive heart failure, diabetes, hip fracture, hyperlipidemia and hypertension. Of those seven conditions for which RAND found underuse of recommended prescription medicines, five are DTC advertised.

The Rand Study, as well as other studies, highlight the underuse of needed medications and other healthcare services in the U.S.

- According to a nationally representative study of 9,090 people aged 18 and up, published in *JAMA*, about 43 percent of participants with recent major depression are getting inadequate therapy.
- A 2004 study published in the *Archives of Internal Medicine*, found that, "In older patients, failures to prescribe indicated medications, monitor medications appropriately, document necessary information, educate patients, and maintain continuity are more common prescribing problems than is use of inappropriate drugs."
- A May/June 2003 study published in the *Journal of Managed Care Pharmacy*, which examined claims data from 3 of the 10 largest health plans in California to determine the appropriateness of prescription medication use based upon widely accepted treatment guidelines, found that "effective medication appears to be underused." Of the four therapeutic areas of study—asthma, CHF, depression, and common cold or upper respiratory tract infections—asthma, CHF, and depression were undertreated. The researchers concluded that "the results are particularly surprising and disturbing when we take into account the fact that three of the conditions studied (asthma, CHF, and depression) are known to produce high costs to the healthcare system."
- According to a study released in May 2005 by the Stanford University School of Medicine, among patients with high cholesterol in moderate and high-risk groups, researchers found fewer than half of patient visits ended with a statin recommendation. Based on the findings, the researchers say physicians should be more aggressive in investigating statin therapy for patients with a high or moderate risk of heart disease, and that patients should ask for their cholesterol levels to be checked regularly.

Increasing Communication between the Doctor and Patient

A vast majority of patients (93 percent) who asked about a drug reported that their doctor "welcomed the questions." Of patients who asked about a drug, 77 percent reported that their relationship with their doctor remained unchanged as a result of the office visit, and 20 percent reported that their relationship improved. In addition, both an FDA survey of physicians (from a random sample of 500 physicians from the American Medical Association's database) and a survey by the nation's oldest and largest African-American medical association, found that DTC advertisements raise disease awareness and bolster doctor–patient ties.

The doctor–patient relationship is enhanced if DTC advertising prompts a patient to talk to his doctor for the first time about a previously undiscussed condition, to comply with a prescribed treatment regimen, or to become aware of a risk or side effect that was otherwise unknown. A 2002 *Prevention Magazine* survey found that 24.8 million Americans spoke with their doctor about a medical condition for the first time as a result of seeing a DTC advertisement.

Similarly, the FDA patient survey on DTC advertising found that nearly one in five patients reported speaking to a physician about a condition for the first time because of a DTC ad.

PhRMA and its member companies believe it is vital that patients, in consultation with their doctors, make decisions about treatments and medicines. Prescribing decisions should be dominated by the doctor's advice. While our member companies direct a large majority of their promotional activities toward physicians, such promotion in no way guarantees medicines will be prescribed.

According to a General Accounting Office report, of the 61.1 million people (33 percent of adults) who had discussions with their physician as a result of a DTC advertisement in 2001, only 8.5 million (5 percent of adults) actually received a prescription for the product, a small percentage of the total volume of prescriptions dispensed. Indeed, an FDA survey of physicians revealed that the vast majority of physicians do not feel pressure to prescribe. According to the survey, 91 percent of physicians said that their patients did not try to influence treatment courses in a way that would have been harmful and 72 percent of physicians, when asked for prescription for a specific brand name drug, felt little or no pressure to prescribe a medicine.

De-stigmatizing Disease

DTC advertising also encourages patients to discuss medical problems that otherwise may not have been discussed because it was either thought to be too personal or that there was a stigma attached to the disease. For example, a Health Affairs article examined the value of innovation and noted that depression medications, known as selective serotonin reuptake inhibitors (SSRIs), that have been DTC advertised, have led to significant treatment expansion. Prior to the 1990s, it was estimated that about half of those persons who met a clinical definition of depression were not appropriately diagnosed, and many of those diagnosed did not receive clinically appropriate treatment. However, in the 1990s with the advent of SSRIs, treatment has been expanded. According to the article, "Manufacturers of SSRIs encouraged doctors to watch for depression and the reduced stigma afforded by the new medications induced patients to seek help." As a result, diagnosis and treatment for depression doubled over the 1990s.

Utilization and DTC Advertising

According to reports and studies, there is no direct relationship between DTC advertising and the price growth of drugs. For example, in comments to the FDA in December 2003, the FTC stated, "[DTC advertising] can empower consumers to manage their own health care by providing information that will help them, with the assistance of their doctors, to make better informed decisions about their treatment options. . . . Consumer receive these benefits from DTC advertising with little, if any, evidence that such advertising increases prescription drug prices." Notably, since January 2000, the CPI component that tracks prescription medicines have been in line with overall medical inflation.

The FTC comments referenced above also note, "DTC advertising accounts for a relatively small proportion of the total cost of drugs, which reinforces the view that such advertising would have a limited, if any, effect on price." Likewise, a study by Harvard University and the Massachusetts Institute of Technology and published by the Kaiser Family Foundation found that DTC advertising accounts for less than 2 percent of the total U.S. spending for prescription medicines.

One study in *The American Journal of Managed Care* looked at whether pharmaceutical marketing has led to an increase in the use of medications by patients with marginal indications. The study found that high-risk individuals were receiving lipid-lowering treatment "consistent with evidence-based practice guidelines" despite the fact that "a substantial portion of patients continue to remain untreated and undertreated. . . ." The study concluded that "greater overall use did not appear to be associated with a shift towards patients with less CV [cardiovascular] risk."

Pharmaceutical utilization is increasing for reasons other than DTC advertising. As the June 2003 study of DTC advertising commissioned by the Kaiser Family Foundation found, "[O]ur estimates indicate that DTCA is important, but not the primary driver of recent growth [in prescription drug spending]."

Other reasons pharmaceutical utilization is increasing, include:

- Improved Medicines—Many new medicines replace higher-cost surgeries and hospital care. In 2004 alone, pharmaceutical companies added 38 new medicines and over the last decade, over 300 new medicines have become available for treating patients. These include important new medicines for some of the most devastating and costly diseases, including: AIDS, cancer, heart disease, Alzheimer's, and diabetes. According to a study prepared for the Department of Health and Human Services, "[n]ew medications are not simply more costly than older ones. They may be more effective or have fewer side effects; some may treat conditions for which no treatment was available."
- New Standards of Medical Practice Encouraging Greater Use of Pharmaceuticals—Clinical standards are changing to emphasize earlier and tighter control of a range of conditions, such as diabetes, hypertension and cardiovascular disease. For example, new recommendations from the two provider groups suggest that early treatment, including lifestyle changes and treatment with two or more types of medications, can significantly reduce the risk of later complications and improve the quality of life for people with type 2 diabetes.
- Greater Treatment of Previously Undiagnosed and Untreated Conditions—According to guidelines developed by the National Heart, Lung, and Blood Institute's National Cholesterol Education Program (NCEP) Adult Treatment Panel (ATP), approximately 36 million adults should be taking medicines to lower their cholesterol, a number that has grown from 13 million just 8 years ago.
- Aging of America—The aging of American translates into greater reliance on pharmaceuticals. For example, congestive heart failure affects an estimated 2 percent of Americans age 40 to 59, more than 5 percent of those aged 60 to 69, and 10 percent of those 70 or more.

While some assume that DTC advertising leads to increased use of newer medicines rather than generic medicines, generics represent just over 50 percent of all prescriptions (generics are historically not DTC advertised). In contrast, in Europe, where DTC advertising is prohibited, the percentage of prescriptions that are generic is significantly lower. Likewise, it is worth noting that while broadcast DTC has been in place since 1997, the rate of growth in drug cost increases has declined in each of the last 5 years and in 2004 was below the rate of growth in overall health care costs.

Economic Value of DTC Advertising

Increased spending on pharmaceuticals often leads to lower spending on other forms of more costly health care. New drugs are the most heavily advertised drugs, a point critics often emphasize. However, the use of newer drugs tends to lower all types of non-drug medical spending, resulting in a net reduction in the total cost of treating a condition. For example, on average replacing an older drug with a drug 15 years newer increases spending on drugs by $18, but reduces overall costs by $111.

The Tufts Center for the Study of Drug Development reports that disease management organizations surveyed believe that increased spending on prescription drugs reduces hospital inpatient costs. "Since prescription drugs account for less than 10 percent of total current U.S. health care spending, while inpatient care accounts for 32 percent, the increased use of appropriate pharmaceutical therapies may help moderate or reduce growth in the costliest component of the U.S. health care system," according to Tufts Center Director Kenneth I. Kaitin.

Opponents also compare the amount of money spent by drug companies on marketing and advertising to the amount they spend on research and development of new drugs. However, in 2004, pharmaceutical manufacturers spent an estimated $4.15 billion on DTC advertising, according to IMS Health, compared to $49.3 billion in total R&D spending by the biopharmaceutical industry, according to Burrill & Company. PhRMA members alone spent $38.8 billion on R&D in 2004.

Conclusion

DTC advertising provides value to patients by making them aware of risks and benefits of new drugs; it empowers patients and enhances the public health; it plays a vital role in addressing a major problem in this country of undertreatment and underdiagnosis of disease; it encourages patients to discuss medical problems with their health care provider that may otherwise not be discussed due to a stigma being attached to the disease; and it encourages patient compliance with physician-directed treatment regimens.

Given the progress that continues to be made in society's battle against disease, patients are seeking more information about medical problems and potential treatments. The purpose of DTC advertising is to foster an informed conversation about health, disease and treatments between patients and their health care practitioners. Our Guiding Principles are an important step in ensuring patients and health care professionals get the information they need to make informed health care decisions.

This concludes my written testimony. I would be happy to answer any questions or to supply any additional material by Members or Committee Staff on this or any other issue.

David A. Kessler and
Douglas A. Levy

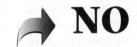 **NO**

Direct-to-Consumer Advertising: Is It Too Late to Manage the Risks?

Pharmaceutical spending on television commercials nearly doubled from $654 million in 2001 to a staggering $1.19 billion in 2005. Nearly one third of the 2005 spending was on only 1 category: sleep medicines.[1] Yet, sleep disorders, however problematic and serious they may be, are almost inconsequential when compared with the major causes of the death in the United States: cardiovascular disease, cancer, and unintentional injuries.[2] No matter how much the industry claims its advertising provides public health benefits, the amount spent promoting drugs for conditions of varying severity begs the question of whether the industry truly is acting for the public benefit.

As Frosch et al. show in this issue,[3] nearly all pharmaceutical ads are based on emotional appeals, not facts, and few provide necessary details about the causes of a medical condition, risk factors, or lifestyle changes that may be appropriate alternatives to pharmaceutical intervention.

Although none of these findings are surprising, they should be disturbing.

As physicians, we know that even the most effective pharmaceutical may not be right for every patient. Physicians consider everything from individual risk factors and medical history to lifestyle and insurance status before writing a prescription. Yet, when patients walk in the door having just seen a television ad showing a miserable allergy sufferer dancing through a weed-filled field, they expect that a simple stroke of a pen onto a prescription pad will solve whatever their problems may be. Patients learn for the first time about conditions they never worried about before and ask physicians for new medicines by trade name because they saw it on television.

Patients have always expected simple answers to complex questions, but direct-to-consumer (DTC) advertising has elevated this problem to new heights, because patients in some ways now rely on Madison Avenue as a provider of health information. There is nothing wrong with pharmaceutical companies communicating directly with consumers, but they should adhere to the standards and ethics of medicine, not the standards and ethics of selling soap or some other consumer product that presents minimal risks.

Pharmaceutical companies like to say that DTC ads make people aware of medical conditions they did not know they had. Industry spokesman Paul Antony told a Senate hearing in 2005, "DTC advertising can be a powerful tool in educating millions of people and improving health."[4]

From *Annals of Family Medicine*, 5 (1), January/February 2007, pp. 4–7. Copyright © 2007 by American Academy of Family Physicians. All rights reserved. Reprinted by permission.

Even if health education is true theoretically, it does not appear to be true in practice. Furthermore, one might question the societal benefit should such communications result in millions more people with conditions being diagnosed that are not major factors in morbidity and mortality. There likely would be strong support for pharmaceutical advertising if it led to millions more conditions diagnosed and people being treated for diabetes or heart disease.

What is equally important is the possibility—the likelihood—that consumers who make health decisions based on what they learn from television commercials ultimately take medicines they may not need, spend money on brand medicines that may be no better than alternatives, or avoid healthy behaviors because they falsely think a medicine is all they need.

In general, the ads that consumers see do not contain the right balance of information to provide any meaningful health education. The facts gleaned from DTC ads are minimal at best, which is an unsurprising consequence of condensing decades of research into a 60-second commercial. Moreover, findings from patients' and physicians' surveys show that the messages that patients take from DTC ads and into their physicians' offices are often wrong.[5] The pharmaceutical companies have done a skillful job of portraying complex medicines in the simplest terms—even if doing so creates inaccurate perceptions in the minds of our patients.

One fact is unquestionable: DTC ads do not effectively or consistently convey important information about product risks and benefits. When the Food and Drug Administration surveyed a sampling of primary care and specialty physicians in 2002, 41% of all physicians said they believed their patients were confused about a drug's efficacy because of DTC ads they saw; 22% of primary care physicians and 13% of specialists said they felt "somewhat" or "very" pressured to prescribe a drug when a patient requested it.[6] Even if physicians resist this pressure, the possibility of risk remains.

Under increased scrutiny, major pharmaceutical companies last year announced new advertising guidelines and pledged to portray serious health conditions seriously and to disclose risks, side effects, and warnings adequately.[7] Although these efforts may be a step in the right direction, physicians, consumers, and policy makers must take further action so that the facts about medicines are not lost in the advertising fog. As Frosch et al. correctly point out, the consequences of poor judgments are quite different for drugs than they are for soap.

References

1. Prescription drugs. *Media Week*. May 1, 2006;SR30.

2. *Health, United States, 2005 With Chartbook on Trends in the Health of Americans*. Hyattsville, Md: National Center for Health Statistics; 2005:195.

3. Frosch DL, Krueger PM, Hornik RC, Cronholm PF, Barg FK. Creating demand for prescription drugs: a content analysis of television direct-to-consumer advertising. *Ann Fam Med*. 2007;5(1):6–13.

4. PhRMA Chief Medical Officer Testifies on DTC Advertising. Washington, DC; 2005: News release publishing PhRMA testimony at Senate hearing. . . .

5. Aikin KJ, Braman AC. Patient and Physician Attitudes and Behaviors Associated With DTC Promotion of Prescription Drugs—Summary of FDA Survey Research Results. Washington, DC: US Department of Health and Human Services. Food and Drug Administration. Center for Drug Evaluation and Research; 2004:63–84.

6. *The Impact of Direct-to-Consumer Drug Advertising on Seniors' Health and Health Care Costs. Senate Special Committee on Aging.* First Session ed. Washington, DC: US Government Printing Office; 2005:30.

7. PhRMA guiding principles direct-to-consumer advertisements about prescription medicines. 2005. . . .

POSTSCRIPT

Does Direct-to-Consumer Drug Advertising Enhance Patient Choice?

From 1996 to 2005, spending on direct-to-consumer advertising increased by 330 percent but still made up only 14 percent of the total promotional spending. Most drug advertising still targets physicians. The number of letters the FDA sent to pharmaceutical manufacturers about violations in their advertising fell from 142 in 1997 to only 21 in 2006 (Julie M. Donohue et al., "A Decade of Direct-to-Consumer Advertising of Prescription Drugs," *New England Journal of Medicine,* August 16, 2007).

Americans watch on average 16 hours of prescription drug advertising a year. A content analysis of these ads found limited information about the causes of a disease or who might be at risk. The ads appeal to the emotional aspect of losing control over some life activities and minimize lifestyle changes as a way to regain control (Dominick L. Frosch et al., "Creating Demand for Prescription Drugs: A Content Analysis of Television Direct-to-Consumer Advertising," *Annals of Family Medicine,* January/February 2007).

Researchers from Harvard University/Massachusetts General Hospital and Harris Interactive conducted a national telephone survey of consumers in 2002 asking about their experience with direct-to-consumer drug advertising. About 35 percent reported that an ad prompted them to have a discussion with a physician about the drug or the condition. A quarter of these patients received a new diagnosis, and nearly three-quarters were given a prescription, with about 43 percent getting a prescription for the advertised drug. About four out of five consumers who got a drug and took it as prescribed reported feeling much or somewhat better (Joel S. Weissman et al., "Consumers' Reports on the Health Effects of Direct-to-Consumer Drug Advertising," *Health Affairs*, February 2003). The same team also surveyed physicians on this issue. They pointed to improved communication and education as a benefit of direct-to-consumer advertising but also felt it led patients to seek unnecessary treatments. When the advertised drug was prescribed, 46 percent of physicians said it was the most effective treatment and 48 percent said that other drugs were equally effective. Among the most common new diagnoses were impotence (15.5 percent), anxiety (9 percent), and arthritis (6.8 percent) (Joel Weissman et al., "Physicians Report on Patient Encounters Involving Direct-to-Consumer Advertising," *Health Affairs*, April 28, 2004).

A more subtle form of consumer persuasion involves news reporting on medication studies, which often fail to report pharmaceutical funding and frequently refer to medications by their brand names instead of their generic counterparts. Since favorable studies get the most press, consumers are indirectly encouraged to ask their physicians for the brand name drug. See Michael Hochman et al., "News Media Coverage of Medication Research," *Journal of the American Medical Association* (October 2, 2008).

Internet References . . .

Euthanasia and Physician-Assisted Suicide: All Sides of the Issues

This site offers a general overview of the controversy concerning physician-assisted suicide as well as statistics and a list of Web sites that represent both sides of the debate.

**http://www.religioustolerance.org/
euthanas.htm**

National Hospice and Palliative Care Organization

This organization's Web site has information about each state's advance directive rules as well as aspects of care of dying people.

http://www.nhpco.org

End-of-Life Dilemmas

*W*hat are the ethical responsibilities associated with death? Doctors are sworn "to do no harm," but this proscription is open to many different interpretations. Death is a natural event that can, in some instances, be hastened to put an end to suffering. Is it ethically necessary to prolong life at all times under all circumstances? Medical personnel as well as families often face these agonizing questions. They are made more agonizing in disaster conditions, when ordinary resources are not available. The right of an individual to decide his or her own fate may conflict with society's interest in maintaining the value of human life or in not wasting valuable resources that could be used to save other lives. This conflict is apparent in the matter of physician-assisted suicide and, in a different way, in the question of "futile" treatment. This section examines some of these anguishing questions.

- Have Advance Directives Failed?

- Is "Palliative Sedation" Ethically Different from Active Euthanasia?

- Should Physicians Be Allowed to Assist in Patient Suicide?

ISSUE 4

Have Advance Directives Failed?

YES: Angela Fagerlin and Carl E. Schneider, from "Enough: The Failure of the Living Will," *Hastings Center Report* (March–April 2004)

NO: Susan E. Hickman, Bernard J. Hammes, Alvin H. Moss, and Susan W. Tolle, from "Hope for the Future: Achieving the Original Intent of Advance Directives," *Hastings Center Report* (November–December 2005)

ISSUE SUMMARY

YES: Psychologist Angela Fagerlin and law professor Carl E. Schneider believe not only that living wills have failed to live up to their advocates' expectations but also that these expectations were unrealistic from the start.

NO: Susan E. Hickman, Bernard J. Hammes, Alvin H. Moss, and Susan W. Tolle, multidisciplinary specialists in end-of-life care, recognize the limitations of traditional advance directives but argue that newer processes of introducing advance directives can achieve their original aims.

Since ancient times people have drawn up wills to determine what should be done with their property, or who should take custody of their children, after they die. In 1969 Luis Kutner, a law professor, proposed a "living will," a document that would determine the course of medical treatment should the signer become unable to express his or her wishes. A typical living will states, "If I am permanently unconscious or there is no reasonable expectation for my recovery from a serious incapacitating or lethal illness or condition, I do not wish to be kept alive by artificial means." The proposal came at a time when the public was just beginning to be aware of the use of machines to keep people breathing and their hearts beating even though there was no possibility of regaining consciousness. In 1975, the Karen Ann Quinlan case, involving a young, permanently unconsciousness woman on a ventilator, focused ethical and legal attention on the unwanted use of medical technology.

In 1976, following the Quinlan case, California enacted the nation's first law approving the use of living wills. Nearly every state in the United States followed suit. Sometimes called "natural death acts," these laws and the wills they approved were so vaguely worded and so difficult to interpret that they were hardly ever effective in achieving their goals. It was difficult, for example, to determine what was meant by "reasonable expectation," "artificial means," or even "lethal illness."

In 1983 the President's Commission for the Study of Ethical Problems in Medicine and Biomedical and Behavioral Research recommended an alternative approach. Rather than signing a document that specified certain treatments that should be forgone, patients were encouraged to name a person who would make health care decisions in their place.

There are several types of advance directives. They can be formally written and legally authorized, or they can be informal communications with family members or health care providers. Much of the legal wrangling about withdrawal of life supports has turned on whether or not the patient expressed such desires while competent. The case of Nancy Cruzan, which eventually went to the U.S. Supreme Court, is one example. The parents of this young Missouri woman, who was permanently unconscious after an automobile accident, sued the state to have her life supports removed, claiming that this is what Nancy herself would have wanted. The state argued that there was no clear and convincing evidence that Nancy would have made the same decision. In 1990 the U.S. Supreme Court ruled that states had an interest in preserving life and could require a high standard of evidence of the patient's expressed preference for withdrawing treatment. The case then went back to the Missouri courts, which this time found the evidence convincing and agreed to allow withdrawal of life support.

To add to the weight of the Supreme Court's decision, in 1991 Congress passed the Patient Self-Determination Act (PSDA), which requires all health care providers reimbursed by Medicare to inform patients about their right to sign advance directives. By this measure Congress intended to promote the use of advance directives in hospitals and nursing homes where elderly patients are often treated.

Despite legislative and judicial approval of advance directives and widespread public opinion supporting them, such documents are still rarely signed by competent patients, and even when signed they are still rarely consulted or implemented. Studies have documented barriers such as lack of appropriate communication and physicians' disregard of the wishes expressed in the directives.

The following selections address the status and future of advance directives from the vantage point of more than 30 years' experience. Angela Fagerlin and Carl E. Schneider want to call halt to the attempt to get people to sign living wills (not health care proxies) because they believe that despite vigorous attempts, the policy has not produced results. Susan E. Hickman and colleagues argue that the original intent of advance directives—to enable patients to gain control over their terminal care—can be achieved by newer, more successful models.

YES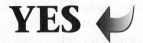

Angela Fagerlin and
Carl E. Schneider

Enough: The Failure of the Living Will

By their fruits ye shall know them.

Enough. The living will has failed, and it is time to say so.

We should have known it would fail: A notable but neglected psychological literature always provided arresting reasons to expect the policy of living wills to misfire. Given their alluring potential, perhaps they were worth trying. But a crescendoing empirical literature and persistent clinical disappointments reveal that the rewards of the campaign to promote living wills do not justify its costs. Nor can any degree of tinkering ever make the living will an effective instrument of social policy.

As the evidence of failure has mounted, living wills have lost some of their friends. We offer systematic support for their change of heart. But living wills are still widely and confidently urged on patients, and they retain the allegiance of many bioethicists, doctors, nurses, social workers, and patients. For these loyal advocates, we offer systematic proof that such persistence in error is but the triumph of dogma over inquiry and hope over experience.

A note about the scope of our contentions: First, we reject only living wills, not durable powers of attorney. Second, there are excellent reasons to be skeptical of living wills on principle. For example, perhaps former selves should not be able to bind latter selves in the ways living wills contemplate.[1] And many people do and perhaps should reject the view of patients, their families, and their communities that informs living wills.[2] But we accept for the sake of argument that living wills desirably serve a strong version of patients' autonomy. We contend, nevertheless, that living wills do not and cannot achieve that goal.

And a stipulation: We do not propose the elimination of living wills. We can imagine recommending them to patients whose medical situation is plain, whose crisis is imminent, whose preferences are specific, strong, and delineable, and who have special reasons to prescribe their care. We argue on the level of public policy: In an attempt to extend patients' exercise of autonomy beyond their span of competence, resources have been lavished to make living wills routine and even universal. This policy has

From *Hastings Center Report,* March/April 2004. Copyright © 2004 by The Hastings Center. Reprinted by permission of the publisher and Angela Fagerlin and Carl E. Schneider.

not produced results that recompense its costs, and it should therefore be renounced.

Living wills are a bioethical idea that has passed from controversy to conventional wisdom, from the counsel of academic journals to the commands of law books, from professors' proposal to professional practice. Advance directives generally are embodied in federal policy by the Patient Self-Determination Act, which requires medical institutions to give patients information about their state's advance directives. In turn, the law of every state provides for advance directives, almost all states provide for living wills, and most states "have at least two statutes, one establishing a living will type directive, the other establishing a proxy or durable power of attorney for health care."[3] Not only are all these statutes very much in effect, but new legislative activity is constant. Senators Rockefeller, Collins, and Specter have introduced bills to "strengthen" the PSDA and living wills,[4] and state legislatures continue to amend living will statutes and to enact new ones.

Courts and administrative agencies too have become advocates of living wills. The Veterans Administration has proposed a rule to encourage the use of advance directives, including living wills.[5] Where legislatures have not granted living wills legal status, some courts have done so as a matter of common law, and where legislatures have granted them legal status, courts have cooperated with eager enthusiasm.[6] Living wills have assumed special importance in states that prohibit terminating treatment in the absence of strong evidence of the patient's wishes.[7] One supreme court summarized a common theme: "[A] written directive would provide the most concrete evidence of the patient's decisions, and we strongly urge all persons to create such a directive."[8]

The grandees of law and medicine also give their benediction to the living will. The AMA's Council on Ethical and Judicial Affairs proclaims: "Physicians should encourage their patients to document their treatment preferences or to appoint a health care proxy with whom they can discuss their values regarding health care and treatment."[9] The elite National Conference of Commissioners on Uniform State Laws continues to promulgate the Uniform Health-Care Decisions Act, a prestigious model statute that has been put into law in a still-growing number of states. Medical journals regularly admonish doctors and nurses to see that patients have advance directives, including living wills.[10] Bar journals regularly admonish lawyers that their clients—*all* their clients—need advance directives, including living wills.[11] Researchers demonstrate their conviction that living wills are important by the persistence of their studies of patients' attitudes toward living wills and ways of inveigling patients to sign them.

Not only do legislatures, courts, administrative agencies, and professional associations promote the living will, but other groups unite with them. The Web abounds in sites advocating the living will to patients.[12] The web site for our university's hospital plugs advance directives and suggests that it "is probably better to have written instructions because then everyone can read them and understand your wishes."[13]

Our own experience in presenting this paper is that its thesis provokes some bioethicists to disbelief and indignation. It is as though they simply cannot bear to believe that living wills might not work. How can anything so intuitively right be proved so infuriatingly wrong? And indeed, bioethicists continue to investigate ways the living will might be extended (to deal with problems of the mentally ill and of minors, for example) and developed for other countries.

Although some sophisticated observers have long doubted the wisdom of living wills,[14] proponents have tended to respond in one of three ways, all of which preserve an important role for living wills. First, proponents have supposed that the principal problem with living wills is that people just won't sign them. These proponents have persevered in the struggle to find ways of getting more people to sign up.[15]

Second, proponents have reasserted the usefulness of the living wills. For example, Norman Cantor, distinguished advocate of living wills, acknowledges that "(s)ome commentators doubt the utility or efficacy of advance directives," (by which he means the living will), but he concludes that "these objections don't obviate the importance of advance directives."[16] Other proponents are daunted by the criticisms of living wills but offer new justifications for them. Linda Emanuel, another eminent exponent of living wills, writes that "living wills can help doctors and patients talk about dying" and can thereby "open the door to a positive, caring approach to death."[17]

Third, some proponents concede the weaknesses of the living will and the advantages of the durable power of attorney and then propose a durable power of attorney that incorporates a living will. That is, the forms they propose for establishing a durable power of attorney invite their authors to provide the kinds of instructions formerly confined to living wills.[18]

None of these responses fully grapples with the whole range of difficulties that confound the policy promoting living wills. In fairness, this is partly because the case against that policy has been made piecemeal and not in a full-fledged and full-throated analysis of the empirical literature on living wills.

In sum, the law has embraced the principle of living wills and cheerfully continues to this moment to expound and expand that principle. Doctors, nurses, hospitals, and lawyers are daily urged to convince their patients and clients to adopt living wills, and patients hear their virtues from many other sources besides. Some advocates of living wills have shifted the grounds for their support of living wills, but they persist in believing that they are useful. The time has come to investigate those policies and those hopes systematically. That is what this article attempts.

We ask an obvious but unasked question: What would it take for a regime of living wills to function as their advocates hope? First, people must have living wills. Second, they must decide what treatment they would want if incompetent. Third, they must accurately and lucidly state that preference. Fourth, their living wills must be available to people making decisions for a patient. Fifth, those people must grasp and heed the living will's instructions. These conditions are unmet and largely unmeetable.

Do People Have Living Wills?

At the level of principle, living wills have triumphed among the public as among the princes of medicine. People widely say they want a living will, and living wills have so much become conventional medical wisdom "that involvement in the process is being portrayed as a duty to physicians and others."[19] Despite this, and despite decades of urging, most Americans lack them.[20] While most of us who need one have a property will, roughly 18 percent have living wills.[21] The chronically or terminally ill are likelier to prepare living wills than the healthy, but even they do so fitfully.[22] In one study of dialysis patients, for instance, only 35 percent had a living will, even though all of them thought living wills a "good idea."[23]

Why do people flout the conventional wisdom? The flouters advance many explanations.[24] They don't know enough about living wills,[25] they think living wills hard to execute,[26] they procrastinate,[27] they hesitate to broach the topic to their doctors (as their doctors likewise hesitate).[28] Some patients doubt they need a living will. Some think living wills are for the elderly or infirm and count themselves in neither group.[29] Others suspect that living wills do not change the treatment people receive; 91 percent of the veterans in one study shared that suspicion.[30] Many patients are content or even anxious to delegate decisions to their families, [31] often because they care less what decisions are made than that they are made by people they trust. Some patients find living wills incompatible with their cultural traditions.[32] Thus in the large SUPPORT and HELP studies, most patients preferred to leave final resuscitation decisions to their family and physician instead of having their own preferences expressly followed (70.8% in HELP and 78.0% in SUPPORT). "This result is so striking that it is worth restating: not even a third of the HELP patients and hardly more than a fifth of the SUPPORT patients "would want their own preferences followed."[33]

If people lacked living wills only because of ignorance, living wills might proliferate with education. But studies seem not to "support the speculations found in the literature that the low level of advance directives use is due primarily to a lack of information and encouragement from health care professionals and family members."[34] Rather, there is considerable evidence "that the elderly's action of delaying execution of advance directives and deferring to others is a deliberate, if not an explicit, refusal to participate in the advance directives process."[35]

The federal government has sought to propagate living wills through the Patient Self-Determination Act,[36] which essentially requires medical institutions to inform patients about advance directives. However, "empirical studies demonstrate that: the PSDA has generally failed to foster a significant increase in advance directives use; it is being implemented by medical institutions and their personnel in a passive manner; and the involvement of physicians in its implementation is lacking."[37] One commentator even thinks "the PSDA's legal requirements have become a ceiling instead of a floor."[38]

In short, people have reasons, often substantial and estimable reasons, for eschewing living wills, reasons unlikely to be overcome by persuasion.

Indeed, persuasion seems quickly to find its limits. Numerous studies indicate that without considerable intervention, approximately 20 percent of us complete living wills, but programs to propagate wills have mixed results.[39] Some have achieved significant if still limited increases in the completion of living wills,[40] while others have quite failed to do so.[41]

Thus we must ask: If after so much propaganda so few of us have living wills, do we really want them, or are we just saying what we think we ought to think and what investigators want to hear?

Do People Know What They Will Want?

Suppose, counterfactually, that people executed living wills. For those documents to work, people would have to predict their preferences accurately. This is an ambitious demand. Even patients making contemporary decisions about contemporary illnesses are regularly daunted by the decisions' difficulty. They are human. We humans falter in gathering information, misunderstand and ignore what we gather, lack well-considered preferences to guide decisions, and rush headlong to choice.[42] How much harder, then, is it to conjure up preferences for an unspecifiable future confronted with unidentifiable maladies with unpredictable treatments?

For example, people often misapprehend crucial background facts about their medical choices. Oregon has made medical policy in fresh and controversial ways, has recently had two referenda on assisted suicide, and alone has legalized it. Presumably, then, its citizens are especially knowledgeable. But only 46 percent of them knew that patients may legally withdraw life-sustaining treatment. Even experience is a poor teacher: "Personal experience with illness . . . and authoring an advance directive . . . were not significantly associated with better knowledge about options."[43]

Nor do people reliably know enough about illnesses and treatments to make prospective life-or-death decisions about them. To take one example from many, people grossly overestimate the effectiveness of CPR and in fact hardly know what it is.[44] For such information, people must rely on doctors. But doctors convey that information wretchedly even to competent patients making contemporaneous decisions. Living wills can be executed without even consulting a doctor,[45] and when doctors are consulted, the conversations are ordinarily short, vague, and tendentious. In the Tulsky study, for example, doctors only described either "dire scenarios . . . in which few people, terminally ill or otherwise, would want treatment" or "situations in which patients could recover with proper treatment."[46]

Let us put the point differently. The conventional—legal and ethical wisdom—insists that candidates for even a flu shot give "informed consent." And that wisdom has increasingly raised the standards for disclosure.[47] If we applied those standards to the information patients have before making the astonishing catalog of momentous choices living wills can embody, the conventional wisdom would be left shivering with indignation.

Not only do people regularly know too little when they sign a living will, but often (again, we're human) they analyze their choices only superficially before placing them in the time capsule. An ocean of evidence affirms that answers are shaped by the way questions are asked. Preferences about treatments are influenced by factors like whether success or failure rates are used,[48] the level of detail employed,[49] and whether longor short-term consequences are explained first.[50] Thus in one study, "201 elderly subjects opted for the intervention 12% of the time when it was presented negatively, 18% of the time when it was phrased as in an advance directive already in use, and 30% of the time when it was phrased positively. Seventy-seven percent of the subjects changed their minds at least once when given the same case scenario but a different description of the intervention."[51]

If patients have trouble with contemporaneous decisions, how much more trouble must they have with prospective ones? For such decisions to be "true," patients' preferences must be reasonably stable. Surprisingly often, they are not. A famous study of eighteen women in a "natural childbirth" class found that preferences about anesthesia and avoiding pain were relatively stable before childbirth, but at "the beginning of active labor (4–5 cm dilation) there was a shift in the preference toward avoiding labor pains. . . . During the transition phase of labor (8–10 cm) the values remained relatively stable, but then . . . the mothers' preferences shifted again at postpartum toward avoiding the use of anesthesia during the delivery of her next child."[52] And not only are preferences surprisingly labile, but people have trouble recognizing that their views have changed.[53] This makes it less likely [that] they will amend their living wills as their opinions develop and more likely that their living wills will treasonously misrepresent their wishes.

Instability matters. The healthy may incautiously prefer death to disability. Once stricken, competent patients can test and reject that preference. They often do.[54] Thus Wilfrid Sheed "quickly learned [that] cancer, even more than polio, has a disarming way of bargaining downward, beginning with your whole estate and then letting you keep the game warden's cottage or badminton court; and by the time it has tried to frighten you to death and threatened to take away your very existence, you'd be amazed at how little you're willing to settle for."[55]

At least sixteen studies have investigated the stability of people's preferences for life-sustaining treatment.[56] A meta-analysis of eleven of these studies found that the stability of patients' preferences was 71 percent (the range was 57 percent to 89 percent).[57] Although stability depended on numerous factors (including the illness, the treatment, and demographic variables), the bottom line is that, over periods as short as two years, almost one-third of preferences for life-sustaining medical treatment changed. More particularly, illness and hospitalization change people's preferences for life-sustaining treatments.[58] In a prospective study, the desire for life-sustaining treatment declined significantly after hospitalization but returned almost to its original level three to six months later.[59] Another study concluded that the "will to live is highly unstable among terminally ill cancer patients."[60] The authors thought their findings "perhaps not surprising, given that only 10–14% of individuals who survive a suicide attempt commit suicide during the next 10 years, which suggests that a desire to die is inherently changeable."

The consistent finding that interest in life-sustaining treatment shifts over time and across contexts coincides tellingly with research charting people's struggles to predict their own tastes, behavior, and emotions even over short periods and under familiar circumstances.[61] People mispredict what poster they will like,[62] how much they will buy at the grocery store,[63] how sublimely they will enjoy an ice cream,[64] and how they will adjust to tenure decisions.[65] And people "miswant" for numerous reasons.[66] They imagine a different event from the one that actually occurs, nurture inaccurate theories about what gives them pleasure,[67] forget they might outwit misery, concentrate on salient negative events and ignore offsetting happier ones,[68] and misgauge the effect of physiological sensations like pain.[69] Given this rich stew of research on people's missteps in predicting their tastes generally, we should expect misapprehensions about end-of-life preferences. Indeed, those preferences should be especially volatile, since people lack experience deciding to die.

Can People Articulate What They Want?

Suppose, *arguendo*, that patients regularly made sound choices about future treatments and write living wills. Can they articulate their choices accurately? This question is crucially unrealistic, of course, because the assumption is false. People have trouble reaching well-considered decisions, and you cannot state clearly on paper what is muddled in your mind. And indeed people do, for instance, issue mutually inconsistent instructions in living wills.[70]

But assume this difficulty away and the problem of articulation persists. In one sense, the best way to divine patients' preferences is to have them write their own living wills to give surrogates the patient's gloriously unmediated voice. This is not a practical policy. Too many people are functionally illiterate,[71] and most of the literate cannot express themselves clearly in writing. It's hard, even for the expert writer. Furthermore, most people know too little about their choices to cover all the relevant subjects. Hence living wills are generally forms that demand little writing. But the forms have failed. For example, "several studies suggest that even those patients who have completed AD forms . . . may not fully understand the function of the form or its language."[72] Living wills routinely baffle patients with their

> "syntactic complexity, concept density, abstractness, organization, coherence, sequence of ideas, page format, length of line of print, length of paragraph, punctuation, illustrations, color, and reader interest." Unfortunately, most advance directive forms . . . often have neither a reasonable scope nor depth. They do not ask all the right questions and they do not ask those questions in a manner that elicits clear responses.[73]

Doctors and lawyers who believe their clients are all above average should ask them what their living will says. One of us (CES) has tried the experiment. The modal answer is, in its entirety: "It says I don't want to be a vegetable."

No doubt the forms could be improved, but not enough to matter. The world abounds in dreadfully drafted forms because writing complex instructions for the future is crushingly difficult. Statutes read horribly because their authors are struggling to (1) work out exactly what rule they want, (2) imagine all the circumstances in which it might apply, and (3) find language to specify all those but only those circumstances. Each task is ultimately impossible, which is why statutes explicitly or implicitly confide their enforcers with some discretion and why courts must interpret—rewrite—statutes. However, these skills and resources are not available to physicians or surrogates.

One might retort that property wills work and that living wills are not that far removed from property wills. But wills work as well as they do to distribute property because their scope is—compared to living wills—narrow and routinized. Most people have little property to distribute and few plausible heirs. As property accumulates and ambitions swell, problems proliferate. Many of them are resolvable because experts—lawyers—exclusively draft and interpret wills. Lawyers have been experimenting for centuries with testamentary language in a process which has produced standard formulas with predictable meanings and standard ways of distributing property into which testators are channeled. Finally, if testators didn't say it clearly enough in the right words and following the right procedures, courts coolly ignore their wishes and substitute default rules.

The lamentable history of the living will demonstrates just how recalcitrant these problems are. There have been, essentially, three generations of living wills. At first, they stated fatuously general desires in absurdly general terms. As the vacuity of overgenerality became clear, advocates of living wills did the obvious: Were living wills too general? Make them specific. Were they "one size fits all"? Make them elaborate questionnaires. Were they uncritically signed? "Require" probing discussions between doctor and patient. However, the demand for specificity forced patients to address more questions than they could comprehend. So, generalities were insufficiently specific and insufficiently considered. Specifics were insufficiently general and perhaps still insufficiently considered. What was a doctor—or lawyer—to do? Behold the "values history," a disquisition on the patient's supposed overarching beliefs from which to infer answers to specific questions.[74] That patients can be induced to trek through these interminable and imponderable documents is unproved and unlikely. That useful conclusions can be drawn from the platitudes they evoke is false. As Justice Holmes knew, "General propositions do not decide concrete cases."[75]

The lessons of this story are that drafting instructions is harder than proponents of living wills seem to believe and that when you move toward one blessing in structuring these documents, you walk away from another. The failure to devise workable forms is not a failure of effort or intelligence. It is a consequence of attempting the impossible.

Where Is the Living Will?

Suppose that, *mirabile dictu*, people executed living wills, knew what they will want, and could say it. That will not matter unless the living will reaches the people responsible for the incompetent patient. Often, it does not. This should be no surprise, for long can be the road from the drafter's chair to the ICU bed.

First, the living will may be signed years before it is used, and its existence and location may vanish in the mists of time.[76] Roughly half of all living wills are drawn up by lawyers and must somehow reach the hospital, and 62 percent of patients do not give their living will to their physician. [77] On admission to the hospital, patients can be too assailed and anxious to recall and mention their advance directives.[78] Admission clerks can be harried, neglectful, and loath to ask patients awkward questions.

Thus when a team of researchers reviewed the charts of 182 patients who had completed a living will before being hospitalized, they found that only 26 percent of the charts accurately recorded information about those directives,[79] and only 16 percent of the charts contained the form. And in another study only 35 percent of the nursing home patients who were transferred to the hospital had their living wills with them.[80]

Will Proxies Read It Accurately?

Suppose, *per impossibile,* that patients wrote living wills, correctly anticipated their preferences, articulated their desires lucidly, and conveyed their document to its interpreters. How acutely will the interpreters analyze their instructions? Living wills are not self-executing: someone must decide whether the patient is incompetent, whether a medical situation described in the living will has arisen, and what the living will then commands.

Usually, the patient's intimates will be central among a living will's interpreters. We might hope that intimates already know the patient's mind, so that only modest demands need be made on their interpreting skills. But many studies have asked such surrogates to predict what treatment the patient would choose.[81] Across these studies, approximately 70 percent of the predictions were correct—not inspiring success for life-and-death decisions.

Do living wills help? We know of only one study that addresses that question. In a randomized trial, researchers asked elderly patients to complete a disease- and treatmentbased or a value-based living will.[82] A control group of elderly patients completed no living will. The surrogates were generally spouses or children who had known the patient for decades. Surrogates who were not able to consult their loved one's living will predicted patients' preferences about 70 percent of the time. Strikingly, surrogates who consulted the living will did no better than surrogates denied it. Nor were surrogates more successful when they discussed living wills with patients just before their prediction.

What is more, a similar study found that primary care physicians' predictions were similarly unimproved by providing them with patients' advance directives.[83] On the other hand, emergency room doctors (complete strangers) given a living will more accurately predicted patients' preferences than ER doctors without one.[84]

Do Living Wills Alter Patient Care?

Our survey of the mounting empirical evidence shows that none of the five requisites to making living wills successful social policy is met now or is likely to be. The program has failed, and indeed is impossible.

That impossibility is confirmed by studies of how living wills are implemented, which show that living wills seem not to affect patients' treatments. For instance, one study concluded that living wills "do not influence the level of medical care overall. This finding was manifested in the quantitatively equal use of diagnostic testing, operations, and invasive hemodynamic monitoring among patients with and without advance directives. Hospital and ICU lengths of stay, as well as health care costs, were also similar for patients with and without advance directive statements."[85] Another study found that in thirty of thirty-nine cases in which a patient was incompetent and the living will was in the patient's medical record, the surrogate decisionmaker was not the person the patient had appointed.[86] In yet a third study, a quarter of the patients received care that was inconsistent with their living will.[87]

But all this is normal. Harry Truman rightly predicted that his successor would "sit here, and he'll say, 'Do this! Do that!' And nothing will happen. Poor Ike—it won't be a bit like the army. He'll find it very frustrating." (Of course, the army isn't like the army either, as Captain Truman surely knew.) Indeed, the whole law of bioethics often seems a whited sepulchre for slaughtered hopes, for its policies have repeatedly fallen woefully short of their purposes. Informed consent is a "fairytale."[88] Programs to increase organ donation have persistently disappointed. Laws regulating DNR orders are hardly better. Legal definitions of brain death are misunderstood by astonishing numbers of doctors and nurses. And so on.[89]

But why don't living wills affect care?[90] Joan Teno and colleagues saw no evidence "that a physician unilaterally decided to ignore or disregard an AD." Rather, there was "a complex interaction of . . . three themes." First (as we have emphasized), "the contents of ADs were vague and difficult to apply to current clinical situations." The imprecision of living wills not only stymies interpreters, it exacerbates their natural tendency to read documents in light of their own preferences. Thus "(e)ven with the therapy-specific AD accompanied by designation of a proxy and prior patient–physician discussion, the proportion of physicians who were willing to withhold therapies was quite variable: cardiopulmonary resuscitation, 100%; administration of artificial nutrition and hydration, 82%; administration of antibiotics, 80%; simple tests, 70%; and administration of pain medication, 13%."[91]

Second, the Teno team found that "patients were not seen as 'absolutely, hopelessly ill,' and thus, it was never considered the time to invoke the AD." Living wills typically operate when patients become terminally ill, but neither doctors nor families lightly conclude patients are dying, especially when that means ending treatment. And understandably. For instance, "on the day before death, the median prognosis for patients with heart failure is still a 50% chance to live 6 more months because patients with heart failure typically die quickly from an unpredictable complication like arrhythmia or infection."[92]

So by the time doctors and families finally conclude the patient is dying, the patient's condition is already so dire that treatment looks pointless quite apart from any living will. "In all cases in which life-sustaining treatment was withheld or withdrawn, this decision was made after a trial of life-sustaining treatment and at a time when the patient was seen as 'absolutely, hopelessly ill' or 'actively dying.' Until patients crossed this threshold, ADs were not seen as applicable." Thus "it is not surprising that our previous research has shown that those with ADs did not differ in timing of DNR orders or patterns of resource utilization from those without ADs."[93]

Third, "family members or the surrogate designated in a [durable power of attorney] were not available, were ineffectual, or were overwhelmed with their own concerns and did not effectively advocate for the patient." Family members are crucial surrogates because they should be: patients commonly want them to be; they commonly want to be; they specially cherish the patient's interests. Doctors ordinarily assume families know the patient's situation and preferences and may not relish responsibility for life-and-death decisions, and doctors intent on avoiding litigation may realize that the only plausible plaintiffs are families. The family, however, may not direct attention to the advance directive and may not insist on its enforcement. In fact, surrogates may be guided by either their own treatment preferences or an urgent desire to keep their beloved alive.[94]

In sum, not only are we awash in evidence that the prerequisites for a successful living wills policy are unachievable, but there is direct evidence that living wills regularly fail to have their intended effect. That failure is confirmed by the numerous convincing explanations for it. And if living wills do not affect treatment, they do not work.

Do Living Wills Have Beneficial Side Effects?

Even if living wills do not effectively promote patients' autonomy, they might have other benefits that justify their costs. There are three promising candidates.

First, living wills might stimulate conversation between doctor and patient about terminal treatment. However, at least one study finds little association between patients' reports of executing an advance directive and their reports of such conversations.[95] Nor do these conversations, when they occur, appear satisfactory.[96] James Tulsky and colleagues asked experienced clinicians who had relationships with patients who were over sixty-five or seriously ill to "discuss advance directives in whatever way you think is appropriate" with them. Although the doctors knew they were being taped, the conversations were impressively short and one-sided: The median discussion "lasted 5.6 minutes (range, 0.9 to 15.0 minutes.) Physicians spoke for a median of 3.9 minutes (range, 0.6 to 10.9 minutes), and patients spoke for the remaining 1.7 minutes (range, 0.3 to 9.6 minutes). . . . Usually, the conversation ended without any specific follow-up plan." The "(p)atients' personal values, goals for care, and reasons for treatment preferences were discussed in 71% of cases and were explicitly elicited by 34% of physicians." But doctors commonly "did not explore the reasons for patient's preferences and merely determined whether they wanted specific interventions."[97]

Nor were the conversations conspicuously informative: "Physicians used vague language to describe scenarios, asking what patients would want if they became 'very, very sick' or 'had something that was very serious.' . . ." Further, "[v]arious qualitative terms were used loosely to describe outcome probabilities." In addition, these brief conversations considered almost exclusively the two ends of the continuum—the most hopeless and the most hopeful cases. Conversations tended to ignore "the more common, less clear-cut predicaments surrounding end-of-life care." True, the patients all thought "their physicians 'did a good job talking about the issues,'" but this only suggests that patients did not understand how little they were told.

The second candidate for beneficial side effect arises from evidence that living wills may comfort patients and surrogates. People with a living will apparently gain confidence that their surrogates will understand their preferences and will implement them comfortably, and the surrogates concur.[98] Improved satisfaction with decisions was also a rare positive effect of the SUPPORT study (which devoted enormous resources to improving end-of-life decisions and care but made dismayingly little difference).[99] In another study, living wills reduced the stress and unhappiness of family members who had recently withdrawn life support from a relative.[100] But even if living wills make patients and surrogates more confident and comfortable, those qualities are apparently unrelated to the accuracy of surrogates' decisions. Thus we are left with the irony that one of the best arguments for a tool for enhancing people's autonomy is that it deceives them into confidence.

Third, because living wills generally constrain treatment, they might reduce the onerous costs of terminal illness. Although several studies associated living wills with small decreases in those costs,[101] several studies have reached the opposite conclusion.[102] The old Scotch verdict, "not proven," seems apt.

The Costs

There is no free living will, and the better (or at least more thorough and careful) the living will, the more it costs. Living wills consume patient's time and energy. When doctors or lawyers help, costs soar. On a broader view, Jeremy Sugarman and colleagues estimated that the Patient Self-Determination Act imposed on all hospitals a start-up cost of $101,569,922 and imposed on one hospital (Johns Hopkins) initial costs of $114,528.[103] These figures omit the expenses, paid even as we write and you read, of administering the program. And this money has bought only *pro forma* compliance.

These are real costs incurred when over 40 million people lack health insurance and when we are spending more of our gross domestic product on health care than comparable countries without buying commensurately better health. If programs to promote and provide living wills showed signs of achieving the goals cherished for them, we would have to decide whether their valuable but incalculable rewards exceeded their diffuse but daunting costs.

However, since those programs have failed, their costs plainly outweigh their benefits.

What Is To Be Done?

Living wills attempt what undertakers like to call "pre-need planning," and on inspection they are as otiose as the mortuary version. Critically, empiricists cannot show that advance directives affect care. This is damning, but were it our only evidence, perhaps we might not be weary in well doing: for in due season we might reap, if we faint not. However, our survey of the evidence suggests that living wills fail not for want of effort, or education, or intelligence, or good will, but because of stubborn traits of human psychology and persistent features of social organization.

Thus when we reviewed the five conditions for a successful program of living wills, we encountered evidence that not one condition has been achieved or, we think, can be. First, despite the millions of dollars lavished on propaganda, most people do not have living wills. And they often have considered and considerable reasons for their choice. Second, people who sign living wills have generally not thought through its instructions in a way we should want for life-and-death decisions. Nor can we expect people to make thoughtful and stable decisions about so complex a question so far in the future. Third, drafters of living wills have failed to offer people the means to articulate their preferences accurately. And the fault lies primarily not with the drafters; it lies with the inherent impossibility of living wills' task. Fourth, living wills too often do not reach the people actually making decisions for incompetent patients. This is the most remediable of the five problems, but it is remediable only with unsustainable effort and unjustifiable expense. Fifth, living wills seem not to increase the accuracy with which surrogates identify patients' preferences. And the reasons we surveyed when we explained why living wills do not affect patients' care suggest that these problems are insurmountable.

The cost-benefit analysis here is simple: If living wills lack detectable benefits, they cannot justify any cost, much less the considerable costs they now exact. Any attempt to increase their incidence and their availability to surrogates must be expensive. And the evidence suggests that broader use of living wills can actually disserve rather than promote patients' autonomy: If, as we have argued, patients sign living wills without adequate reflection, lack necessary information, and have fluctuating preferences anyway, then living wills will not lead surrogates to make the choices patients would have wanted. Thus, as Pope suggests, the "PSDA, rather than promoting autonomy has 'done a disservice to most real patients and their families and caregivers.' It has promoted the execution of uninformed and under-informed advance directives, and has undermined, not protected, self-determination."[104]

If living wills have failed, we must say so. We must say so to patients. If we believe our declamations about truth-telling, we should frankly warn patients how faint is the chance that living wills can have their intended effect. More broadly, we should abjure programs intended to cajole everyone into signing living wills. We should also repeal the PSDA, which was passed with arrant and arrogant indifference to its effectiveness and its costs and which today imposes accumulating paperwork and administrative expense for paltry rewards.[105]

Of course we recognize the problems presented by the decisions that must be made for incompetent patients, and our counsel is not wholly negative. Patients anxious to control future medical decisions should be told about durable powers of attorney. These surely do not guarantee patients that their wishes will blossom into fact, but nothing does. What matters is that powers of attorney have advantages over living wills. First, the choices that powers of attorney demand of patients are relatively few, familiar, and simple. Second, a regime of powers of attorney requires little change from current practice, in which family members ordinarily act informally for incompetent patients. Third, powers of attorney probably improve decisions for patients, since surrogates know more at the time of the decision than patients can know in advance. Fourth, powers of attorney are cheap; they require only a simple form easily filled out with little advice. Fifth, powers of attorney can be supplemented by legislation (already in force in some states) akin to statutes of intestacy. These statutes specify who is to act for incompetent patients who have not specified a surrogate. In short, durable powers of attorney are—as these things go—simple, direct, modest, straightforward, and thrifty.

In social policy as in medicine, plausible notions can turn out to be bad ideas. Bad ideas should be renounced. Bloodletting once seemed plausible, but when it demonstrably failed, the course of wisdom was to abandon it, not to insist on its virtues and to scrounge for alternative justifications for it. Living wills were praised and peddled before they were fully developed, much less studied. They have now failed repeated tests of practice. It is time to say, "enough."

Disclaimer

This report and its conclusions are the opinions of the authors and do not necessarily represent those of the Department of Veterans Affairs.

References

1. R. Dresser, "Missing Persons: Legal Perceptions of Incompetent Patients," *Rutgers Law Review* 46 (1994): 609–695.

2. J. Lynn, "Why I Don't Have a Living Will," *Law, Medicine & Health Care* 19, nos. 1-2 (1991): 101–104.

3. C.P. Sabatino, "End-of-Life Legal Trends," *ABA Commission on Legal Problems of the Elderly 2,* (2000).

4. Health Care Assurance of 2001. S. 26. 107th Congress ed; 2001; The Advance Planning and Compassionate Care Act of 1999. S. 628. 106th Congress ed; 1999.

5. 38 CFR Part 17 RIN. 2900-AJ28. November 2, 1998.

6. Knight v. Beverly Health Care. 820 S2d 92; 2001.

7. See *Conservatorship of Wendland*, where the California Supreme Court construed the state's Health Care Decisions Law as "requiring clear

and convincing evidence of a conscious conservatee's wish to justify withholding life-sustaining treatment" but held that decision did not affect patients who had left "formal directions for health care." 28 P.3d 151; 2001.

8. In re Martin. 538 NW2d 399; Mich 1995.

9. Council on Ethical and Judicial Affairs of the American Medical Association, *Surrogate Decision Making* E8.081. http://www.ama-assn.org

10. P.J. Aitken, "Incorporating Advance Care Planning into Family Practice," *American Family Physician,"* 59 (1999): 605–620; A.O. Calvin and A.P. Clark, "How Are You Facilitating Advance Directives in Your Clinical Nurse Specialist Practice?" *Clinical Nurse Specialist* 16, no. 6 (2002): 292–94.

11. A document that "[g]ives person responsible for making medical decisions greater information, specificity and insight about your specific health-care related decisions, wishes, and objectives" is "A MUST FOR NEARLY EVERYONE" (P. A. Meints, "A Trust and Estate Planning Questionnaire for Families with Minor Children," *The Practical Tax Lawyer* 16, no. 1, [2001]: 33). Providing living wills has also become a pro bono activity. "Wills on Wheels was established by a committee of paralegals and consulting attorneys determined to provide . . . low-income adults with simple wills and living wills" (J.M. Price, "pro Bono and Paralegals: Helping to Make a Difference" *Colorado Lawyer* (September 30, 2000), 55–56.

12. See www.aarp.org/confacts/programs/endoflife.html.

13. The form's critical paragraph reads; "My desires concerning medical treatment are—." Then it leaves fourteen bland lines the patient may fill in. Available at www.med.umich.edu/1libr/aha/umlegal04.htm.

14. R. Dresser, "Precommitment: A Misguided Strategy for Securing Death with Dignity," *Texas Law Review* 81 (2003): 1823–1847.

15. A.R. Eiser and M.D. Weiss, "The Underachieving Advance Directive: Recommendations for Increasing Advance Directive Completion," *American Journal of Bioethics* 1 (2001): 1–5.

16. N.L. Cantor, "Twenty-five Years after Quinlan: A Review of the Jurisprudence of Death and Dying," *Journal of Law, Medicine & Ethics* 29 (2001): 182–96.

17. L. Emanuel, "Living Wills Can Help Doctors and Patients Talk about Dying," *Western Journal of Medicine* 173 (2000): 368.

18. For example, the form provided by a consortium of the American Bar Association, the American Medical Association, and the American Association of Retired Persons "combines and expands the traditional Living Will and Health Care Power of Attorney into a single, comprehensive document" (http://www.ama-assn.org/public/booklets/livgwill.htm).

19. D.M. High, "Why Are Elderly People Not Using Advance Directives?" *Journal of Aging and Health* 5, no. 4 (1993): 497–515.

20. L.L. Emanuel, "Advance Directives for Medical Care; Reply." *NEJM* 325 (1991): 1256; N.L. Cantor, "Making Advance Directives Meaningful," *Psychology, Public Policy, and Law* 4, no. 3 (1998): 629–52; D.M. Cox and G.A. Sachs, "Advance Directives and the Patient Self-Determination Act," *Clinics in Geriatric Medicine* 10 (1994): 431–43; G.A.D. Havens, "Differences in the Execution/Nonexecution of Advance Directives by Community

Dwelling Adults," *Research in Nursing and Health* 23 (2000): 319–33; D.M. High, "Advance Directives and the Elderly: A Study of Intervention Strategies to Increase Use," *Gerontologist* 33, no. 3 (1993): 342–49; S.H. Miles, R. Koepp, and E.P. Weber, "Advance End-of-Life Treatment Planning: A Research Review," *Archives of Internal Medicine* 156, no. 10 (1996): 1062–1068; S.R. Steiber, "Right to Die: Public Balks at Deciding for Others," *Hospitals* 61 (1987): 572; J. Teno et al., "Do Advance Directives Provide Instructions that Direct Care? SUPPORT Investigators. Study to Understand Prognoses and Preferences for Outcomes and Risks of Treatment," *Journal of the American Geriatrics Society* 45, no. 4 (1997): 508–512.

21. Emanuel, "Advance Directives for Medical Care; Reply."

22. Miles, Koepp, and Weber, "Advance End-of-Life Treatment Planning"; J.L. Holley et al., "Factors Influencing Dialysis Patients' Completion of Advance Directives," *American Journal of Kidney Diseases* 30, no. 3 (1997): 356–60; L.C. Hanson and E. Rodgman, "The Use of Living Wills at the End of Life: A National Study," *Archives of Internal Medicine* 156, no. 9 (1996): 1018–1022; J.M. Teno et al., "Do Advance Directives Provide Instructions that Direct Care? SUPPORT Investigators. Study to Understand Prognoses and Preferences for Outcomes and Risks of Treatment," *Journal of the American Geriatrics Society* 45, no. 4 (1997): 508–512.

23. Holley et al., "Factors Influencing Dialysis Patients' Completion of Advance Directives."

24. Cox and Sachs, "Advance Directives and the Patient Self-Determination Act"; Miles, Koepp, and Weber, "Advance End-of-Life Treatment Planning"; D.M. High, "All in the Family: Extended Autonomy and expectations in Surrogate Health Care Decision-Making," *Gerontologist* 28 (suppl) (1988): 46–51.

25. L.L. Emanuel and E.J. Emanuel, "The Medical Directive: A New Comprehensive Advance Care Document," *JAMA* 261 (1989): 3288–93.

26. High, "Advance Directives and the Elderly"; J.M. Roe et al., "Durable Power of Attorney for Health care: A Survey of Senior Center Participants," *Archives of Internal Medicine* 152 (1992): 292–96.

27. High, "Why Are Elderly People Not Using Advance Directives?"; Roe et al., "Durable Power of Attorney for Health care."

28. High, "Why Are Elderly People Not Using Advance Directives?"; Roe et al., "Durable Power of Attorney for Health care"; E.J. Emanuel, L.L. Emanuel, and D. Orentlicher, "Advance Directives," *JAMA* 266 (1991): 2563–63; G.A. Sachs, C.B. Stocking, and S.H. Miles, "Empowerment of the older patient? A Randomized, Controlled Trial to Increase Discussion and Use of Advance Directives," *Journal of the American Geriatrics Society* 40, no. 3 (1992): 269–73; L.L. Brunetti, S.D. Carperos, and R.E. Westlund, "Physicians' Attitudes towards Living Wills and Cardiopulmonary Resuscitation," *Journal of General Internal Medicine* 6 (1991): 323–29; T.E. Finucane et al., "Planning with Elderly Outpatients for Contingencies of Severe Illness: A Survey and Clinical Trial," *Journal of General Internal Medicine* 3, no. 4 (1988): 322–25; B. Lo, G.A. McLeod, and G. Saika, "Patient Attitudes to Discussing Life-sustaining Treatment," *Archives of Internal Medicine* 146, no. 8 (1986): 1613–15; R. Yamada et al., "A Multimedia Intervention on Cardiopulmonary Resuscitation and Advance Directives," *Journal of General Internal Medicine* 14 (1999): 559–63.

29. Cox and Sachs, "Advance Directives and the Patient Self-Determination Act"; L.L. Emanuel and E. Emanuel, "Advance Directives," *Annals of Internal Medicine* 116 (1992): 348–49; B.B. Ott, "Advance Directives: The Emerging Body of Research," *American Journal of Critical Care* 8 (1999): 514–19.

30. J. Sugarman, M. Weinberger, and G. Samsa, "Factors Associated with Veterans' Decisions about Living Wills," *Archives of Internal Medicine* 152 (1992): 343–47.

31. Cox and Sachs, "Advance Directives and the Patient Self-Determination Act"; Holley et al., "Factors Influencing Dialysis Patients' Completion of Advance Directives," High, "All in the Family"; Roe et al., "Durable Power of Attorney for Health care"; Ott, "Advance Directives"; N.A. Hawkins et al., "Do Patients Want to Micro-manage Their Own Deaths? Process Preferences, Values and Goals in End-of-Life Medical Decision Making," Unpublished manuscript. P.B. Terry et al., "End-of-Life Decision Making: When Patients and Surrogates Disagree," *Journal of Clinical Ethics* 10, no. 4 (1999): 286–93.

32. J. Carrese and L. Rhodes, "Western Bioethics on the Navajo Reservation: Benefit or Harm?" *JAMA* 274 (1995): 826–29; L.J. Blackhall et al., "Ethnicity and Attitudes toward Patient Autonomy," *JAMA* 274 (1995): 820–25.

33. C.M. Puchalski et al., Patients Who Want their Family and Physician to Make Resuscitation Decisions for Them: Observations from SUPPORT and HELP; *JAGS* 48 (2000): S84.

34. High, "Why Are Elderly People Not Using Advance Directives?"

35. Ibid.

36. Patient Self-Determination Act of 1990. of the Omnibus Reconsiliation Act of 1990.

37. J.L. Yates and H.R. Glick, "The Failed Patient Self-Determination Act and Policy Alternatives for the Right to Die," *Journal of Aging and Social Policy* 29 (1997): 29, 31.

38. M.T. Pope, "The Maladaptation of Miranda to Advance Directives: A Critique of the Implementation of the Patient Self-Determination Act," *Health Matrix* 9 (1999): 139.

39. Cox and Sachs, "Advance Directives and the Patient Self-Determinaction Act."

40. J. Hare and C. Nelson, "Will Outpatients Complete Living Wills? A Comparison of Two Interventions," *Journal of General Internal Medicine* 6 (1991): 41–46.

41. Yamada et al., "A Multimedia Intervention on Cardiopulmonary Resuscitation and Advance Directives"; G.A. Sachs, S.H. Miles, and R.A. Levin, "Limiting Resuscitation: Emerging Policy in the Emergency Medical System," *Annals of Internal Medicine* 114 (1991): 151–54.

42. C.E. Schneider, *The Practice of Autonomy: Patients, Doctors, and Medical Decisions* (New York: Oxford University Press, 1998).

43. M.J. Silveira et al., "Patient's Knowledge of Options at the End of Life: Ignorance in the Face of Death," *JAMA* 284 (2000): 2483, 2486–87.

44. Yamada et al., "A Multimedia Intervention on Cardiopulmonary Resuscitation and Advance Directives"; S.H. Miles, "Advanced Directives to Limit

Treatment: The Need for Portability," *Journal of the American Geriatrics Society* 35, no. 1 (1987): 74–76; K.M. Coppola et al., "Perceived Benefits and Burdens of Life-Sustaining Treatments: Differences among Elderly Adults, Physicians, and Young Adults," *Journal of Ethics, Law, and Aging* 4, no. 1 (1998): 3–13.

45. Roe et al., "Durable Power of Attorney for Health care."

46. J.A. Tulsky et al., "Opening the Black Box: How Do Physicians Communicate about Advance Directives?" *Annals of Internal Medicine* 129 (1998): 441, 444.

47. C.E. Schneider and M. Farrell, *Information, Decisions, and the Limits of Informed Consent* (New York: Oxford University Press, 2000).

48. B.J. McNeil et al., "On the Elicitation of Preferences for Alternative Therapies," *NEJM* 306 (1982): 1259–62.

49. T.R. Malloy et al., "The Influence of Treatment Descriptions on Advance Medical Directive Decisions," *Journal of the American Geriatrics Society* 40, no. 12 (1992): 1255–60; D.J. Mazur and D.H. Hickman, "Patient Preferences: Survival versus Quality-of-Life Considerations," *Journal of General Internal Medicine* 8, no. 7 (1993): 374–77; D.J. Mazur and J.F. Merz, "How Age, Outcome Severity, and Scale Influence General Medicine Clinic Patients' Interpretations of Verbal Probability Terms" (See comments), *Journal of General Internal Medicine* 9 (1994): 268–71.

50. Miles, Koepp, and Weber, "Advance End-of-Life Treatment Planning."

51. Ott, "Advance Directives."pp. 514, 517.

52. J.J. Christensen-Szalanski, "Discount Functions and the Measurement of Patients' Values: Women's Decisions during Childbirth," *Medical Decision Making* 4, no. 1 (1984): 47–58.

53. R.M. Gready et al., "Actual and Perceived Stability of Preferences for Life-Sustaining Treatment," *Journal of Clinical Ethics* 11, no. 4 (2000): 334–46.

54. A. Upadya et al, "Patient, Physician, and Family Member Understanding of Living Wills," *American Journal of Respiratory and Critical Care Medicine* 166 (2002): 1433.

55. W. Sheed, *In Love with Daylight: A Memoir of Recovery* (New York: Simon and Schuster, 1995): 14.

56. Gready et al., "Actual and Perceived Stability of Preferences for Life-Sustaining Treatment"; J.T. Berger and D. Majerovitz, "Stability of Preferences for Treatment among Nursing Home Residents," *Gerontologist* 28, no. 2 (1998): 217–23; S. Carmel and E. Mutran, "Stability of Elderly Persons' Expressed Preferences regarding the Use of Life-Sustaining Treatments," *Social Science and Medicine* 49, no. 3 (1999): 303–311; M. Danis et al., "Stability of Choices about Life-Sustaining Treatments," *Annals of Internal Medicine* 120, no. 7 (1994): 567–73; P.H. Ditto et al., "A Prospective Study of the Effects of Hospitalization on Life-Sustaining Treatment Preferences: Context Changes Choices," Unpublished manuscript; P.H. Ditto et al., "The Stability of Older Adults' Preferences for Life-Sustaining Medical Treatment," Unpublished manuscript; E.J. Emanuel, "Commentary on Discussions about Life-Sustaining Treatments," *Journal of Clinical Ethics* 5, no. 3 (1994): 250–51; L.L. Emanuel et al., "Advance Directives: Stability of Patients' Treatment Choices," *Archives of Internal Medicine* 154 (1994):

209–217; M.A. Everhart and R.A. Pearlman, "Stability of Patient Preferences regarding Life-Sustaining Treatments," *Chest* 97 (1990): 159–64; L. Ganzini et al., "The Effect of Depression Treatment on Elderly Patients' Preferences for Life-Sustaining Medical Therapy," *American Journal of Psychiatry* 151, no. 11 (1994): 1631–36; N. Kohut et al., "Stability of Treatment Preferences: Although Most Preferences Do Not Change, Most People Change Some of their Preferences," *Journal of Clinical Ethics* 8, no. 2 (1997): 124–35; M.D. Silverstein et al., "Amyotrophic Lateral Sclerosis and Life-Sustaining Therapy: Patients' Desires for Information, Participation in Decision Making, and Life-Sustaining Therapy," *Mayo Clinic Proceedings* 66 (1991): 906–913; J.S. Weissman et al., "The Stability of Preferences for Life-Sustaining Care among Persons with AIDS in the Boston Health Study," *Medical Decision Making* 19 (1999): 16–26; K.M. Coppola et al., "Are Life-Sustaining Treatment Preferences Stable over Time? An Analysis of the Literature," unpublished manuscript.

57. Coppola et al., "Are Life-Sustaining Treatment Preferences Stable over Time?"

58. Danis et al., "Stability of Choices about Life-Sustaining Treatments"; Ditto et al., "A Prospective Study of the Effects of Hospitalization"; Weissman et al., "The Stability of Preferences for Life-Sustaining Care."

59. Ditto et al., "A Prospective Study of the Effects of Hospitalization."

60. H.M. Chochinov et al., "Will to Live in the Terminally Ill," *Lancet* 354 (1999): 816, 818.

61. D.T. Gilbert and T.D. Wilson, "Miswanting: Some Problems in the Forecasting of Future Affective States," in *Feeling and Thinking: The Role of Affect in Social Cognition,* ed. J.P. Forgas (New York: Cambridge University Press, 2000): 178–97; C.H. Griffith 3rd et al., "Knowledge and Experience with Alzheimer's Disease: Relationship to Resuscitation Preference," *Archives of Family Medicine* 4, no. 9 (1995): 780–84; T.M. Osberg and J.S. Shrauger, "Self-prediction: Exploring the Parameters of Accuracy," *Journal of Personality and Social Psychology* 51, no. 5 (1986): 1044–57.

62. Griffith 3rd et al., "Knowledge and Experience with Alzheimer's Disease."

63. Gilbert and Wilson, "Miswanting."

64. D. Kahneman and J. Snell, "Predicting a Changing Taste: Do People Know What They Will Like?" *Journal of Behavioral Decision Making* 5, no. 3 (1992): 187–200.

65. Gilbert and Wilson, "Miswanting."

66. Ibid.

67. G. Loewenstein and D. Schkade, "Wouldn't It Be Nice? Predicting future feelings," in *Hedonic Psychology: Scientific Approaches to Enjoyment, Suffering and Wellbeing,"* ed. N. Schwartz and D. Kahneman (New York: Russell Sage Foundation, 1997).

68. D. Schkade, Does Living in California Make People Happy? A Focusing Illusion in Judgements of Life Satisfaction," *Psychological Science* 9 (1998): 340–46.

69. Loewenstein and Schkade, "Wouldn't It Be Nice?"

70. A.S. Brett, "Limitations of Listing Specific Medical Interventions in Advance Directives," *JAMA* 266 (1991): 825–28.

71. I.S. Kirsch et al., *Adult Literacy in America: A First Look at the Results of the National Adult Literacy Survey,* U.S. Department of Education; August 1993; NCES 93275.

72. Cox and Sachs, "Advance Directives and the Patient Self-Determination Act"; Miles, Koepp, and Weber, "Advance End-of-Life Treatment Planning"; Silveira et al., "Patient's Knowledge of Options at the End of Life"; Coppola et al., "Perceived Benefits and Burdens of Life-Sustaining Treatments."

73. Pope, "The Maladaptation of Miranda to Advance Directives." pp. 139, 165–66.

74. D.J. Doukas and L.B. McCullough, "The Values History: The Evaluation of the Patient's Values and Advance Directives," *Journal of Family Practice* 32, no. 2 (1991): 145–53.

75. Lochner v. New York N. 198 U.S. 45: Supreme Court of the United States; 1905.

76. H.J. Silverman et al., "Implementation of the Patient Self-Determination Act in a Hospital Setting: An Initial Evaluation," *Archives of Internal Medicine* 155, no. 5 (1995: 502–510.

77. Roe et al., "Durable Power of Attorney for Health Care."

78. R.S. Morrison et al., "The Inaccessibility of Advance Directives on Transfer from Ambulatory to Acute Care Settings," *JAMA* 274 (1995): 478–82.

79. Ibid.

80. M. Danis et al., "A Prospective Study of the Impact of Patient Preferences on Life-Sustaining Treatment and Hospital Cost," *Critical Care Medicine* 24, 11 (1996): 1811–17.

81. J.A. Druley et al., "Physicians' Predictions of Elderly Outpatients' Preferences for Life-Sustaining Treatment," *Journal of Family Practice* 37 (1993): 469–75; J. Hare, C. Pratt, and C. Nelson, "Agreement between Patients and Their Self-Selected Surrogates on Difficult Medical Decisions," *Archives of Internal Medicine* 152, no. 5 (1992): 1049–1054; P.M. Layde et al., "Surrogates' Predictions of Seriously Ill Patients' Resuscitation Preferences," *Archives of Family Medicine* 4, no. 6 (1995): 518–23; J.G. Ouslander, A.J. Tymchuk, and B. Rahbar, "Health Care Decisions among Elderly Long-term Care Residents and Their Potential Proxies," *Archives of Internal Medicine* 149 no. 6 (1989): 1367–72; A.B. Seckler et al., "Substituted Judgment: How Accurate Are Proxy Predictions?" *Annals of Internal Medicine* 115 (1991): 92–98; D.P. Sulmasy et al., "The Accuracy of Substituted Judgments in Patients with Terminal Diagnoses," *Annals of Internal Medicine* 128, no. 8 (1998): 621–29; R.F. Uhlmann, R.A. Pearlman, and K.C. Cain, "Physicians' and Spouses' Predictions of Elderly Patients' Resuscitation Preferences," *Journal of Gerontology* 43, no. 5 (1988): M115–M121; R.F. Uhlmann, R.A. Pearlman, and K.C. Cain, "Understanding of Elderly Patients' Resuscitation Preferences by Physicians and Nurses," *Western Journal of Medicine* 150 (1989): 705–707; N.R. Zweibel and C.K. Cassell, "Treatment Choices at the End of Life: A Comparison of Decisions by Older Patients and Their Physician-Selected Proxies," *Gerontologist* 29, no. 5 (1989): 615–21.

82. L. Emanuel, "The Health Care Directive: Learning How to Draft Advance Care Documents," *Journal of the American Geriatrics Society* 39, no. 12

(1991): 1221–28; P.H. Ditto et al., "Fates Worse than Death: The Role of Valued Life Activities in Health-State Evaluations," *Health Psychology* 15, no. 5 (1996): 332–43.

83. K.M. Coppola et al., "Accuracy of Primary Care and Hospital-based Physicians' Predictions of Elderly Outpatients' Treatment Preferences with and without Advance Directives," *Archives of Internal Medicine* 161, no. 3 (2001): 431–40.

84. Ibid.

85. M.D. Goodman, M. Tarnoff, and G.J. Slotman, "Effect of Advance Directives on the Management of Elderly Critically Ill Patients," *Critical Care Medicine* 26, no. 4 (1998): 701–704.

86. Morrison et al., "The Inaccessibility of Advance Directives."

87. M. Danis and J.M. Garrett, "Advance Directives for Medical Care: Reply," *NEJM* 325 (1991): PP NO?.

88. J. Katz, "Informed Consent—A Fairy Tale? Law's vision," *University of Pittsburgh Law Review* 39, no. 2 (1977): 137–74; C.H. Braddock 3rd et al., "Informed Decision Making in Outpatient Practice: Time to Get Back to Basics," *JAMA* 282, no. 24 (1999): 2313–20.

89. C.E. Schneider, "The Best-Laid Plans," *Hastings Center Report* 30, no. 4 (2000): 24–25; C.E. Schneider, "Gang Aft Agley," *Hastings Center Report* 31, no. 1 (2001): 27–28.

90. Teno et al., "Do Advance Directives Provide Instructions that Direct Care?"

91. W.R. Mower and L.J. Baraff, "Advance Directives: Effect of Type of Directive on Physicians' Therapeutic Decisions," *Archives of Internal Medicine* 153 (1993): 375, 378.

92. J. Lynn, "Learning to Care for People with Chronic Illness Facing the End of Life," *JAMA* 284 (2000): 2508–09.

93. J. Teno et al., "The Illusion of End-of-Life Resource Savings with Advance Directives. SUPPORT Investigators. Study to Understand Prognoses and Preferences for Outcomes and Risks of Treatment," *Journal of the American Geriatrics Society* 45, no. 4 (1997): 513–18.

94. A. Fagerlin et al., "Projection in Surrogate Decisions about Life-Sustaining Medical Treatments," *Health Psychology* 20, no. 3 (2001): 166–75.

95. J. Virmani, L.J. Schneiderman, and R.M. Kaplan, "Relationship of Advance Directives to Physician-Patient Communication," *Archives of Internal Medicine* 154 (1994): 909–913.

96. J.A. Tulsky, M.A. Chesney, B. Lo, "How Do Medical Residents Discuss Resuscitation with Patients?" *Journal of General Internal Medicine* 10 no. 8 (1995): 436–42.

97. Tulsky et al., "Opening the Black Box." pp. 441, 445.

98. P.H. Ditto et al., "Advance Directives as Acts of Communication: A Randomized Controlled Trial, *Archives of Internal Medicine* 161, no. 3 (2001): 421–30.

99. R. Baker et al., "Family Satisfaction with End-of-Life Care in Seriously Ill Hospitalized Adults," *Journal of the American Geriatrics Society* 48, no 5 (suppl) (2000): S61–S69.

100. V.P. Tilden et al., "Family Decisionmaking to Withdraw Life-Sustaining Treatments from Hospitalized Patients," *Nursing Research* 50, no. 2 (2001): 105–115.

101. Miles, Koepp, and Weber, "Advance End-of-Life Treatment Planning."

102. Teno et al., "The Illusion of End-of-Life Resource Savings with Advance Directives"; E.J. Emanuel and L.L. Emanuel, "The Economics of Dying: The Illusion of Cost Savings at the End of Life," *NEJM* 330 (1994): 540–44; L.J. Schneiderman et al., "Effects of Offering Advance Directives on Medical Treatments and Costs," *Annals of Internal Medicine* 117, no. 7 (1992): 599–606.

103. J. Sugarman et al., "The Cost of Ethics Legislation: A Look at the Patient Self-Determination Act," *Kennedy Institute of Ethics Journal* 3, no. 4 (1993): 387–99.

104. Pope, "The Maladaptation of Miranda to Advance Directives." pp. 139, 167.

105. Yates and Glick, "The Failed Patient Self-Determination Act"; Sugarman et al., "The Cost of Ethics Legislation."

Susan E. Hickman, Bernard J. Hammes,
Alvin H. Moss, and Susan W. Tolle

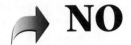 **NO**

Hope for the Future: Achieving the Original Intent of Advance Directives

The development of new, life-prolonging medical technologies in the 1970s aroused concern among Americans about the indiscriminant use of aggressive, life-prolonging treatments. Highly public cases such as those of Karen Ann Quinlan and Nancy Cruzan drew attention to the importance of end of life care planning for healthy adults. Advance directives were developed as a way for people to retain control over their medical care by specifying their treatment values and choices and by naming someone to make medical decisions once they were no longer able to do so. Over the past several decades, it has become clear that statutory advance directives alone have not been as successful as originally hoped in giving patients control over their end of life care. However, the initial goal of advance directives was laudable and is worth preserving. Promising new models have evolved from practice and research that move us closer to achieving the original intent of advance directives.

Most traditional advance directives, such as statutory living wills and surrogate appointments, were created by legislative processes that set specific requirements about content and established rules regarding their use to define the rights of adults to forgo medical treatment, to protect providers who honor these decisions, and to appoint an authorized surrogate decision-maker. Statutory living wills are a tool for patients to express preferences about medical treatments that can be used if a person is no longer able to make his or her own decisions. These documents typically focus on potentially life-prolonging treatments in a very limited set of circumstances, such as when a person is faced with "imminent death regardless of treatment" or is in a "persistent vegetative state." In most states, a person can also designate a surrogate to make decisions in the event the patient loses decisional capacity. Depending on state law, a surrogate may be called a health care proxy or agent, medical power of attorney, or durable power of attorney for health care.

Limitations of Traditional Advance Directives

Despite the hope that traditional advance directives would ensure that patient preferences are honored, numerous studies have found that only a minority (20 to 30 percent) of American adults have an advance directive and that these documents have limited effects on treatment decisions near the end of life, though more recent research suggests use may be higher at the end of life. In addition to a low completion rate, there are many reasons why traditional advance directives are less successful than originally hoped. These reasons include the following:

(1) The focus is often on a patient's legal right to refuse unwanted medical treatments, reflecting the legislative origins of traditional advance directives. Those who complete such documents generally do not receive assistance in understanding or discussing their underlying goals and values.

(2) The instructions given in these documents and the scenarios provided for discussion are generally either too vague to be clear (for example, "If I am close to death") or too medically specific to be helpful in common clinical situations (for example, "If I am in a persistent vegetative state").

(3) Vague instructions result in conversations that produce equally vague expressions of wishes such as "Do not keep me alive with machines" or "Let me die if I am a vegetable."

(4) Once advance directives are completed, planning is typically considered finished. A systematic effort to reopen the conversation as a person's health declines is rarely made. The only repeated question that a patient might hear is, "Do you have an advance directive?" as required by the Patient Self-Determination Act.

(5) Traditional advance directives are seen as a right of the patient, with little attention given to routinely integrate planning into the clinical care of patients.

(6) Traditional advance directives are based on the assumption that autonomy is the primary mode of decision-making for most people. However, many people in the United States, particularly those from non-Western cultures, conceptualize the broader social network as the basis of treatment decisions, not the wishes and needs of the individual. Patients may also choose to delegate their autonomy to a family member, religious leader, or others, and defer discussions about prognosis and treatments for cultural or other reasons.

(7) In selecting a surrogate, a patient authorizes someone to speak on his or her behalf; however, advance directives typically do not include directions for the surrogate or health care professionals about treatment preferences unless special instructions are also provided. Additional information about values and goals is important to assist surrogates in decision-making during stressful times.

(8) Some patients may wish for their surrogates' or families' interests to be taken into account in decision-making rather than expecting

the surrogate to base decisions solely on the wishes of the patient using a substituted judgment standard. Research suggests that many patients do not expect surrogates to rigidly follow their traditional advance directives, but rather intend for surrogates to exercise judgment to determine the course of care when there is insufficient information available or for extenuating circumstances.

In response to the difficulties with traditional legalistic advance directives, clinicians and researchers have developed new models that preserve the original goal of advance directives while addressing their shortcomings. One well-known example is "Five Wishes," a document that incorporates a surrogate appointment with a range of wishes about medical, personal, spiritual, and emotional needs (www.agingwithdignity.org). Five Wishes offers advantages over traditional advance directives because it covers a range of issues typically not found in statutory living wills or health care power of attorney documents, such as how comfortable a person wants to be or how he or she wishes to be treated if unable to speak for him or herself. Five Wishes meets the legal requirements for advance directives in thirty-seven states and the District of Columbia. Unfortunately, there are no published research studies to support the efficacy of Five Wishes in guiding surrogates and health care professionals or in ensuring that wishes are honored.

"Let Me Decide" is a recently developed Canadian program with empirical data to support its effectiveness (www.newgrangepress.com). The program was studied in a randomized, controlled trial of 1,292 residents at a group of regional nursing homes and hospitals in Ontario. Residents and their family members had an opportunity to document a range of health care choices regarding levels of care, nutritional support, and cardiopulmonary resuscitation. The program was implemented systematically and nursing home staff received training in how to integrate the advance directive into clinical care. Results indicate that the intervention group had a higher prevalence of planning. Additionally, plans were more specific, residents were less likely to die in the hospital, fewer resources were used, and families were more satisfied with the process than were family members in the control facilities using more traditional advance care planning.[1]

In La Crosse, Wisconsin, "Respecting Choices" began in 1991 as part of a community-wide care planning system (www.gundersenlutheran.com/eolprograms). Local health care systems developed institutional policies to ensure that written advance directives were always available in their medical records when needed. Components of the program include staff education about the program and advance care planning; clearly defined roles and expectations of physicians; training for advanced care planning facilitators; routine public and patient engagement in advanced care planning; clinically relevant advance directives incorporated into clinical care; and written protocols so that emergency personnel can follow physician orders that reflect patient preferences. Quality improvement projects were undertaken to measure outcomes and to improve parts of the system when they did not perform in the way intended.[2]

A study of the Respecting Choices program evaluated La Crosse County deaths over an eleven-month period (524 in all). Eighty-five percent of all decedents had some type of a written advance directive at the time of death; 96 percent of written plans were found in the medical record where the person died; and treatment decisions made in the last weeks of life were consistent with written instructions in 98 percent of the deaths where an advance directive existed. Decedents with written advance directives were also significantly less likely to die in the hospital (31 percent versus 68 percent, p=0.001). Respecting Choices is now being implemented by more than fifty-five communities and organizations in the United States and Canada and is being piloted nationwide in Australia.

One of the most studied systems of advance care planning and documentation is the "Physician Orders for Life-Sustaining Treatment" paradigm, originally developed in Oregon (www.polst.org) and complementary to Respecting Choices (in fact, the Respecting Choices program strongly advocates use of the POLST paradigm to document physician orders in the out-of-hospital setting). The POLST form is designed for patients with serious illness and advanced frailty. The centerpiece of the program is the POLST document, a brightly colored medical order form that converts patient treatment preferences into written medical orders based on a conversation among health care professionals, the patient, and/ or surrogates about treatment goals. The form transfers with patients across care settings to ensure that wishes are honored throughout the health care system. The POLST form is an example of an actionable advance directive that is specific and effective immediately. In a prospective study at eight nursing homes, residents whose POLST forms included a do not resuscitate (DNR) order and an order for comfort measures only were followed for one year. None received unwanted intensive care, ventilator support, or cardiopulmonary resuscitation.[3]

In contrast to the varied out-of-hospital DNR orders used around the country, the POLST paradigm provides patients the opportunity to document treatment goals and preferences for interventions across a range of treatment options, permitting greater individualization.[4] Research suggests that the POLST form accurately represents patient treatment preferences the majority of the time[5] and that treatments at the end of life tend to match orders.[6] A majority of nursing homes and hospices in Oregon use the voluntary POLST Program, and POLST is widely recognized by emergency medical services.[7] At least thirteen states have adapted versions of the POLST program, including Oregon, Washington, West Virginia, Utah, and parts of Wisconsin, New York, Pennsylvania, North Carolina, New Hampshire, Tennessee, and Michigan, reflecting a high degree of acceptance by health care professionals. Each state has made minor alterations to the document to accommodate local regulations and statutes. A National POLST Paradigm Task Force formed in 2004 to support national growth of the program.

Elements of Successful Advance Directive Programs

The newer, more successful, clinically based advance directive programs share key elements: a facilitated process, documentation, proactive but appropriately staged timing, and the development of systems and processes that ensure planning occurs.

First, successful advance directive programs are not limited to the content or rules relating to legal documents. Instead, an individualized plan is developed through a process of interaction with the patient that is specific not only to the patient's values and goals, but also to his or her relationships, culture, and medical condition. Advance care planning should focus on defining "good" care for each patient, rather than on simply listing the right to refuse treatment or promoting individual autonomy. A skilled facilitator can enhance advance care planning by engaging those who are close to the patient so that they understand, support, and follow the plans that are made. The process permits shared or delegated decision-making depending on the beliefs and preferences of the patient. Facilitators should encourage patients and surrogates to discuss how much leeway a surrogate has in decision-making.

Second, for advance directive programs to be implemented successfully as a patient moves between different treatment settings, documentation of wishes, goals, and plans is essential. This documentation should include the identity of a designated surrogate. Ideally, this documentation would be in the form of actionable advance directives that direct treatment with specific medical orders reflecting a patient's current treatment preferences—in contrast to traditional advance directives that address preferences in hypothetical future scenarios. To be truly effective, the actionable advance directive form must be standardized and recognized throughout the broader health care system, and it must provide clear, specific language that is actionable in all settings to which a patient might be transferred. The power of actionable advance directives is most completely realized in a system in which all institutional entities that interact with the patient (health care personnel in emergency medical services, emergency departments, hospitals, nursing homes, hospices, home health care, and others) recognize the actionable advance directive form and are authorized to follow its written orders.

Third, successful advance directive programs also require proactive but appropriately staged timing: some discussion should anticipate health care decisions, but much of it must be revisited as the patient's prognosis becomes known. For an otherwise healthy patient, the presumption is that the treatment goal is to return to his or her prior state of health. Individuals who fit this description do not need an advance directive to guide initial treatment. However, healthy adults can benefit from the process of advance care planning to prepare for sudden, severe illness or injury. Healthy adults should appoint a trusted family member or friend to serve as a health care surrogate who can act as a strong advocate in the event that they are unable to speak for themselves. Healthy adults should also discuss with their surrogates whether and when a permanent loss of neurological function would be so bad that the goals of medical care would change from prolonging life to providing comfort, and they should address the degree of leeway that they grant to the surrogate.

In people with advanced chronic disease and frailty, planning should expand to include discussion of changing treatment goals. Success rates for interventions decline as disease and frailty progress, and patients' evaluations of the desirability of interventions often change in the face of this new reality. Patients and families look to health care professionals to initiate conversations about end of life care planning, and it seems most relevant to broach the topic in the context of a limited prognosis. Once the prognosis has been discussed, health care professionals (but not necessarily physicians) trained to facilitate advance care planning discussions can help guide patients so that plans are specific not only to the patient's experiences, values, and goals, but also to the patient's health condition, culture, and personal relationships. This planning should focus on treatment goals in scenarios likely to occur in the course of that person's chronic disease. Completion of an actionable advance directive may be particularly helpful at this time.

Finally, perhaps the most crucial elements of more successful advance directive programs are policies, procedures, and teamwork within each part of the health care system that ensures advance care planning and implementation occurs. Plans need to be clear and should reflect the individual's values and goals. Plans should be updated over time and available when needed; whenever possible, plans should be honored. A successful model requires the establishment of systems at many levels to achieve these goals. Health care organizations can create policies and procedures to assure that any written plan is available when needed. The roles and responsibilities of different health professionals must be clearly defined so that each person knows his or her part and can perform it. Furthermore, optimal performance of each player's role benefits from periodic assessment, which requires that health organizations conduct quality improvement initiatives to ensure that the implemented system achieves the desired outcomes. Organizations should be prepared to gather the necessary information to improve the system when and where it falls short.

For advance directives to be effective, they need to be integrated into each part of the system of care, including emergency medical service protocols and regulations. State statutes vary regarding traditional advance directives, surrogate appointment, and other relevant factors, such as emergency medical technicians' scope of practice. Therefore, state end of life coalitions consisting of key stakeholders (emergency medicine, long-term care, hospice, nurses, physicians, and health lawyers, among others) may need to identify and overcome state-specific regulatory, legal, and cultural barriers to the implementation of optimal advance care planning.

The original intent of advance directives to enable patients to retain control over their terminal care once they lose decision-making capacity was not fully achieved through the use of the traditional advance directives. New, more successful models address the limitations of the traditional models yet remain true to the concept's original intent. The key elements of these new models are advance care planning in a system with specially trained personnel; highly visible, standardized order forms that are immediately actionable; proactive, appropriately staged timing; ongoing evaluation and quality improvement.

For these new models to be used more broadly, systems to implement them will need to be established in each state and within every health organization. These systems need to ensure that traditional and actionable advance directives are written at the appropriate time, that they are recognized, and that they are honored. Given the initial success of these models, it is reasonable to believe that the original goal of advance directives—to ensure respect for patients' treatment wishes at the end of life—can and will be more completely realized in the future.

References

1. D.W. Molloy et al., "Systematic Implementation of an Advance Directive Program in Nursing Homes: A Randomized Controlled Trial," *Journal of the American Medical Association* 283, no. 11 (2000): 1437–44.

2. B.J. Hammes and B.L. Rooney, "Death and End-of-Life Planning in One Midwestern Community," *Archives of Internal Medicine* 158 (1998): 383–90.

3. S.W. Tolle et al., "A Prospective Study of the Efficacy of the Physician Orders for Life Sustaining Treatment," *Journal of the American Geriatrics Society* 46, no. 9 (1998): 1097–1102.

4. S.E. Hickman et al., "Use of the POLST (Physician Orders for Life-Sustaining Treatment) Program in Oregon: Beyond Resuscitation Status," *Journal of the American Geriatrics Society* 52 (2004): 1424–29.

5. J.L. Meyers et al., "Use of the Physician Orders for Life-Sustaining Treatment (POLST) Form to Honor the Wishes of Nursing Home Residents for End of Life Care: Preliminary Results of a Washington State Pilot Project," *Journal of Gerontological Nursing* 30, no. 9 (2004): 37–46.

6. M.A. Lee et al., "Physician Orders for Life-Sustaining Treatment (POLST): Outcomes in a PACE Program," *Journal of the American Geriatrics Society* 48 (2002): 1219–25.

7. T.A. Schmidt et al., "The Physician Orders for Life-Sustaining Treatment (POLST) Program: Oregon Emergency Medical Technicians' Practical Experiences and Attitudes," *Journal of the American Geriatrics Society* 52 (2004): 1430–34.

POSTSCRIPT

Have Advance Directives Failed?

The case of Terri Schiavo, a Florida woman who was in a persistent vegetative state from 1990 until her death in March 2005, garnered more media attention and political involvement than did the similar case of Nancy Cruzan, 30 years earlier. Cruzan's family was united in their effort to remove her feeding tube. In contrast, Schiavo's husband Michael began efforts to remove her feeding tube in 1998, declaring that this was his wife's wish should she be in a permanent non-responsive condition, but her parents, Robert and Mary Schindler, vehemently opposed this action. The case was tried in the legal system and in the court of public opinion through extensive media coverage and political actions. In the end Michael Schiavo prevailed and the feeding tube was removed, but Terri Schiavo's death did not end the controversy. In March 2006, three books were published presenting different sides of the controversy: Michael Schiavo and Michael Hirsh published *Terri: The Truth* (Dutton); "Terri's Family" (her parents, brother, and sister) published *A Life That Matters: The Legacy of Terri Schiavo—A Lesson for Us All* (Warner Books); and Arthur L. Caplan, James J. McCartney, and Dominic A. Sisti published *The Case of Terri Schiavo: Ethics at the End of Life* (Prometheus).

All 50 states and the District of Columbia have laws on advance directives; however, they differ in the limits they place on the substitute decision maker's power to refuse life-sustaining treatment, specifically artificial nutrition and hydration. See Muriel T. Gillick, "Advance Care Planning," *The New England Journal of Medicine* (February 11, 2005) for a review.

The President's Council on Bioethics' 2006 report *Taking Care: Ethical Caregiving in an Aging Society* argues that advance directives do not account for the possibility that a person might change his or her mind, and that surrogate decision makers should not be bound by patients' prior declarations. The report is available at: http://bioethics.georgetown.edu/pcbe/reports/taking_care/taking_care.pdf.

Nancy M. P. King argues in favor of advance directives in *Making Sense of Advance Directives*, rev. ed. (Georgetown University Press, 1996). Among her major points are that advance directives are only one procedural mechanism for implementing an individual's constitutional right to make decisions concerning his or her own body. See also Robert S. Olick, *Taking Advance Directives Seriously: Prospective Autonomy and Decisions Near the End of Life* (Georgetown University Press, 2001) and Lawrence P. Ulrich and Mark J. Hanson, eds., *The Patient Self-Determination Act: Meeting the Challenge in Patient Care* (Georgetown University Press, 2001). In "What I Learned from Schiavo," *Hastings Center Report* (November–December 2007), estate law attorney Gerald W. Witherspoon offers advice about advance directives, including the importance of selecting a trusted person as the proxy or surrogate decision maker and making clear this person's authority to prevent challenges.

ISSUE 5

Is "Palliative Sedation" Ethically Different from Active Euthanasia?

YES: American Medical Association, from "Sedation to Unconsciousness in End-of-Life Care," *Report of the Council on Ethical and Judicial Affairs* (June 2008)

NO: Margaret P. Battin, from "Terminal Sedation: Pulling the Sheet Over Our Eyes," *Hastings Center Report* (September–October 2008)

ISSUE SUMMARY

YES: The American Medical Association affirms that in cases of extreme suffering the physician's duty to relieve pain and suffering includes palliative sedation—using drugs that result in unconsciousness and may hasten death.

NO: Philosopher Margaret P. Battin believes that palliative or terminal sedation is an unsatisfying compromise that offers no greater protection against abuse than do institutional safeguards established for direct physician aid in dying.

One persistent theme in bioethics is appropriate care and decision making at the end of life. Beginning with the case of Karen Ann Quinlan (see Introduction) and continuing through many highly publicized cases, philosophers, theologians, physicians, policymakers, and patients and family members have struggled with questions about what ethical standards should be used in determining how to use modern medical technology humanely and who should make those decisions. The most publicized cases have concerned young women—Karen Ann Quinlan, Nancy Cruzan, and Terry Schiavo. All suffered traumatic events that put them into long-term, nonresponsive states. But these situations arise even more frequently when individuals with chronic conditions, often frail and elderly, undergo a long period of debilitation before they reach the end of life.

Euthanasia—physician participation in administration of drugs that will result in death—is banned in all states. Only Oregon and Washington have laws that allow physicians under certain circumstances to prescribe but not administer lethal drugs to people at the end of life (see Issue 6).

To respect individual autonomy—the right to choose what medical interventions one would or would not accept—many attempts have been made to encourage people to express their wishes through advance directives. As the selections in Issue 4 demonstrate, most people do not sign advance directives or in any way indicate their preferences for care at the end of life. Family members are often left to make these decisions based on what they think the patient would have wanted.

Beginning in the 1970s, hospices became an option for people who did not want aggressive medical care. The hospice movement started in Great Britain and emphasized comfort and spiritual care. Today there are over 5,000 hospices in the United States. Contrary to popular perception, which sees hospice as a place where people go to die, most hospice care is provided at home. There are, in addition, some freestanding hospices and hospice units in acute care hospitals and nursing homes. Medicare (the federal health insurance program for people over 65) has a special hospice benefit for people whose life expectancy is 6 months or less. Most people, however, come to hospice very late in the course of their disease, with a median length of stay of 26 days. They and their families fail to obtain the full benefit of the multidisciplinary hospice approach to care.

For many people, one of the drawbacks to hospice is the requirement to give up treatments that are intended to cure the disease. (Medications that ease pain and symptoms are permitted.) Palliative care has become an option in these situations. Palliative care has many of the same goals as hospice—relief of symptoms, multidisciplinary care of the whole person, family involvement—but also allows curative treatments. Importantly, it is available to individuals at any stage of disease. Most palliative care today is provided in hospitals, and there is no special insurance benefit for palliative care at home.

What then is "palliative" or "terminal" sedation and where does it fit in this array of options? Sedation—administering drugs that are to relieve pain or symptoms without causing loss of consciousness—is part of ordinary medical care (unless the patient objects). Depending on the severity of the patient's pain or symptoms, palliative care may include higher levels of medications, which may result in loss of consciousness but is not the intended result. The major controversy concerns the use of drugs in levels that are intended to cause loss of consciousness and are maintained at that level until the patient dies.

In the following selections, the American Medical Association's Council on Judicial and Ethical Affairs maintains that palliative sedation, within guidelines, is an acceptable extension of the physician's duty to relieve pain and suffering. Philosopher Margaret P. Battin does not object to palliative sedation itself but declares that it is not ethically different from more direct means of ending a patient's life.

YES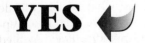

American Medical
Association

Sedation to Unconsciousness in End-of-Life Care

Introduction

The duty to relieve pain and suffering is central to the physician's role as healer and is an obligation physicians have to their patients. Palliative care is universally accepted as a multidisciplinary approach to prevent and relieve suffering of patients with life-limiting illnesses. In this setting, palliative sedation is an important technique for combating extreme suffering; however, there is much debate over the use of palliative sedation to unconsciousness because of its potential to be misconstrued as active euthanasia. Even when done properly, it may still provoke moral objection due to the mistaken perception of a risk of hastening death. . . .

This report examines the ethics of the palliative use of sedation to unconsciousness as an intervention of last resort for a terminally ill patient to reduce severe, refractory pain or other distressing clinical symptoms that have not been relieved by aggressive symptom-specific palliation. This report will not dwell on the specific ethics of withholding or withdrawing life-sustaining medical treatment, euthanasia, or physician-assisted suicide, all of which are addressed in the AMA's *Code of Medical Ethics,* but may differentiate palliative sedation to unconsciousness from such interventions for the purposes of clarification.

Background

. . . Palliative care is an integral part of the treatment regimen of terminally ill patients. However, even with the highest standards of care and attempts at palliation, it is estimated that between 5% and 35% of patients receiving palliative care in hospice programs experience severe pain and other intractable symptoms in the last week of life.[1] . . .

Clinical Issues

Palliative sedation to unconsciousness is only appropriate for terminally ill patients "as an intervention of last resort to reduce severe, refractory pain or other distressing clinical symptoms that have not been relieved by aggressive symptom-specific palliation." Specifically, such clinical symptoms include pain, nausea and vomiting, shortness of breath, agitated delirium, and dyspnea. Additionally, palliative sedation to unconsciousness has been indicated for patients who exhibit urinary retention due to clot formation, gastrointestinal pain, uncontrolled bleeding, and myoclonus.[2] Severe psychological distress may also warrant palliative sedation to unconsciousness when potentially treatable mental health conditions have been excluded.[2] Purely existential suffering may be defined as the experience of agony and distress that results from living in an unbearable state of existence including, for example, death anxiety, isolation, and loss of control. Some have proposed that such suffering in and of itself should also be recognized as an appropriate indication for palliative sedation to unconsciousness, but this remains controversial.[3] However, the Council concurs with those who argue that existential suffering, distinct from previously listed clinical symptoms, is not an appropriate indication for treatment with palliative sedation to unconsciousness, because the causes of this type of suffering are better addressed by other interventions.[4] For example, palliative sedation to unconsciousness is not the way to address suffering created by social isolation and loneliness; rather such suffering should be addressed by providing the patient with needed social support. For patients whose suffering is existential, it is necessary to show compassion and enlist the support of the patient's broader social and spiritual network in order to address issues which are beyond the scope of clinical care.[5]

Ethical Considerations

As described above, a wide spectrum of actions can be taken to relieve the various forms of suffering a terminally ill patient may experience at the end of life. When the usual armamentarium of medical interventions has been exhausted, choices still remain; these range from letting the terminal illness take its course without further intervention to unacceptable choices, such as euthanasia. Actions that are solely intended to hasten the death of patients, such as physician-assisted suicide or euthanasia, are ethically and medically unacceptable (both are "fundamentally incompatible with the physician's role as healer"). In contrast, the withholding and withdrawing of life-sustaining treatment, when done based on the patient's autonomous refusal of unwanted care, and allowing the natural course of disease to take place, are ethically and medically appropriate. Palliative sedation to unconsciousness is intended to relieve patient suffering and, like withholding or withdrawing life support, may also allow the natural process of terminal disease to take place. A recent review of studies of opiate and sedative use in palliative care concluded that there is no evidence to support shortened survival of terminally ill patients who were sedated.[6,7]

Though evidence suggests that opiate and sedative use in the palliative care setting rarely if ever hastens patient death, ethical issues of "intention" and "proportionality" remain of concern. When exploring the ethics of palliative sedation and differentiating it from those of physician-assisted suicide and euthanasia, it is paramount to consider the primary intention of the measure being utilized. Although intended to relieve suffering, physician-assisted suicide and euthanasia achieve this by bringing about death, where palliative sedation is intended to relieve suffering by providing proportionate sedation. Death due to the course of a terminal illness is anticipated in a patient who receives palliative sedation to unconsciousness. However, bringing about the patient's death is not the intent of the sedation.[8] Although intent cannot be observed directly, it can be gauged in part by examining the medical record. Repeated doses or continuous infusions are indicators of proportionate palliative sedation, whereas one large dose or rapidly accelerating doses out of proportion to the level of immediate patient suffering may signify lack of knowledge or an inappropriate intention to hasten death.[3] These questions about intent demonstrate the importance of careful documentation in the medical record of purpose and strategy for patients receiving any palliative care including palliative sedation to unconsciousness.

The doctrine of double effect illuminates how intent makes some forms of end-of-life care morally permissible and others unacceptable. The principle of double effect is applied to situations where it is impossible to avoid all harmful actions. It requires that the good effect (relieving severe suffering) must outweigh the bad effect (potential to unintentionally hasten death), and that the bad effect (ending the patient's life) cannot be the means of achieving the good effect (relieving suffering).[9] Proportionality is also a central tenant of the principle of double effect; the level of sedation sought (and the associated risk of hastening death) must be in direct relationship with, and justified by,[10,11] the level of unacceptable suffering the patient is experiencing. The greater the patient's pain or suffering, the more a physician must be willing to sedate a patient in order to reduce and hopefully eliminate the unacceptable symptoms. The combination and amount of sedative must be just sufficient, but not more so, to relieve distressing clinical symptoms.[3] Furthermore, the concepts of proportionality and justification help to differentiate palliative sedation from physician-assisted suicide and euthanasia since in the case of palliative sedation the physician aims only to sedate to a level of unconsciousness and no further.[12]

It is also important to consider palliative sedation to unconsciousness from the perspectives of autonomy, beneficence, and non-maleficence. Similar to the ethical argument made for withholding or withdrawing life-sustaining medical treatment where the principle of patient autonomy requires that physicians respect the decision of a patient who possesses decision-making capacity to forgo life-sustaining treatment, autonomous decision-making dictates that a fully informed patient should also be able to choose palliative sedation. A designated surrogate decision-maker would also be able to choose palliative sedation for a patient who lacks decision-making capacity and meets the criteria for receiving sedation at the end of life. Requests for palliative sedation to unconsciousness (by patients or their surrogates) that do not fit within acceptable clinical parameters identified by the definition of palliative sedation are inappropriate. The principle of beneficence dictates taking necessary steps to relieve pain and suffering. When discussing the possibility of palliative sedation, it is necessary to fully inform the patient or surrogate about the various levels of sedation and whether intermittent sedation or continuous sedation to unconsciousness is an appropriate option. Patients and their surrogate decision-makers, with guidance from their physicians, should separately decide whether they will continue to receive any life-sustaining treatments and whether they want to maintain, withhold or withdraw life-sustaining interventions (including nutrition and hydration). . . .

Recommendation

The Council on Ethical and Judicial Affairs recommends that the following be adopted. . . .

The duty to relieve pain and suffering is central to the physician's role as healer and is an obligation physicians have to their patients. Palliative sedation to unconsciousness is the administration of sedative medication to the point of unconsciousness in a terminally ill patient. It is an intervention of last resort to reduce severe, refractory pain or other distressing clinical symptoms that do not respond to aggressive symptom-specific palliation. It is an accepted and appropriate component of end-of-life care under specific, relatively rare circumstances. When symptoms cannot be diminished through all other means of palliation, including symptom-specific treatments, it is the ethical obligation of a physician to offer palliative sedation to unconsciousness as an option for the relief of intractable symptoms. When considering the use of palliative sedation, the following ethical guidelines are recommended:

1. Patients may be offered palliative sedation when they are in the final stages of terminal illness. The rationale for all palliative care measures should be documented in the medical record.
2. Palliative sedation to unconsciousness may be considered for those terminally ill patients whose clinical symptoms have been unresponsive to aggressive, symptom-specific treatments.
3. Physicians should ensure that the patient and/or the patient's surrogate have given informed consent for palliative sedation to unconsciousness.
4. Physicians should consult with a multidisciplinary team, including an expert in the field of palliative care, to ensure that symptom-specific treatments have been sufficiently employed and that palliative sedation to unconsciousness is now the most appropriate course of treatment.
5. Physicians should discuss with their patients considering palliative sedation the care plan relative to degree and length (intermittent or constant) of sedation, and the specific expectations for continuing, withdrawing or withholding future life-sustaining treatments.
6. Once palliative sedation is begun, a process must be implemented to monitor for appropriate care.
7. Palliative sedation is not an appropriate response to suffering that is primarily existential, defined as the experience of agony and distress that may arise from such issues as death anxiety, isolation and loss of control. Existential suffering is better addressed by other

interventions. For example, palliative sedation is not the way to address suffering created by social isolation and loneliness; such suffering should be addressed by providing the patient with needed social support.

8. Palliative sedation must never be used to intentionally cause a patient's death.

References

1. Quill, T. E., Byock, I. R., for the ACP-ASIM End-of-Life Care Consensus Panel. Responding to intractable terminal suffering: the role of terminal sedation and voluntary refusal of food and fluids. *Ann Intern Med.* 2000;132:408–414.

2. National Ethics Committee, Veterans Health Administration. The Ethics of palliative sedation as a therapy of last resort. *Am J Hosp Palliat Med.* 2007;23(6):483–491.

3. de Graeff A, Dean M. Palliative sedation therapy in the last weeks of life: a literature review and recommendations for standards. *J Palliat Med.* 2007 Feb;10(1):67–85.

4. Taylor BR, McCann RM. Controlled sedation for physical and existential suffering? *J of Palliat Med.* 2005;8(1):144–147.

5. Snyder L, Sulmasy DP, for the Etchis and Human Rights Committee, ACP-ASIM. Physician-assisted suicide—Position paper. *Ann Intern Med.* 2001;135:208–216.

6. Charter S, Viola R, Paterson J. Sedation for intractable distress in dying—A survey of experts. *Palliat Med.* 1998;12:255–296.

7. Morita T, Chinone Y, Ikenaga M, Miyoshi M, Nakaho T, Nishitateno K et al. Efficacy and safety of palliative sedation therapy: A multicenter, prospective, observational study conducted on specialized palliative care units in Japan. *J Pain Symptom Manage.* 2005;30(4):320–8.

8. Quill TE, Lo B, Brock DW. Palliative options of last resort: a comparison of voluntary stopping eating and drinking, terminal sedation, physician assisted suicide, and voluntary active euthanasia. *JAMA.* 1997;278(23):2099–2104.

9. Quill TE, Dresser R, Brock DW. The rule of double effect—a critique of its role in end-of-life decision making. *N Eng J Med.* 1997;337:1768–1771.

10. Cantor NL, Thomas GC. The legal bounds of physician conduct hastening death. *Buffalo L Rev.* 2000;48(1):83–173.

11. Kollas CD, Boyer-Kollas B, Kollas JW. Criminal prosecutions of physicians providing palliative or end-of-life care. *J Palliat Med.* 2008;11(3):233–241.

12. Emanuel E. Ethics in pain management: an introductory overview. *Pain Med.* 2001:2(2)112–6.

Margaret P. Battin 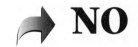 **NO**

Terminal Sedation: Pulling the Sheet Over Our Eyes

Terminal sedation—also called "palliative sedation," "continuous deep sedation," or "primary deep continuous sedation"—has become a new favorite in end-of-life care, a seeming compromise in the debate over physician-assisted dying. Like all compromises, it offers something to each side of a dispute. But it is not a real down-the-middle compromise. It sells out on most of the things that may be important—to both sides. To corrupt an already awkward metaphor, terminal sedation pulls the sheet over our eyes. Terminal sedation may still be an important option in end-of-life care, but we should not present it as the only option in difficult deaths.

Proponents of assisted dying point to autonomy and mercy. The principle of autonomy holds that people are entitled to be the architects, as much as possible, of how they die. (Of course, autonomy has limits—one cannot inflict harm on others—and when one is no longer competent, values and interests may be expressed only indirectly; advance directives or surrogate decision-makers must be brought into play. But the principle itself is clear enough.) The principle of mercy requires that pain and suffering be relieved to the extent possible. These two principles operate in tandem to underwrite physician-assisted dying: physician assistance in bringing about death is to be provided just when the person voluntarily seeks it and just when it serves to avoid pain and suffering or the prospect of them. *Both* requirements must be met.

Opponents base their objections to physician-assisted dying on two other concerns. One is the sanctity of life, a religious or secular absolute respect for life that is held to entail the wrongness of killing, suicide, and murder. This principled objection holds regardless of whether a patient seeks assistance in dying in the face of pain and suffering. The second objection is that physician-assisted dying might lead to abuse. This concern is often spelled out in two ways: physician-assisted dying risks undercutting the integrity of the medical profession, and institutional or social pressures might make people victims of assisted dying they did not want.

These latter objections operate independently. One could be opposed to aid in dying on sanctity-of-life grounds even without fearing the slippery slope, and one could worry about the slippery slope without accepting the sanctity-of-life concerns. Often, however, these two concerns are fused in a

From *Hastings Center Report*, September/October 2008, pp. 27–30. Copyright © 2008 by The Hastings Center. Reprinted by permission of the publisher and Margaret P. Battin.

general objection—a joint claim that it is wrong for doctors to kill and that if doctors *do* kill, even in sympathetic cases like that of the seriously suffering and already dying patient who begs for help, then they might start killing in other, more worrisome cases as well. In short, it's autonomy *and* mercy on the one side, sanctity of life *and/or* the possibility of abuse on the other. That's the standoff over physician-assisted dying, argued in a kaleidoscope of ways over the past several decades.

Terminal sedation is often proffered as an alternative last resort measure that can overcome these practical and ideological disputes. In the 1997 cases *Washington v. Glucksberg* and *Vacco v. Quill*, the Supreme Court recognized the legality of providing pain relief in palliative care even if doing so might shorten life, provided the intention was to relieve pain. But careful scrutiny of terminal sedation—particularly sedation to unconsciousness, in which nutrition and hydration are withheld—suggests that it is not much of a compromise after all.

An Inadequate Compromise

Consider how terminal sedation fails to meet the concerns that underlie the dispute.

Autonomy

Consent of the person affected is central to the concept of autonomy, but it is not and—as a consequence of some political interpretations—*cannot* be honored in decisions to use terminal sedation. First, terminal sedation is often used for patients suffering from severe pain, for whom pain management has failed, but if pain is severe enough, reflective, unimpaired consent may no longer be possible. Decision-making must be deflected to a second party. (Of course, voluntary, informed consent is often challenged by pain: consider women in the throes of labor consenting to an epidural or a caesarean, or trauma victims consenting to surgery.)

More importantly, even when the decision is made in advance of the onset of intense pain, the focus of consent is obscured. Terminal sedation may end pain, but it also ends life. It does so in two ways: it immediately ends sentient life and the possibility for social interaction, and then, because artificial nutrition and hydration are usually withheld, it also ends biological life. But because the assumption is that sedation is used just to end pain, without the *intention* of ending life, the patient cannot be asked for consent to end his or her life, but only to relieve his or her pain. Of course, the consent process could include some mention of the possibility that relieving pain might inadvertently shorten life, but if the acknowledgment that life will be ended is stronger than that, the question of what is intended will arise. Thus, the focus of consent is on avoiding pain, but it should be on causing death.

The new euphemism, "palliative sedation," now often used instead of the more distressing "terminal sedation," only reinforces this problem. By avoiding the word "terminal" and hence any suggestion that death may be coming, the most important feature of this practice is obscured and terminal sedation is confused with "palliative care." Thus, the patient cannot consent to the really significant decision—whether his or her life shall be ended now. Autonomy is therefore undercut whether the patient's capacity for reflection is impaired by severe pain or not.

Mercy

Terminal sedation is typically used only at the very end of the downhill course, and only when the patient's pain has become extreme and other palliative measures are not effective. A broad study of pooled data over the last forty years on pain in cancer found that 59 percent of patients on anticancer treatment and 64 percent of patients with advanced metastatic disease experience pain.[1] Agitation, delirium, dyspnea, seizures, urinary and fecal retention, and nausea and protracted vomiting are also problems. Bernard Lo and Gordon Rubenfeld, writing in the *Journal of the American Medical Association,* discuss a forty-nine-year-old cancer patient given very high doses of morphine who developed myoclonus: seizures in the extremities and eventually in the whole body, producing intense pain.[2] As they say of palliative sedation for her and other dying patients: "We turn to it when everything else hasn't worked."

Terminal sedation to unconsciousness can certainly provide relief from such suffering, but some patients wish to avoid this long downhill course—especially the last stages of it. The use of terminal sedation "to relieve pain" presupposes that the patient is *already* experiencing pain. It provides no rationale for sedating a patient who is not currently in pain. Thus, the rationale for the use of terminal sedation in effect *requires* that the patient suffer.

The Sanctity of Life

The dispute over the principle of the wrongness of killing, or the sanctity of life, has focused mainly on ending a person's life before it would "naturally" end. Terminal sedation does not honor this principle. Rather, it unarguably causes death, and it does so in a way that is not "natural."

It is important to be perfectly clear about the process. Terminal sedation commonly involves two components: (1) inducing sedation, and (2) withholding the administration of fluids and nutrition. The first is not intrinsically lethal,[3] but the second is, if pursued long enough. Patients who are sedated to the degree involved in terminal sedation cannot eat or drink, and without "artificial" nutrition and hydration will necessarily die, virtually always before they would have died otherwise. Patients are sometimes sedated to unconsciousness with food and fluids continued—a practice that extends the dying period (and the cost), but this is not the usual form.

The death itself is not "natural," either. The airy, rather romantic notion of "natural" death usually refers to death that results from an underlying disease, but in terminal sedation death typically results from or is accelerated by dehydration. This is not "natural" dehydration; it is induced by a physician. If respect for the sanctity of life means that a patient's life should not be caused to end, but rather that death must occur only as the result of the underlying disease process, then terminal sedation does not honor this principle.

The Possibility of Abuse

This concern takes two general forms: (1) concern that the integrity of the medical profession will be undercut, and (2) concern that various familial, institutional, or social pressures will maneuver the patient into death when that would have been neither her choice nor in accord with her interests. Yet there is nothing in the practice of terminal sedation that offers greater protection against the possibility of abuse in either of these forms than does direct physician-assisted dying. Is the integrity of the medical profession likely to be undercut? There are many vivid forms of this charge leveled against direct physician-assisted dying—that physicians are overworked, anxious to cover their mistakes, unwilling to work with patients they dislike, biased against patients of certain class or racial backgrounds, beholden to cost pressures from their HMOs, and so on—but there is no reason to assume that terminal sedation would be less subject to these abuses than direct aid in dying. Indeed, direct aid in dying, at least as it is legally practiced in Oregon, requires a series of safeguards—confirmation of a terminal diagnosis, oral and written consent, a waiting period, and more—that do not come into play in terminal sedation. Terminal sedation has no institutional safeguards built in.

What about the sorts of familial, institutional, or social pressures that opponents claim would maneuver a patient into choosing death when that would not have been his choice? In terminal sedation, the choice a patient faces is already obscured: it is not framed as a choice of death versus life, but only as pain versus the relief of pain—a seemingly far easier choice to make, and hence one presumably far more easily shaped by external pressures from greedy family members, overworked or intolerant physicians, or the agents of cost-conscious institutions. *You don't need to suffer like this* is all they need to say.

In short, terminal sedation offers no greater protection against abuse than do the institutional safeguards established for (direct) physician aid in dying.

The Case in Favor of Terminal Sedation

Several writers in the field have argued, as I have, that terminal sedation fails to satisfy fully any of the major principles on either side of the aid in dying disputes. Timothy Quill, describing in close detail the "ambiguity of clinical intentions," has pointed out that it is virtually impossible for the clinician administering terminal sedation to intend palliation but not intend that death occur.[4] David Orentlicher lambasted the 1997 Supreme Court decision in *Washington v. Glucksberg* and *Vacco v. Quill* for "rejecting physician-assisted suicide, embracing euthanasia."[5] Tim Quill, Rebecca Dresser, and Dan Brock have skewered the Court's tortuous use of double-effect reasoning in supporting the practice of terminal sedation while rejecting voluntary, patient-requested physician-assisted suicide.[6]

Just the same, a case may be made for terminal sedation. It offers a definitive response to uncontrollable suffering. The gradual induction of death over the several days or more that terminal sedation takes may appeal to some patients and their families, especially if this slow process is perceived as gentler and easier for the patient, and as permitting the family more time to absorb the reality of their loss. It may also be perceived as less final than physician-assisted death: some forms of palliative sedation involve lightening up on the level of sedation periodically—for example, once a day—to see if the patient is still suffering.

The argument in favor of terminal sedation is one of perceptions: it may *feel* natural (even if it is not), it may *feel* safer (even if it offers less protection from abuse), it may *feel* like something the patient can openly choose (even if the choice is constructed in a way that obscures its real nature), and it may *feel* to the physician as if it is more in keeping with medical codes that prohibit killing (even if it still brings about death). We live in a society that tolerates many obfuscations and hypocrisies, and this may be another one we ought to embrace.

The Need for Guidelines

But we should do so with caution, and with a measure of skepticism about efforts to promote it. Some months before the November ballot that would include the state of Washington's measure I-1000, which is modeled on Oregon's Death with Dignity Act, the American Medical Association Council on Ethical and Judicial Affairs issued a report on "Sedation to Unconsciousness in End-of-Life Care."[7] This report makes an earnest effort to try to preclude many of the practical and ethical difficulties with palliative sedation. For example, the report acknowledges the importance of patient or surrogate consent. It insists that the patient's symptoms really warrant this measure. It emphasizes the importance of interdisciplinary consultation and careful monitoring. And it distinguishes between physical and existential suffering, insisting that palliative sedation may be appropriate in the former but that measures like social supports are to be used for the latter.

However, in its effort to distinguish palliative sedation (it avoids the expression "terminal sedation") from euthanasia, the report undercuts its own courage in addressing these difficult issues by trying to argue that palliative sedation (the permissible strategy) has nothing in common with euthanasia (the impermissible strategy). It does not distinguish between voluntary euthanasia (legal in the Netherlands and Belgium), nonvoluntary euthanasia (of a patient no longer capable of expressing his wishes or of giving legal consent), and involuntary euthanasia (against the patient's wishes). It fails to notice that the Dutch and the Nazi senses of "euthanasia" are entirely different, and that one could welcome the former while reviling the latter.

The AMA report distinguishes palliative sedation from euthanasia (or physician-assisted suicide or aid in dying) on the basis of intention—an application of the well-worn principle of double effect—and then attempts to infer intent from the pattern of practice. "One large dose" or "rapidly accelerating doses" of morphine may signify a bad intention—seeking to cause death—whereas "repeated doses or continuous infusions" are benign. This is naive in the extreme. It's the slyest courtier who poisons the emperor gradually; what could equally well be inferred from repeated doses and continuous infusions is a clever attempt to cover one's tracks. Nor is it clear what counts as "large doses" or other treatment measures in this simplistic dichotomy.

Is a fentanyl patch in a fentanyl-naive patient "rapidly accelerating" or "continuously infusing" when opioid tolerance may be in question? If a hydromorphone infusion for a patient with myoclonus is increased overnight from forty milligrams per hour to one hundred, does the increase count as "rapidly accelerating"? Are one hundred milligram boluses of hydromorphone given every fifteen to thirty minutes on top of a one hundred milligram/hour infusion considered to be "large doses," or are they merely "repeated" doses? What about the doses involved in initiating palliative sedation for this patient: a loading dose of phenobarbital and maintenance on a continuous phenobarbital infusion, together with intravenous dantrolene to lessen the myoclonus? In the case of the forty-nine-year-old cancer patient discussed by Lo and Rubenfeld, the patient died within approximately four hours of the initiation of palliative sedation. Indeed, the average survival in terminal sedation cases is just 1.5 to 3.1 days.[8]

What is astonishing is the AMA's attempt to try to differentiate between different sorts of clinical intentions on the basis of observed practice, when it is simply not possible—nor morally defensible—to draw this false bright line between them. These unworkable distinctions can only exacerbate the unease and legal dread in physicians who work to ease their patients' dying.

It's not that palliative sedation/sedation to unconsciousness/terminal sedation is wrong. It's that it can be practiced hypocritically, as the AMA report seems to ensure. Because there is so much anxiety that it might be confused with euthanasia, the features that it shares with euthanasia are obscured or sanitized. This is where the sheet is pulled over our eyes. The implausible effort to draw a completely bright line between continuous terminal sedation and euthanasia makes the practice of terminal sedation both more dangerous and more dishonest than it should be—and makes what can be a decent and humane practice morally problematic.

Another factor that hasn't been adequately explored is where terminal sedation ought to fit on a spectrum of end-of-life options: much of the "compromise" discussion seems to suggest that terminal sedation is the one and only way to deal with difficult deaths. But there are many last resort options, including patient-elected cessation of eating and drinking and direct physician-assisted dying. Terminal sedation is not an acceptable "compromise" if it overshadows these alternatives.

There is no reason why everyone facing a predictable, potentially difficult death should die in the same way. Knowing that pain is likely in some diseases and that even with the best palliative care not all pain can be relieved, some patients will prefer to avoid the worst, so to speak, and choose an earlier, gentler way out. Some will want to hang on as long as possible, in spite of everything. There is no reason that terminal sedation should not be recognized as an option, but there are excellent reasons why it should not be seen as the *only* option—or even the best option—for easing a bad death.

References

1. M.H. van den Beuken-van Everdingen et al., "Prevalence of Pain in Patients with Cancer: A Systematic Review of the Last 40 Years," *Annals of Oncology* 18, no. 9 (2007): 1437–49.

2. B. Lo and G. Rubenfeld, "Palliative Sedation in Dying Patients: 'We Turn to It When Everything Else Hasn't Worked,'" *Journal of the American Medical Association* 294 (2005): 1810–16.

3. For an analysis of data from the National Hospice Outcomes Project concerning whether opioids used in terminal illness cause death, see R.K. Portenoy et al., "Opioid Use and Survival at the End of Life: A Survey of a Hospice Population," *Journal of Pain and Symptom Management* 32, no. 6 (2006): 532–40.

4. T.E. Quill, "The Ambiguity of Clinical Intentions," *New England Journal of Medicine* 329 (1993): 1039–40.

5. D. Orentlicher, "The Supreme Court and Terminal Sedation: Rejecting Assisted Suicide, Embracing Euthanasia," *Hastings Constitutional Law Quarterly* 24, no. 4 (1997): 947–68.

6. T.E. Quill, R. Dresser, and D.W. Brock, "The Rule of Double Effect: A Critique of Its Role in End-of-Life Decision Making," *New England Journal of Medicine* 227 (1997): 1768–71.

7. American Medical Association Council on Ethical and Judicial Affairs, CEJA Report 5-A-08, "Sedation to Unconsciousness in End-of-Life Care."

8. C. Vena, K. Kuebler, and S.E. Schrader, "The Dying Process," in K. Kuebler, M.P. David, and C.C. Moore, eds., *Palliative Practices* (St. Louis, Mo.: Elsevier Mosby, 2005), 346, citing data from 1998 and 2000. See also Veterans Affairs National Ethics Teleconference, Terminal Sedation, August 27, 2002, online at http://www.ethics.va.gov/ETHICS/docs/net/NET_Topic_20020827_Terminal_Sedation.doc.

POSTSCRIPT

Is "Palliative Sedation" Ethically Different from Active Euthanasia?

Several Web sites carry posts opposing palliative sedation, some equating it to abortion or euthanasia. See, for example, http://www.hospicepatients.org, sponsored by the Hospice Patients Alliance, a "watchdog" organization.

In "Last-Resort Options for Palliative Sedation," Timothy E. Quill, Bernard Lo, Dan W. Brock, and Alan Meisel recommend that palliative care and hospice programs develop clear policies about various levels of palliative sedation, including mechanisms for training and ensuring clinician competency (*Annals of Internal Medicine*, September 15, 2009).

Two of the authors of this article (Timothy E. Quill, and Ira Byock, MD), writing for the American College of Physicians–American Society of Internal Medicine End-of-Life Consensus Panel, assert that terminal sedation and voluntary refusal of hydration and nutrition are options that substantially increase patients' choices ("Responding to Intractable Terminal Suffering: The Role of Terminal Sedation and Voluntary Refusal of Food and Fluids," *Annals of Internal Medicine*, March 7, 2000).

After reviewing organizational guidelines around palliative sedation, Jeffrey Berger concluded that "current guidelines treat palliative sedation to unconsciousness as an effective medical treatment for terminally ill patients who need relief from severe symptoms, yet also restrict its use in ways that are extraordinary for medical treatments." He proposes loosening the guidelines that require imminent death and the failure of other aggressive measures ("Rethinking Guidelines for the Use of Palliative Sedation," *Hastings Center Report*, May–June 2010).

Erich H. Loewy, a physician, offers a personal commentary in "Terminal Sedation, Self-Starvation, and Orchestrating the End of Life," *Archives of Internal Medicine* (February 12, 2001). He believes that when end-of-life care is skillfully orchestrated by a well-trained and practiced team, "few persons will want to take refuge in these options of last resort." He says that there is an enormous difference between allowing people to end their lives in this way and encouraging it.

ISSUE 6

Should Physicians Be Allowed to Assist in Patient Suicide?

YES: Marcia Angell, from "The Supreme Court and Physician-Assisted Suicide—The Ultimate Right," *The New England Journal of Medicine* (January 2, 1997)

NO: Kathleen M. Foley, from "Competent Care for the Dying Instead of Physician-Assisted Suicide," *The New England Journal of Medicine* (January 2, 1997)

ISSUE SUMMARY

YES: Physician Marcia Angell asserts that a physician's main duties are to respect patient autonomy and to relieve suffering, even if that sometimes means assisting in a patient's death.

NO: Physician Kathleen M. Foley counters that if physician-assisted suicide becomes legal, it will begin to substitute for interventions that otherwise might enhance the quality of life for dying patients.

Since the early 1980s, physicians, lawyers, philosophers, and judges have examined questions about withholding life-sustaining treatment. Their deliberations have resulted in a broad consensus that competent adults have the right to make decisions about their medical care, even if those decisions seem unjustifiable to others and even if they result in death. Furthermore, the right of individuals to name others to carry out their prior wishes or to make decisions if they should become incompetent is now well established. Thirty-eight states now have legislation allowing advance directives (commonly known as "living wills").

The debate in specific cases continues (see, for example, Issue 5 on palliative sedation), but on the whole, patients' rights to self-determination have been bolstered by 80 or more legal cases, dozens of reports, and statements made by medical societies and other organizations.

As often occurs in bioethical debate, the resolution of one issue only highlights the lack of resolution about another. There is clearly no consensus about either euthanasia or physician-assisted suicide.

Like truth telling, euthanasia is an old problem given new dimensions by the ability of modern medical technology to prolong life. The word itself is Greek (literally, *happy death*) and the Greeks wrestled with the question of whether, in some cases, people would be better off dead. But the Hippocratic Oath in this instance was clear: "I will neither give a deadly drug to anybody if asked for it, nor will I make a suggestion to that effect." On the other hand, if the goal of medicine is not simply to prolong life but to reduce suffering, at some point the question of what measures should be taken or withdrawn will inevitably arise. The problem is: When death is inevitable, how far should one go in hastening it?

The majority of cases in which euthanasia is raised as a possibility are among the most difficult ethical issues to resolve, for they involve the conflict between a physician's duty to preserve life and the burden on the patient and the family that is created by fulfilling that duty. One common distinction is between *active* euthanasia (that is, some positive act such as administering a lethal injection) and *passive* euthanasia (that is, an inaction such as deciding not to administer antibiotics when the patient has a severe infection). Another common distinction is between *voluntary* euthanasia (that is, the patient wishes to die and consents to the action that will make it happen) and *involuntary—or better, nonvoluntary*—euthanasia (that is, the patient is unable to consent, perhaps because he or she is in a coma).

The two selections that follow address a particularly controversial aspect of this issue. Is it ethical for a physician to assist in a hopelessly ill patient's suicide? Marcia Angell argues that sometimes hastening death should be an option for physicians although "reluctantly as a last resort." Angell states that a physician must consider patient autonomy and suffering when deciding upon care. Kathleen M. Foley contends that the medical profession should take the lead in developing guidelines for the end of life. This means that one must not confuse compassion for a patient's suffering with competence in care.

YES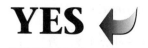

Marcia Angell

The Supreme Court and Physician-Assisted Suicide—The Ultimate Right

The importance and contentious issue of physician-assisted suicide, now being argued before the U.S. Supreme Court, is the subject of the following two editorials. Writing in favor of permitting assisted suicide under certain circumstances is the Journal's executive editor, Dr. Marcia Angell. Arguing against it is Dr. Kathleen Foley, co-chief of the Pain and Palliative Care Service of Memorial Sloan-Kettering Cancer Center in New York. We hope these two editorials, which have in common the authors' view that care of the dying is too often inadequate, will help our readers in making their own judgments.

—Jerome P. Kassirer, M.D.

The U.S. Supreme Court will decide later this year whether to let stand decisions by two appeals courts permitting doctors to help terminally ill patients commit suicide.[1] The Ninth and Second Circuit Courts of Appeals last spring held that state laws in Washington and New York that ban assistance in suicide were unconstitutional as applied to doctors and their dying patients.[2,3] If the Supreme Court lets the decisions stand, physicians in 12 states, which include about half the population of the United States, would be allowed to provide the means for terminally ill patients to take their own lives, and the remaining states would rapidly follow suit. Not since *Roe* v. *Wade* has a Supreme Court decision been so fateful.

The decision will culminate several years of intense national debate, fueled by a number of highly publicized events. Perhaps most important among them is Dr. Jack Kevorkian's defiant assistance in some 44 suicides since 1990, to the dismay of many in the medical and legal establishments, but with substantial public support, as evidenced by the fact that three juries refused to convict him even in the face of a Michigan statute enacted for that purpose. Also since 1990, voters in three states have considered ballot initiatives that would legalize some form of physician-assisted dying, and in 1994 Oregon became the first state to approve such a measure.[4] (The Oregon law was stayed pending a court challenge.) Several surveys indicate that roughly two thirds of the American public now support physician-assisted suicide,[5,6] as do more than half the doctors in the United States,[6,7] despite the fact that influential physicians' organizations are opposed. It seems clear that many Americans are now so concerned about

From *The New England Journal of Medicine*, January 2, 1997, pp. 50–53. Copyright © 1997 by Massachusetts Medical Society. All rights reserved. Reprinted by permission.

the possibility of a lingering, high-technology death that they are receptive to the idea of doctors' being allowed to help them die.

In this editorial I will explain why I believe the appeals courts were right and why I hope the Supreme Court will uphold their decisions. I am aware that this is a highly contentious issue, with good people and strong arguments on both sides. The American Medical Association (AMA) filed an amicus brief opposing the legalization of physician-assisted suicide,[8] and the Massachusetts Medical Society, which owns the *Journal,* was a signatory to it. But here I speak for myself, not the *Journal* or the Massachusetts Medical Society. The legal aspects of the case have been well discussed elsewhere, to me most compellingly in Ronald Dworkin's essay in the *New York Review of Books.*[9] I will focus primarily on the medical and ethical aspects.

I begin with the generally accepted premise that one of the most important ethical principles in medicine is respect for each patient's autonomy, and that when this principle conflicts with others, it should almost always take precedence. This premise is incorporated into our laws governing medical practice and research, including the requirement of informed consent to any treatment. In medicine, patients exercise their self-determination most dramatically when they ask that life-sustaining treatment be withdrawn. Although others may sometimes consider the request ill-founded, we are bound to honor it if the patient is mentally competent—that is, if the patient can understand the nature of the decision and its consequences.

A second starting point is the recognition that death is not fair and is often cruel. Some people die quickly, and others die slowly but peacefully. Some find personal or religious meaning in the process, as well as an opportunity for a final reconciliation with loved ones. But others, especially those with cancer, AIDS, or progressive neurologic disorders, may die by inches and in great anguish, despite every effort of their doctors and nurses. Although nearly all pain can be relieved, some cannot, and other symptoms, such as dyspnea, nausea, and weakness, are even more difficult to control. In addition, dying sometimes holds great indignities and existential suffering. Patients who happen to require some treatment to sustain their lives, such as assisted ventilation or dialysis, can hasten death by having the life-sustaining treatment withdrawn, but those who are not receiving life-sustaining treatment may desperately need help they cannot now get.

If the decisions of the appeals courts are upheld, states will not be able to prohibit doctors from helping such patients to die by prescribing a lethal dose of a drug and advising them on its use for suicide. State laws barring euthanasia (the administration of a lethal drug by a doctor) and assisted suicide for patients who are not terminally ill would not be affected. Furthermore, doctors would not be *required* to assist in suicide; they would simply have that option. Both appeals courts based their decisions on constitutional questions. This is important, because it shifted the focus of the debate from what the majority would approve through the political process, as exemplified by the Oregon initiative, to a matter of fundamental rights, which are largely immune from the political process. Indeed, the Ninth Circuit Court drew an explicit analogy between suicide and abortion, saying that both were personal choices protected by the

Constitution and that forbidding doctors to assist would in effect nullify these rights. Although states could regulate assisted suicide, as they do abortion, they would not be permitted to regulate it out of existence.

It is hard to quarrel with the desire of a greatly suffering, dying patient for a quicker, more humane death or to disagree that it may be merciful to help bring that about. In those circumstances, loved ones are often relieved when death finally comes, as are the attending doctors and nurses. As the Second Circuit Court said (in the case of *Quill v. Vacco*), the state has no interest in prolonging such a life. Why, then, do so many people oppose legalizing physician-assisted suicide in these cases? There are a number of arguments against it, some stronger than others, but I believe none of them can offset the overriding duties of doctors to relieve suffering and to respect their patients' autonomy. Below I list several of the more important arguments against physician-assisted suicide and discuss why I believe they are in the last analysis unpersuasive.

Assisted suicide is a form of killing, which is always wrong. In contrast, withdrawing life-sustaining treatment simply allows the disease to take its course.   There are three methods of hastening the death of a dying patient: withdrawing life-sustaining treatment, assisting suicide, and euthanasia. The right to stop treatment has been recognized repeatedly since the 1976 case of Karen Ann Quinlan[10] and was affirmed by the U.S. Supreme Court in the 1990 Cruzan decision[11] and the U.S. Congress in its 1990 Patient Self-Determination Act.[12] Although the legal underpinning is the right to be free of unwanted bodily invasion, the purpose of hastening death was explicitly acknowledged. In contrast, assisted suicide and euthanasia have not been accepted; euthanasia is illegal in all states, and assisted suicide is illegal in most of them.

Why the distinctions? Most would say they turn on the doctor's role: whether it is passive or active. When life-sustaining treatment is withdrawn, the doctor's role is considered passive and the cause of death is the underlying disease, despite the fact that switching off the ventilator of a patient dependent on it looks anything but passive and would be considered homicide if done without the consent of the patient or a proxy. In contrast, euthanasia by the injection of a lethal drug is active and directly causes the patient's death. Assisting suicide by supplying the necessary drugs is considered somewhere in between, more active than switching off a ventilator but less active than injecting drugs, hence morally and legally more ambiguous.

I believe, however, that these distinctions are too doctor-centered and not sufficiently patient-centered. We should ask ourselves not so much whether the doctor's role is passive or active but whether the *patient's* role is passive or active. From that perspective, the three methods of hastening death line up quite differently. When life-sustaining treatment is withdrawn from an incompetent patient at the request of a proxy or when euthanasia is performed, the patient may be utterly passive. Indeed, either act can be performed even if the patient is unaware of the decision. In sharp contrast, assisted suicide, by definition, cannot occur without the patient's knowledge and participation. Therefore, it must be active—that is to say, voluntary. That is a crucial distinction, because it provides an inherent safeguard against abuse that is not present with the other two methods of hastening death. If the loaded term "kill" is to be used, it is not the doctor who kills, but the patient. Primarily because euthanasia can be performed without the patient's participation, I oppose its legalization in this country.

Assisted suicide is not necessary. All suffering can be relieved if care givers are sufficiently skillful and compassionate, as illustrated by the hospice movement. I have no doubt that if expert palliative care were available to everyone who needed it, there would be few requests for assisted suicide. Even under the best of circumstances, however, there will always be a few patients whose suffering simply cannot be adequately alleviated. And there will be some who would prefer suicide to any other measures available, including the withdrawal of life-sustaining treatment or the use of heavy sedation. Surely, every effort should be made to improve palliative care, as I argued 15 years ago,[13] but when those efforts are unavailing and suffering patients desperately long to end their lives, physician-assisted suicide should be allowed. The argument that permitting it would divert us from redoubling our commitment to comfort care asks these patients to pay the penalty for our failings. It is also illogical. Good comfort care and the availability of physician-assisted suicide are no more mutually exclusive than good cardiologic care and the availability of heart transplantation.

Permitting assisted suicide would put us on a moral "slippery slope." Although in itself assisted suicide might be acceptable, it would lead inexorably to involuntary euthanasia. It is impossible to avoid slippery slopes in medicine (or in any aspect of life). The issue is how and where to find a purchase. For example, we accept the right of proxies to terminate life-sustaining treatment, despite the obvious potential for abuse, because the reasons for doing so outweigh the risks. We hope our procedures will safeguard patients. In the case of assisted suicide, its voluntary nature is the best protection against sliding down a slippery slope, but we also need to ensure that the request is thoughtful and freely made. Although it is possible that we may someday decide to legalize voluntary euthanasia under certain circumstances or assisted suicide for patients who are not terminally ill, legalizing assisted suicide for the dying does not in itself make these other decisions inevitable. Interestingly, recent reports from the Netherlands, where both euthanasia and physician-assisted suicide are permitted, indicate that fears about a slippery slope there have not been borne out.[14, 15, 16]

Assisted suicide would be a threat to the economically and socially vulnerable. The poor, disabled, and elderly might be coerced to request it. Admittedly, overburdened families or cost-conscious doctors might pressure vulnerable patients to request suicide, but similar wrongdoing is at least as likely in the case of withdrawing life-sustaining treatment, since that decision can be made by proxy. Yet, there is no evidence of widespread abuse. The Ninth Circuit Court recalled that it was feared *Roe* v. *Wade* would lead to coercion of poor and uneducated women to request abortions, but that did not happen. The concern that coercion is more likely in this era of managed care, although understandable, would hold suffering patients hostage to the deficiencies of our health care system. Unfortunately, no human endeavor is immune to abuses. The question is not whether a perfect system can be devised, but whether abuses are likely to be sufficiently rare to be offset by the benefits to patients who otherwise would be condemned to face the end of their lives in protracted agony.

Depressed patients would seek physician-assisted suicide rather than help for their depression. Even in the terminally ill, a request for assisted suicide might signify treatable depression, not irreversible suffering.   Patients suffering greatly at the end of life may also be depressed, but the depression does not necessarily explain their decision to commit suicide or make it irrational. Nor is it simple to diagnose depression in terminally ill patients. Sadness is to be expected, and some of the vegetative symptoms of depression are similar to the symptoms of terminal illness. The success of antidepressant treatment in these circumstances is also not ensured. Although there are anecdotes about patients who changed their minds about suicide after treatment,[17] we do not have good studies of how often that happens or the relation to antidepressant treatment. Dying patients who request assisted suicide and seem depressed should certainly be strongly encouraged to accept psychiatric treatment, but I do not believe that competent patients should be *required* to accept it as a condition of receiving assistance with suicide. On the other hand, doctors would not be required to comply with all requests; they would be expected to use their judgment, just as they do in so many other types of life-and-death decisions in medical practice.

Doctors should never participate in taking life. If there is to be assisted suicide, doctors must not be involved.   Although most doctors favor permitting assisted suicide under certain circumstances, many who favor it believe that doctors should not provide the assistance.[6, 7] To them, doctors should be unambiguously committed to life (although most doctors who hold this view would readily honor a patient's decision to have life-sustaining treatment withdrawn). The AMA, too, seems to object to physician-assisted suicide primarily because it violates the profession's mission. Like others, I find that position too abstract.[18] The highest ethical imperative of doctors should be to provide care in whatever way best serves patients' interests, in accord with each patient's wishes, not with a theoretical commitment to preserve life no matter what the cost in suffering.[19] If a patient requests help with suicide and the doctor believes the request is appropriate, requiring someone else to provide the assistance would be a form of abandonment. Doctors who are opposed in principle need not assist, but they should make their patients aware of their position early in the relationship so that a patient who chooses to select another doctor can do so. The greatest harm we can do is to consign a desperate patient to unbearable suffering—or force the patient to seek out a stranger like Dr. Kevorkian. Contrary to the frequent assertion that permitting physician-assisted suicide would lead patients to distrust their doctors, I believe distrust is more likely to arise from uncertainty about whether a doctor will honor a patient's wishes.

Physician-assisted suicide may occasionally be warranted, but it should remain illegal. If doctors risk prosecution, they will think twice before assisting with suicide.   This argument wrongly shifts the focus from the patient to the doctor. Instead of reflecting the condition and wishes of patients, assisted suicide would reflect the courage and compassion of their doctors. Thus, patients with doctors like Timothy Quill, who described in a 1991 *Journal* article how he helped a patient take her life,[20] would get the help they need and want, but similar patients with less steadfast doctors would not. That makes no sense.

People do not need assistance to commit suicide. With enough determination, they can do it themselves.   This is perhaps the cruelest of the arguments against physician-assisted suicide. Many patients at the end of life are, in fact, physically unable to commit suicide on their own. Others lack the resources to do so. It has sometimes been suggested that they can simply stop eating and drinking and kill themselves that way. Although this method has been described as peaceful under certain conditions,[21] no one should count on that. The fact is that this argument leaves most patients to their suffering. Some, usually men, manage to commit suicide using violent methods. Percy Bridgman, a Nobel laureate in physics who in 1961 shot himself rather than die of metastatic cancer, said in his suicide note, "It is not decent for Society to make a man do this to himself."[22]

My father, who knew nothing of Percy Bridgman, committed suicide under similar circumstances. He was 81 and had metastatic prostate cancer. The night before he was scheduled to be admitted to the hospital, he shot himself. Like Bridgman, he thought it might be his last chance. At the time, he was not in extreme pain, nor was he close to death (his life expectancy was probably longer than six months). But he was suffering nonetheless— from nausea and the side effects of antiemetic agents, weakness, incontinence, and hopelessness. Was he depressed? He would probably have freely admitted that he was, but he would have thought it beside the point. In any case, he was an intensely private man who would have refused psychiatric care. Was he overly concerned with maintaining control of the circumstances of his life and death? Many people would say so, but that was the way he was. It is the job of medicine to deal with patients as they are, not as we would like them to be.

I tell my father's story here because it makes an abstract issue very concrete. If physician-assisted suicide had been available, I have no doubt my father would have chosen it. He was protective of his family, and if he had felt he had the choice, he would have spared my mother the shock of finding his body. He did not tell her what he planned to do, because he knew she would stop him. I also believe my father would have waited if physician-assisted suicide had been available. If patients have access to drugs they can take when they choose, they will not feel they must commit suicide early, while they are still able to do it on their own. They would probably live longer and certainly more peacefully, and they might not even use the drugs.

Long before my father's death, I believed that physician-assisted suicide ought to be permissible under some circumstances, but his death strengthened my conviction that it is simply a part of good medical care—something to be done reluctantly and sadly, as a last resort, but done nonetheless. There should be safeguards to ensure that the decision is well considered and consistent, but they should not be so daunting or violative of privacy that they become obstacles instead of protections. In particular, they should be directed not toward reviewing the reasons for an autonomous decision, but only toward ensuring that the decision is indeed autonomous. If the Supreme Court upholds the decisions of the appeals courts, assisted suicide will not be forced on either patients or doctors, but it will be a choice for those patients who need it and those doctors willing to help. If, on the other hand, the Supreme Court overturns the lower courts' decisions, the issue will continue to be grappled with state by state, through the political process. But sooner or later, given the need and the widespread public support, physician-assisted suicide will be demanded of a compassionate profession.

References

1. Greenhouse L. High court to say if the dying have a right to suicide help. New York Times. October 2, 1996:A1.

2. Compassion in Dying v. Washington, 79 F.3d 790 (9th Cir. 1996).

3. Quill v. Vacco, 80 F.3d 716 (2d Cir. 1996).

4. Annas GJ. Death by prescription—the Oregon initiative. N Engl J Med 1994;331:1240–3.

5. Blendon RJ, Szalay US, Knox RA. Should physicians aid their patients in dying? The public perspective. JAMA 1992;267:2658–62.

6. Bachman JG, Alcser KH, Doukas DJ, Lichtenstein RL, Corning AD, Brody H. Attitudes of Michigan physicians and the public toward legalizing physician-assisted suicide and voluntary euthanasia. N Engl J Med 1996;334:303–9.

7. Lee MA, Nelson HD, Tilden VP, Ganzini L, Schmidt TA, Tolle SW. Legalizing assisted suicide—views of physicians in Oregon. N Engl J Med 1996;334:310–5.

8. Gianelli DM. AMA to court: no suicide aid. American Medical News. November 25, 1996:1, 27, 28.

9. Dworkin R. Sex, death, and the courts. New York Review of Books. August 8, 1996.

10. In re: Quinlan, 70 N.J. 10, 355 A.2d 647 (1976).

11. Cruzan v. Director, Missouri Department of Health, 497 U.S. 261, 110 S.Ct. 2841 (1990).

12. Omnibus Budget Reconciliation Act of 1990, P.L. 101–508, sec. 4206 and 4751, 104 Stat. 1388, 1388–115, and 1388–204 (classified respectively at 42 U.S.C. 1395cc(f) (Medicare) and 1396a(w) (Medicaid) (1994)).

13. Angell M. The quality of mercy. N Engl J Med 1982;306:98–9.

14. van der Maas PJ, van der Wal G, Haverkate I, et al. Euthanasia, physician-assisted suicide, and other medical practices involving the end of life in the Netherlands, 1990–1995. N Engl J Med 1996;335:1699–705.

15. van der Wal G, van der Maas PJ, Bosma JM, et al. Evaluation of the notification procedure for physician-assisted death in the Netherlands. N Engl J Med 1996;335:1706–11.

16. Angell M. Euthanasia in the Netherlands—good news or bad? N Engl J Med 1996;335:1676–8.

17. Chochinov HM, Wilson KG, Enns M, et al. Desire for death in the terminally ill. Am J Psychiatry 1995;152:1185–91.

18. Cassel CK, Meier DE. Morals and moralism in the debate over euthanasia and assisted suicide. N Engl J Med 1990;323:750–2.

19. Angell M. Doctors and assisted suicide. Ann R Coll Physicians Surg Can 1991;24:493–4.

20. Quill TE. Death and dignity—a case of individualized decision making. N Engl J Med 1991;324:691–4.

21. Lynn J, Childress JF. Must patients always be given food and water? Hastings Cent Rep 1983;13(5):17–21.

22. Nuland SB. How we die. New York: Alfred A. Knopf, 1994:152.

Kathleen M. Foley 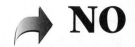 **NO**

Competent Care for the Dying Instead of Physician-Assisted Suicide

While the Supreme Court is reviewing the decisions by the Second and Ninth Circuit Courts of Appeals to reverse state bans on assisted suicide, there is a unique opportunity to engage the public, health care professionals, and the government in a national discussion of how American medicine and society should address the needs of dying patients and their families. Such a discussion is critical if we are to understand the process of dying from the point of view of patients and their families and to identify existing barriers to appropriate, humane, compassionate care at the end of life. Rational discourse must replace the polarized debate over physician-assisted suicide and euthanasia. Facts, not anecdotes, are necessary to establish a common ground and frame a system of health care for the terminally ill that provides the best possible quality of living while dying.

The biased language of the appeals courts evinces little respect for the vulnerability and dependency of the dying. Judge Stephen Reinhardt, writing for the Ninth Circuit Court, applied the liberty-interest clause of the Fourteenth Amendment, advocating a constitutional right to assisted suicide. He stated, "The competent terminally ill adult, having lived nearly the full measure of his life, has a strong interest in choosing a dignified and humane death, rather than being reduced to a state of helplessness, diapered, sedated, incompetent."[1] Judge Roger J. Miner, writing for the Second Circuit Court of Appeals, applied the equal-rights clause of the Fourteenth Amendment and went on to emphasize that the state "has no interest in prolonging a life that is ending."[2] This statement is more than legal jargon. It serves as a chilling reminder of the low priority given to the dying when it comes to state resources and protection.

The appeals courts' assertion of a constitutional right to assisted suicide is narrowly restricted to the terminally ill. The courts have decided that it is the patient's condition that justifies killing and that the terminally ill are special—so special that they deserve assistance in dying. This group alone can receive such assistance. The courts' response to the New York and Washington cases they reviewed is the dangerous form of affirmative action in the name of compassion. It runs the risk of further devaluing the lives of terminally ill patients and may provide the excuse for society to abrogate its responsibility for their care.

Both circuit courts went even further in asserting that physicians are already assisting in patients' deaths when they withdraw life-sustaining treatments such as respirators or administer high doses of pain medication that hasten death. The appeals courts argued that providing a lethal prescription to allow a terminally ill patient to commit suicide is essentially the same as withdrawing life-sustaining treatment or aggressively treating pain. Judicial reasoning that eliminates the distinction between letting a person die and killing runs counter to physicians' standards of palliative care.[3] The courts' purported goal in blurring these distinctions was to bring society's legal rules more closely in line with the moral value it places on the relief of suffering.[4]

In the real world in which physicians care for dying patients, withdrawing treatment and aggressively treating pain are acts that respect patients' autonomous decisions not to be battered by medical technology and to be relieved of their suffering. The physician's intent is to provide care, not death. Physicians do struggle with doubts about their own intentions.[5] The courts' arguments fuel their ambivalence about withdrawing life-sustaining treatments or using opioid or sedative infusions to treat intractable symptoms in dying patients. Physicians are trained and socialized to preserve life. Yet saying that physicians struggle with doubts about their intentions in performing these acts is not the same as saying that their intention is to kill. In palliative care, the goal is to relieve suffering, and the quality of life, not the quantity, is of utmost importance.

Whatever the courts say, specialists in palliative care do not think that they practice physician-assisted suicide or euthanasia.[6] Palliative medicine has developed guidelines for aggressive pharmacologic management of intractable symptoms in dying patients, including sedation for those near death.[3, 7, 8] The World Health Organization has endorsed palliative care as an integral component of a national health care policy and has strongly recommended to its member countries that they not consider legalizing physician-assisted suicide and euthanasia until they have addressed the needs of their citizens for pain relief and palliative care.[9] The courts have disregarded this formidable recommendation and, in fact, are indirectly suggesting that the World Health Organization supports assisted suicide.

Yet the courts' support of assisted suicide reflects the requests of the physicians who initiated the suits and parallels the numerous surveys demonstrating that a large proportion of physicians support the legalization of physician-assisted suicide.[10, 11, 12, 13, 14, 15] A smaller proportion of physicians are willing to provide such assistance, and an even smaller proportion are willing to inject a lethal dose of medication with the intent of killing a patient (active voluntary euthanasia). These survey data reveal a gap between the attitudes and behavior of physicians; 20 to 70 percent of physicians favor the legalization of physician-assisted suicide, but only 2 to 4 percent favor active voluntary euthanasia, and only approximately 2 to 13 percent have actually aided patients in dying, by either providing a prescription or administering a lethal injection. The limitations of these surveys, which are legion, include inconsistent definitions of physician-assisted suicide and euthanasia, lack of information about nonrespondents, and provisions for maintaining confidentiality that have led to inaccurate reporting.[13, 16] Since physicians' attitudes toward alternatives to assisted suicide have not been studied, there is a void in our knowledge about the priority that physicians place on physician-assisted suicide.

The willingness of physicians to assist patients in dying appears to be determined by numerous complex factors, including religious beliefs, personal values, medical specialty, age, practice setting, and perspective on the use of financial resources.[13, 16, 17, 18, 19] Studies of patients' preferences for care at the end of life demonstrate that physicians' preferences strongly influence those of their patients.[13] Making physician-assisted suicide a medical treatment when it is so strongly dependent on these physician-related variables would result in a regulatory impossibility.[19] Physicians would have to disclose their values and attitudes to patients to avoid potential conflict.[13] A survey by Ganzini et al. demonstrated that psychiatrists' responses to requests to evaluate patients were highly determined by their attitudes.[13] In a study by Emanuel et al., depressed patients with cancer said they would view positively those physicians who acknowledged their willingness to assist in suicide. In contrast, patients with cancer who were suffering from pain would be suspicious of such physicians.[11]

In this controversy, physicians fall into one of three groups. Those who support physician-assisted suicide see it as a compassionate response to a medical need, a symbol of nonabandonment, and a means to reestablish patients' trust in doctors who have used technology excessively.[20] They argue that regulation of physician-assisted suicide is possible and, in fact, necessary to control the actions of physicians who are currently providing assistance surreptitiously.[21] The two remaining groups of physicians oppose legalization.[19, 22, 23, 24] One group is morally opposed to physician-assisted suicide and emphasizes the need to preserve the professionalism of medicine and the commitment to "do no harm." These physicians view aiding a patient in dying as a form of abandonment, because a physician needs to walk the last mile with the patient, as a witness, not as an executioner. Legalization would endorse justified killing, according to these physicians, and guidelines would not be followed, even if they could be developed. Furthermore, these physicians are concerned that the conflation of assisted suicide with the withdrawal of life support or adequate treatment of pain would make it even harder for dying patients, because there would be a backlash against existing policies. The other group is not ethically opposed to physician-assisted suicide and, in fact, sees it as acceptable in exceptional cases, but these physicians believe that one cannot regulate the unregulatable.[19] On this basis, the New York State Task Force on Life and the Law, a 24-member committee with broad public and professional representation, voted unanimously against the legalization of physician-assisted suicide.[24] All three groups of physicians agree that a national effort is needed to improve the care of the dying. Yet it does seem that those in favor of legalizing physician-assisted suicide are disingenuous in their use of this issue as a wedge. If this form of assistance with dying is legalized, the courts will be forced to broaden the assistance to include active voluntary euthanasia and, eventually, assistance in response to requests from proxies.

One cannot easily categorize the patients who request physician-assisted suicide or euthanasia. Some surveys of physicians have attempted to determine retrospectively the prevalence and nature of these requests.[10] Pain, AIDS, and neurodegenerative disorders are the most common conditions in patients requesting assistance in dying. There is a wide range in the age of such patients, but many are younger persons with AIDS.[10] From the limited data available, the factors most commonly involved in requests for assistance are concern about future loss of control, being or becoming a burden to others, or being unable to care for oneself and fear of severe pain.[10] A small number of recent studies have directly asked terminally ill patients with cancer or AIDS about their desire for death.[25, 26, 27] All these studies show that the desire for death is closely associated with depression and that pain and lack of social support are contributing factors.

Do we know enough, on the basis of several legal cases, to develop a public policy that will profoundly change medicine's role in society?[1, 2] Approximately 2.4 million Americans die each year. We have almost no information on how they die and only general information on where they die. Sixty-one percent die in hospitals, 17 percent in nursing homes, and the remainder at home, with approximately 10 to 14 percent of those at home receiving hospice care.

The available data suggest that physicians are inadequately trained to assess and manage the multifactorial symptoms commonly associated with patients' requests for physician-assisted suicide. According to the American Medical Association's report on medical education, only 5 of 126 medical schools in the United States require a separate course in the care of the dying.[28] Of 7048 residency programs, only 26 percent offer a course on the medical and legal aspects of care at the end of life as a regular part of the curriculum. According to a survey of 1068 accredited residency programs in family medicine, internal medicine, and pediatrics and fellowship programs in geriatrics, each resident or fellow coordinates the care of 10 or fewer dying patients annually.[28] Almost 15 percent of the programs offer no formal training in terminal care. Despite the availability of hospice programs, only 17 percent of the training programs offer a hospice rotation, and the rotation is required in only half of those programs; 9 percent of the programs have residents or fellows serving as members of hospice teams. In a recent survey of 55 residency programs and over 1400 residents, conducted by the American Board of Internal Medicine, the residents were asked to rate their perception of adequate training in care at the end of life. Seventy-two percent reported that they had received adequate training in managing pain and other symptoms; 62 percent, that they had received adequate training in telling patients that they are dying; 38 percent, in describing what the process will be like; and 32 percent, in talking to patients who request assistance in dying or a hastened death (Blank L: personal communication).

The lack of training in the care of the dying is evident in practice. Several studies have concluded that poor communication between physicians and patients, physicians' lack of knowledge about national guidelines for such care, and their lack of knowledge about the control of symptoms are barriers to the provision of good care at the end of life.[23, 29, 30]

Yet there is now a large body of data on the components of suffering in patients with advanced terminal disease, and these data provide the basis for treatment algorithms.[3] There are three major factors in suffering: pain and other physical symptoms, psychological distress, and existential distress (described as the experience of life without meaning). It is not only the patients who suffer but also their families and the health care professionals attending them. These experiences of suffering are often closely and inextricably related. Perceived distress in any one of the three groups amplifies distress in the others.[31, 32]

Pain is the most common symptom in dying patients, and according to recent data from U.S. studies, 56 percent of outpatients with cancer, 82 percent of outpatients with AIDS, 50 percent of hospitalized patients with various diagnoses, and 36 percent of nursing home residents have inadequate management of pain during the course of their terminal illness.[33, 34, 35, 36] Members of minority groups and women, both those with cancer and those with AIDS, as well as the elderly, receive less pain treatment than other groups of patients. In a survey of 1177 physicians who had treated a total of more than 70,000 patients with cancer in the previous six months, 76 percent of the respondents cited lack of knowledge as a barrier to their ability to control pain.[37] Severe pain that is not adequately controlled interferes with the quality of life, including the activities of daily living, sleep, and social interactions.[33, 38]

Other physical symptoms are also prevalent among the dying. Studies of patients with advanced cancer and of the elderly in the year before death show that they have numerous symptoms that worsen the quality of life, such as fatigue, dyspnea, delirium, nausea, and vomiting.[36, 38]

Along with these physical symptoms, dying patients have a variety of well-described psychological symptoms, with a high prevalence of anxiety and depression in patients with cancer or AIDS and the elderly.[27, 39] For example, more than 60 percent of patients with advanced cancer have psychiatric problems, with adjustment disorders, depression, anxiety, and delirium reported most frequently. Various factors that contribute to the prevalence and severity of psychological distress in the terminally ill have been identified.[39] The diagnosis of depression is difficult to make in medically ill patients[3, 26, 40]; 94 percent of the Oregon psychiatrists surveyed by Ganzini et al. were not confident that they could determine, in a single evaluation, whether a psychiatric disorder was impairing the judgment of a patient who requested assistance with suicide.[13]

Attention has recently been focused on the interaction between uncontrolled symptoms and vulnerability to suicide in patients with cancer or AIDS.[41] Data from studies of both groups of patients suggest that uncontrolled pain contributes to depression and that persistent pain interferes with patients' ability to receive support from their families and others. Patients with AIDS have a high risk of suicide that is independent of physical symptoms. Among New York City residents with AIDS, the relative risk of suicide in men between the ages of 20 and 59 years was 36 times higher than the risk among men without AIDS in the same age group and 66 times higher than the risk in the general population.[41] Patients with AIDS who committed suicide generally did so within nine months after receiving the diagnosis; 25 percent had made a previous suicide attempt, 50 percent had reported severe depression, and 40 percent had seen a psychiatrist within four days before committing suicide.

As previously noted, the desire to die is most closely associated with the diagnosis of depression.[26, 27] Suicide is the eighth leading cause of death in the United States, and the incidence of suicide is higher in patients with cancer or AIDS and in elderly men than in the general population. Conwell and Caine reported that depression was underdiagnosed by primary care physicians in a cohort of elderly patients who subsequently committed suicide; 75 percent of the patients had seen a primary care physician during the last month of life but had not received a diagnosis of depression.[22]

The relation between depression and the desire to hasten death may vary among subgroups of dying patients. We have no data, except for studies of a small number of patients with cancer or AIDS. The effect of treatment for depression on the desire to hasten death and on requests for assistance in doing so has not been examined in the medically ill population, except for a small study in which four of six patients who initially wished to hasten death changed their minds within two weeks.[26]

There is also the concern that certain patients, particularly members of minority groups that are estranged from the health care system, may be reluctant to receive treatment for their physical or psychological symptoms because of the fear that their physicians will, in fact, hasten death. There is now some evidence that the legalization of assisted suicide in the Northern Territory of Australia has undermined the Aborigines' trust in the medical care system[42]; this experience may serve as an example for the United States, with its multicultural population.

The multiple physical and psychological symptoms in the terminally ill and elderly are compounded by a substantial degree of existential distress. Reporting on their interviews with Washington State physicians whose patients had requested assistance in dying, Back et al. noted the physicians' lack of sophistication in assessing such nonphysical suffering.[10]

In summary, there are fundamental physician-related barriers to appropriate, humane, and compassionate care for the dying. These range from attitudinal and behavioral barriers to educational and economic barriers. Physicians do not know enough about their patients, themselves, or suffering to provide assistance with dying as a medical treatment for the relief of suffering. Physicians need to explore their own perspectives on the meaning of suffering in order to develop their own approaches to the care of the dying. They need insight into how the nature of the doctor-patient relationship influences their own decision making. If legalized, physician-assisted suicide will be a substitute for rational therapeutic, psychological, and social interventions that might otherwise enhance the quality of life for patients who are dying. The medical profession needs to take the lead in developing guidelines for good care of dying patients. Identifying the factors related to physicians, patients, and the health care system that pose barriers to appropriate care at the end of life should be the first step in a national dialogue to educate health care professionals and the public on the topic of death and dying. Death is an issue that society as a whole faces, and it requires a compassionate response. But we should not confuse compassion with competence in the care of terminally ill patients.

References

1. Reinhardt, Compassion in Dying v. State of Washington, 79 F. 3d 790 9th Cir. 1996.

2. Miner, Quill v. Vacco 80 F. 3d 716 2nd Cir. 1996.

3. Doyle D, Hanks GWC, MacDonald N. The Oxford textbook of palliative medicine. New York: Oxford University Press, 1993.

4. Orentlicher D. The legalization of physician-assisted suicide. N Engl J Med 1996;335:663–7.

5. Wilson WC, Smedira NG, Fink C, McDowell JA, Luce JM. Ordering and administration of sedatives and analgesics during the withholding and withdrawal of life support from critically ill patients. JAMA 1992; 267:949–53.

6. Foley KM. The relationship of pain and symptom management to patient requests for physician-assisted suicide. J Pain Symptom Manage 1991;6:289–97.

7. Cherny NI, Coyle N, Foley KM. Guidelines in the care of the dying patient. Hematol Oncol Clin North Am 1996;10:261–86.

8. Cherny NI, Portenoy RK. Sedation in the management of refractory symptoms: guidelines for evaluation and treatment. J Palliat Care 1994;10(2): 31–8.

9. Cancer pain relief and palliative care. Geneva: World Health Organization, 1989.

10. Back AL, Wallace JI, Starks HE, Pearlman RA. Physician-assisted suicide and euthanasia in Washington State: patient requests and physician responses. JAMA 1996;275:919–25.

11. Emanuel EJ, Fairclough DL, Daniels ER, Clarridge BR. Euthanasia and physician-assisted suicide: attitudes and experiences of oncology patients, oncologists, and the public. Lancet 1996;347:1805–10.

12. Lee MA, Nelson HD, Tilden VP, Ganzini L, Schmidt TA, Tolle SW. Legalizing assisted suicide—views of physicians in Oregon. N Engl J Med 1996;334: 310–5.

13. Ganzini L, Fenn DS, Lee MA, Heintz RT, Bloom JD. Attitudes of Oregon psychiatrists toward physician-assisted suicide. Am J Psychiatry 1996; 153:1469–75.

14. Cohen JS, Fihn SD, Boyko EJ, Jonsen AR, Wood RW. Attitudes toward assisted suicide and euthanasia among physicians in Washington State. N Engl J Med 1994;331:89–94.

15. Doukas DJ, Waterhouse D, Gorenflo DW, Seid J. Attitudes and behaviors on physician-assisted death: a study of Michigan oncologists. J Clin Oncol 1995;13:1055–61.

16. Morrison S, Meier D. Physician-assisted dying: fashioning public policy with an absence of data. Generations. Winter 1994:48–53.

17. Portenoy RK, Coyle N, Kash K, et al. Determinants of the willingness to endorse assisted suicide: a survey of physicians, nurses, and social workers. Psychosomatics (in press).

18. Fins J. Physician-assisted suicide and the right to care. Cancer Control 1996;3:272–8.

19. Callahan D, White M. The legalization of physician-assisted suicide: creating a regulatory Potemkin Village. U Richmond Law Rev 1996;30:1–83.

20. Quill TE. Death and dignity—a case of individualized decision making. N Engl J Med 1991;324:691–4.

21. Quill TE, Cassel CK, Meier DE. Care of the hopelessly ill—proposed clinical criteria for physician-assisted suicide. N Engl J Med 1992;327:1380–4.

22. Conwell Y, Caine ED. Rational suicide and the right to die—reality and myth. N Engl J Med 1991;325:1100–3.

23. Foley KM. Pain, physician assisted suicide and euthanasia. Pain Forum 1995;4:163–78.

24. When death is sought: assisted suicide and euthanasia in the medical context. New York: New York State Task Force on Life and the Law, May 1994.

25. Brown JH, Henteleff P, Barakat S, Rowe CJ. Is it normal for terminally ill patients to desire death? Am J Psychiatry 1986;143:208–11.

26. Chochinov HM, Wilson KG, Enns M, et al. Desire for death in the terminally ill. Am J Psychiatry 1995;152:1185–91.

27. Breitbart W, Rosenfeld BD, Passik SD. Interest in physician-assisted suicide among ambulatory HIV-infected patients. Am J Psychiatry 1996;153:238–42.

28. Hill TP. Treating the dying patient: the challenge for medical education. Arch Intern Med 1995;155:1265–9.

29. Callahan D. Once again reality: now where do we go? Hastings Cent Rep 1995;25(6):Suppl:S33–S36.

30. Solomon MZ, O'Donnell L, Jennings B, et al. Decisions near the end of life: professional views on life-sustaining treatments. Am J Public Health 1993;83:14–23.

31. Cherny NI, Coyle N, Foley KM. Suffering in the advanced cancer patient: definition and taxonomy. J Palliat Care 1994;10(2):57–70.

32. Cassel EJ. The nature of suffering and the goals of medicine. N Engl J Med 1982;306:639–45.

33. Cleeland CS, Gonin R, Hatfield AK, et al. Pain and its treatment in outpatients with metastatic cancer. N Engl J Med 1994;330:592–6.

34. Breitbart W, Rosenfeld BD, Passik SD, McDonald MV, Thaler H, Portenoy RK. The undertreatment of pain in ambulatory AIDS patients. Pain 1996; 65:243–9.

35. The SUPPORT Principal Investigators. A controlled trial to improve care for seriously ill hospitalized patients. JAMA 1995;274:1591–8.

36. Seale C, Cartwright A. The year before death. Hants, England: Avebury, 1994.

37. Von Roenn JH, Cleeland CS, Gonin R, Hatfield AK, Pandya KJ. Physician attitudes and practice in cancer pain management: a survey from the Eastern Cooperative Oncology Group. Ann Intern Med 1993;119:121–6.

38. Portenoy RK. Pain and quality of life: clinical issues and implications for research. Oncology 1990;4:172–8.

39. Breitbart W. Suicide risk and pain in cancer and AIDS patients. In: Chapman CR, Foley KM, eds. Current and emerging issues in cancer pain. New York: Raven Press, 1993.

40. Chochinov H, Wilson KG, Enns M, Lander S. Prevalence of depression in the terminally ill: effects of diagnostic criteria and symptom threshold judgments. Am J Psychiatry 1994;151:537–40.

41. Passik S, McDonald M, Rosenfeld B, Breitbart W. End of life issues in patients with AIDS: clinical and research considerations. J Pharm Care Pain Symptom Control 1995;3:91–111.

42. NT "success" in easing rural fear of euthanasia. The Age. August 31, 1996:A7.

POSTSCRIPT

Should Physicians Be Allowed to Assist in Patient Suicide?

In 1997, Oregon became the first state to implement a law legalizing physician-assisted suicide. The Death with Dignity Act was originally passed in 1994, but its implementation was delayed until 1997, when it was upheld by a large majority of voters. Under this law, a person who is mentally competent and suffering from a terminal illness (likely to die within 6 months) may receive lethal drugs from a physician. The person has to consult two doctors and wait 15 days before obtaining the drugs. Similar laws were enacted in Washington (2008) and Montana (2010).

Based on 10 years of experience, very few patients in Oregon actually use the option of requesting physician-assisted suicide, and the number has remained stable since 2002. In 2009, for example, 59 Oregon residents died after taking medications prescribed under the Death with Dignity Act, including 6 who had received medications in 2008. In 2009, 55 physicians wrote a total of 95 prescriptions for lethal doses of medications. Those most likely to request drugs were married, white, more highly educated, and had cancer as a primary diagnosis. Physicians reported that patient request stemmed from concerns related to loss of autonomy, decreasing ability to participated in enjoyable activities, and loss of dignity, rather than unbearable pain. Nearly all the patients were enrolled in hospice and had health insurance. The full report from the Oregon Department of Human Services is available at http://oregon .gov/DHS/ph/pas/docs/year12.pdf. Based on Washington's first year of experience, the patient population and concerns are similar to Oregon's.

Researchers led by Susan Tolle in Oregon found that, regardless of legalization, many more people consider physician-assisted suicide than follow through with it. The complexity of the process to obtain a lethal drug—a safeguard against misuse—also may be a barrier to those who do not fulfill their intentions (Susan W. Tolle et al., "Characteristics and Proportion of Dying Oregonians Who Personally Consider Physician-Assisted Suicide," *Journal of Clinical Ethics*, Summer 2004).

In "Legal Regulation of Physician-Assisted Death—The Latest Report Cards" (*New England Journal of Medicine*, May 10, 2007), Timothy E. Quill concludes that legalization has resulted in more open conversation and careful evaluation of end-of-life options.

In November 2008, voters in the state of Washington approved a measure similar to Oregon's law. In 1991, voters rejected a bill that would allow doctors to administer the lethal medications; the 2008 version requires patients to take the medications on their own.

In the Netherlands, euthanasia—defined as "the intentional termination of the life of a patient at his or her request by a physician"—was legalized in 2002. The practice had occurred before 2002 without repercussions for the physician. About 9,700 requests are made each year. Those who oppose the practice claim that not all requests are voluntary.

A review of the impact in Oregon and the Netherlands of physician-assisted suicide on "vulnerable" groups such as the elderly, women, people with low educational status, racial and ethnic minorities, and people with psychiatric illness found no evidence that these groups were disproportionately involved. The only people with a heightened risk were people with AIDS. Those who received physician-assisted suicide were more likely to be better educated, have more economic and social resources, and professional status (Margaret P. Battin et al., "Legal Physician-Assisted Dying in Oregon and the Netherlands: Evidence Concerning the Impact on Patients in 'Vulnerable' Groups," *Journal of Medical Ethics,* 2007).

Physician-Assisted Dying: The Case for Palliative Care and Patient Choice, edited by Timothy E. Quill and Margaret P. Battin, is a collection of articles that present the case for the legalization of physician-assisted dying (Johns Hopkins University Press, 2004). Opposing the practice are the authors in *The Case Against Assisted Suicide,* edited by Kathleen E. Foley and Herbert Hendin (Johns Hopkins University Press, 2002). See also Arthur L. Caplan, Lois Snyder, and Kathy Feber-Langendoen, "The Role of Guidelines in the Practice of Physician-Assisted Suicide," *Annals of Internal Medicine* (March 21, 2000). The entire issue is devoted to this subject.

Internet References . . .

NARAL Online

This is the home page of the National Abortion and Reproductive Rights Action League (NARAL), an organization that works to promote reproductive freedom and dignity for women and their families.

http://www.naral.org

The Lindesmith Center—Drug Policy Foundation

This site offers articles concerning the issue of punishing pregnant drug users as well as articles about the case of *Cornelia Whitner v. State of South Carolina*. Search under "pregnant drug users" to access these articles.

http://www.lindesmith.org/news/

Students for Life

This organization run by students at Simon Fraser University in Vancouver, Canada, lists Web sites representing the diversity of pro-life views.

http://www.studentsforlife.org

UNIT 3

Choices in Reproduction

*F*ew bioethical issues could be of greater personal and social significance than questions concerning reproduction. Advances in medical technology, such as in vitro fertilization and egg donation have opened new possibilities for infertile couples, while challenging traditional notions of family. Some advances in genetic manipulation, such as cloning, are still in the experimental stage and raise complex ethical issues. Another type of technological advance, the ability to see images of the developing fetus, has enhanced our understanding of both normal growth and birth defects. This technology has provided evidence of the impact of the mother's behavior on fetal development. While many behaviors of pregnant women expose fetuses to risk, and while fathers' exposure to chemicals and other toxic substances also affect fetuses, attention has focused mainly on the mothers' use of illegal drugs. Preventing risk to fetuses raises troubling questions concerning the role of police and the courts in medical matters and the best way to assist drug-addicted women. The most polarized question remains the morality of abortion, where common ground is elusive. The issues in this section come to grips with some of the most perplexing and fundamental questions that confront medical practitioners, individual women and their partners, and society in general.

- Is Abortion Immoral?
- Should a Pregnant Woman Be Punished for Exposing Her Fetus to Risk?

ISSUE 7

Is Abortion Immoral?

YES: Patrick Lee and Robert P. George, from "The Wrong of Abortion," in Andrew Cohen and Christopher Heath Wellman, eds., *Contemporary Debates in Applied Ethics* (Blackwell, 2005)

NO: Margaret Olivia Little, from "The Morality of Abortion," in Bonnie Steinbock, John D. Arras, and Alex John London, eds., *Ethical Issues in Modern Medicine* (McGraw-Hill, 2003)

ISSUE SUMMARY

YES: Philosopher Patrick Lee and professor of jurisprudence Robert P. George assert that human embryos and fetuses are complete (though immature) human beings and that intentional abortion is unjust and objectively immoral.

NO: Philosopher Margaret Olivia Little believes that the moral status of the fetus is only one aspect of the morality of abortion. She points to gestation as an intimacy, motherhood as a relationship, and creation as a process to advance a more nuanced approach.

Abortion is the most divisive bioethical issue of our time. The issue has been a persistent one in history, but in the past 30 years or so the debate has polarized. One view—known as "pro-life"—sees abortion as the wanton slaughter of innocent life. The other view—"pro-choice"—considers abortion as an option that must be available to women if they are to control their own reproductive lives. According to the pro-life view, women who have access to "abortion on demand" put their own selfish whims ahead of an unborn child's right to life. According to the pro-choice view, women have the right to choose to have an abortion—especially if there is an overriding reason, such as preventing the birth of a child with a severe genetic defect or one conceived as a result of rape or incest.

Behind these strongly held convictions, as political scientist Mary Segers has pointed out, are widely differing views of what determines value (that is, whether value is inherent in a thing or ascribed to it by human beings), the relation between law and morality, and the use of limits of political solutions to social problems, as well as the value of scientific progress. Those who condemn abortion as immoral generally follow a classical tradition in which abortion is a public matter because it involves our conception of how we should live together in an ideal society. Those who accept the idea of abortion, on the other hand, generally share the liberal, individualistic ethos of contemporary society. They believe that abortion is a private choice, and that public policy should reflect how citizens actually behave, not some unattainable ideal.

This is what we know about abortion practices in America today: Abortion has been legal since the 1973 Supreme Court decision of *Roe v. Wade* declared that a woman has a constitutional right to privacy, which includes an abortion. According to the National Center on Health Statistics, abortion at eight weeks or less gestation is seven times safer than childbirth, although there are some unknown risks—primarily the effect of repeated abortions on subsequent pregnancies.

In the past 30 years, the demographic profile of women who have abortions has changed significantly, according to a review of the Centers for Disease Control and Prevention by the Guttmacher Institute, a private research organization. Relatively fewer white childless teenagers are choosing abortion, while more low-income women of color in their 20s and 30s who already have children are having abortions. Overall the abortion rate dropped 33 percent from 1974 to 2004, from a high of 29 abortions for every thousand women aged 15-44 to 20 per thousand in 2004. Some of the reasons are the use of long-acting hormonal contraceptives, a lower pregnancy rate among teenagers, and growing use of emergency contraception (see Issue 21). The typical woman having an abortion is between the ages of 20 and 30, has never married, lives in a metropolitan area, and is a Christian (42.8 percent Protestant, 27.4 percent Catholic, 7.6 percent "other," and 22.7 percent "none").

The following two selections offer thoughtful and reasoned but opposing views on abortion. Patrick Lee and Robert P. George conclude that being a mother generates a special responsibility and that the sacrifice morally required of the mother is less burdensome than the harm that would be done by expelling the child, causing his or her death, to escape that responsibility. They see abortion as objectively immoral. Margaret Olivia Little believes that if we acknowledge gestation as an intimacy, motherhood as a relationship, and creation as a process, we will be better able to appreciate the moral textures of abortion.

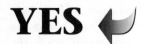

YES ↵

**Patrick Lee and
Robert P. George**

The Wrong of Abortion

Much of the public debate about abortion concerns the question whether deliberate feticide ought to be unlawful, at least in most circumstances. We will lay that question aside here in order to focus first on the question: is the choice to have, to perform, or to help procure an abortion morally wrong?

We shall argue that the choice of abortion is objectively immoral. By "objectively" we indicate that we are discussing the choice itself, not the (subjective) guilt or innocence of someone who carries out the choice: someone may act from an erroneous conscience, and if he is not at fault for his error, then he remains subjectively innocent, even if his choice is objectively wrongful.

The first important question to consider is: what is killed in an abortion? It is obvious that some living entity is killed in an abortion. And no one doubts that the moral status of the entity killed is a central (though not the only) question in the abortion debate. We shall approach the issue step by step, first setting forth some (though not all) of the evidence that demonstrates that what is killed in abortion—a human embryo—is indeed a human being, then examining the ethical significance of that point.

Human Embryos and Fetuses Are Complete (though Immature) Human Beings

It will be useful to begin by considering some of the facts of sexual reproduction. The standard embryology texts indicate that in the case of ordinary sexual reproduction the life of an individual human being begins with complete fertilization, which yields a genetically and functionally distinct organism, possessing the resources and active disposition for internally directed development toward human maturity.[1] In normal conception, a sex cell of the father, a sperm, unites with a sex cell of the mother, an ovum. Within the chromosomes of these sex cells are the DNA molecules which constitute the information that guides the development of the new individual brought into being when the sperm and ovum fuse. When fertilization occurs, the 23 chromosomes of the sperm unite with the 23 chromosomes of the ovum. At the end of this process there is produced an entirely new and distinct organism, originally a single cell. This organism, the human embryo, begins to grow by the normal process of cell division—it divides into 2 cells, then 4, 8, 16, and so on (the divisions are not simultaneous, so there is a 3-cell stage, and so on). This embryo gradually develops all of the organs and organ systems necessary for the full functioning of a mature human being. His or her development (sex is determined from the beginning) is very rapid in the first few weeks. For example, as early as eight or ten weeks of gestation, the fetus has a fully formed, beating heart, a complete brain (although not all of its synaptic connections are complete— nor will they be until sometime *after* the child is born), a recognizably human form, and the fetus feels pain, cries, and even sucks his or her thumb.

There are three important points we wish to make about this human embryo. First, it is from the start *distinct* from any cell of the mother or of the father. This is clear because it is growing in its own distinct direction. Its growth is internally directed to its own survival and maturation. Second, the embryo is *human:* it has the genetic makeup characteristic of human beings. Third, and most importantly, the embryo is a *complete* or *whole* organism, though immature. The human embryo, from conception onward, is fully programmed actively to develop himself or herself to the mature stage of a human being, and, *unless prevented by disease or violence, will actually do so, despite possibly significant variation in environment* (in the mother's womb). None of the changes that occur to the embryo after fertilization, for as long as he or she survives, generates a new direction of growth. Rather, *all* of the changes (for example, those involving nutrition and environment) either facilitate or retard the internally directed growth of this persisting individual.

Sometimes it is objected that if we say human embryos are human beings, on the grounds that they have the potential to become mature humans, the same will have to be said of sperm and ova. This objection is untenable. The human embryo is radically unlike the sperm and ova, the sex cells. The sex cells are manifestly not *whole* or *complete* organisms. They are not only genetically but also functionally identifiable as parts of the male or female potential parents. They clearly are destined either to combine with an ovum or sperm or die. Even when they succeed in causing fertilization, they do not survive; rather, their genetic material enters into the composition of a distinct, new organism.

Nor are human embryos comparable to somatic cells (such as skin cells or muscle cells), though some have tried to argue that they are. Like sex cells, a somatic cell is functionally only a part of a larger organism. The human embryo, by contrast, possesses from the beginning the internal resources and active disposition to develop himself or herself to full maturity; all he or she needs is a suitable environment and nutrition. The direction of his or her growth *is not extrinsically determined,* but the embryo is internally directing his or her growth toward full maturity.

So, a human embryo (or fetus) is not something distinct from a human being; he or she is not an individual of any non-human or intermediate species. Rather, an embryo (and fetus) is a human being at a certain (early) stage of development—the embryonic (or fetal) stage. In abortion, what is killed is a human being, a whole living member of the species *homo sapiens,* the same *kind* of entity as you or I, only at an earlier stage of development. . . .

The Argument That Abortion Is Justified as Non-Intentional Killing

Some "pro-choice" philosophers have attempted to justify abortion by denying that all abortions are intentional killing. They have granted (at least for the sake of argument) that an unborn human being has a right to life but have then argued that this right does not entail that the child *in utero* is morally entitled to the use of the mother's body for life support. In effect, their argument is that, at least in many cases, abortion is not a case of intentionally killing the child, but a choice not to provide the child with assistance, that is, a choice to expel (or "evict") the child from the womb, despite the likelihood or certainty that expulsion (or "eviction") will result in his or her death (Little, 1999; McDonagh, 1996; Thomson, 1971).

Various analogies have been proposed by people making this argument. The mother's gestating a child has been compared to allowing someone the use of one's kidneys or even to donating an organ. We are not *required* (morally or as a matter of law) to allow someone to use our kidneys, or to donate organs to others, even when they would die without this assistance (and we could survive in good health despite rendering it). Analogously, the argument continues, a woman is not morally required to allow the fetus the use of her body. We shall call this "the bodily rights argument."

It may be objected that a woman has a special responsibility to the child she is carrying, whereas in the cases of withholding assistance to which abortion is compared there is no such special responsibility. Proponents of the bodily rights argument have replied, however, that the mother has not voluntarily assumed responsibility for the child, or a personal relationship with the child, and we have strong responsibilities to others only if we have voluntarily assumed such responsibilities (Thomson, 1971) or have consented to a personal relationship which generates such responsibilities (Little, 1999). True, the mother may have voluntarily performed an act which she knew may result in a child's conception, but that is distinct from consenting to gestate the child if a child is conceived. And so (according to this position) it is not until the woman consents to pregnancy, or perhaps not until the parents consent to care for the child by taking the baby home from the hospital or birthing center, that the full duties of parenthood accrue to the mother (and perhaps the father).

In reply to this argument we wish to make several points. We grant that in some few cases abortion is not intentional killing, but a choice to expel the child, the child's death being an unintended, albeit foreseen and (rightly or wrongly) accepted, side effect. However, these constitute a small minority of abortions. In the vast majority of cases, the death of the child *in utero* is precisely the object of the abortion. In most cases the end sought is to avoid being a parent; but abortion brings that about only by bringing it about that the child dies. Indeed, the attempted abortion would be considered by the woman requesting it and the abortionist performing it to have been *unsuccessful* if the child survives. In most cases abortion *is* intentional killing. Thus, even if the bodily rights argument succeeded, it would justify only a small percentage of abortions.

Still, in some few cases abortion is chosen as a means precisely toward ending the condition of pregnancy, and the woman requesting the termination of her pregnancy would not object if somehow the child survived. A pregnant woman may have less or more serious reasons for seeking the termination of this condition, but if that is her objective, then the child's death resulting from his or her expulsion will be a side effect, rather than the means chosen. For example, an actress may wish not to be pregnant because the pregnancy will change her figure during a time in which she is filming scenes in which having a slender appearance is important; or a woman may dread the discomforts, pains, and difficulties involved in pregnancy. (Of course, in many abortions there may be mixed motives: the parties making the choice may intend both ending the condition of pregnancy and the death of the child.)

Nevertheless, while it is true that in some cases abortion is not intentional killing, it remains misleading to describe it simply as choosing not to provide bodily life support. Rather, it is actively expelling the human embryo or fetus from the womb. There is a significant moral difference between *not doing* something that would assist someone, and *doing* something that causes someone harm, even if that harm is an unintended (but foreseen) side effect. It is more difficult morally to justify the latter than it is the former. Abortion is the *act* of extracting the unborn human being from the womb—an extraction that usually rips him or her to pieces or does him or her violence in some other way.

It is true that in some cases causing death as a side effect is morally permissible. For example, in some cases it is morally right to use force to stop a potentially lethal attack on one's family or country, even if one foresees that the force used will also result in the assailant's death. Similarly, there are instances in which it is permissible to perform an act that one knows or believes will, as a side effect, cause the death of a child *in utero*. For example, if a pregnant woman is discovered to have a cancerous uterus, and this is a proximate danger to the mother's life, it can be morally right to remove the cancerous uterus with the baby in it, even if the child will die as a result. A similar situation can occur in ectopic pregnancies. But in such cases, not only is the child's death a side effect, but the mother's life is in proximate danger. It is worth noting also that in these cases *what is done* (the means) is the correction of a pathology (such as a cancerous uterus, or a ruptured uterine tube). Thus, in such cases, not only the child's death, but also the ending of the pregnancy, are side effects. So, such acts are what traditional casuistry referred to as *indirect* or *non-intentional*, abortions.

But it is also clear that not every case of causing death as a side effect is morally right. For example, if a man's daughter has a serious respiratory disease and the father is told that his continued smoking in her presence will cause her death, it would obviously be immoral for him to continue the smoking. Similarly, if a man works for a steel company in a city with significant levels of air pollution, and his child has a serious respiratory problem making the air pollution a danger to her life, certainly he should move to another city. He should move, we would say, even if that meant he had to resign a prestigious position or make a significant career change.

In both examples, (a) the parent has a special responsibility to his child, but (b) the act that would cause the child's death would avoid a harm to the parent but cause a significantly worse harm to his child. And so, although the harm done would be a side effect, in both cases the act that caused the death would be an *unjust* act, and morally wrongful *as such*. The special responsibility of parents to their children requires that they *at least* refrain from performing acts that cause terrible harms to their children in order to avoid significantly lesser harms to themselves.

But (a) and (b) also obtain in intentional abortions (that is, those in which the removal of the child is directly sought, rather than the correction of a life-threatening pathology) even though they are not, strictly speaking, intentional killing. First, the mother has a special responsibility to her child, in virtue of being her biological mother (as does the father in virtue of his paternal relationship). The parental relationship itself—not just the voluntary acceptance of that relationship—gives rise to a special responsibility to a child.

Proponents of the bodily rights argument deny this point. Many claim that one has full parental responsibilities only if one has voluntarily assumed them. And so the child, on this view, has a right to care from his or her mother (including gestation) only if the mother has accepted her pregnancy, or perhaps only if the mother (and/or the father?) has in some way voluntarily begun a deep personal relationship with the child (Little, 1999).

But suppose a mother takes her baby home after giving birth, but the only reason she did not get an abortion was that she could not afford one. Or suppose she lives in a society where abortion is not available (perhaps very few physicians are willing to do the grisly deed). She and her husband take the child home only because they had no alternative. Moreover, suppose that in their society people are not waiting in line to adopt a newborn baby. And so the baby is several days old before anything can be done. If they abandon the baby and the baby is found, she will simply be returned to them. In such a case the parents have not voluntarily assumed responsibility; nor have they consented to a personal relationship with the child. But it would surely be wrong for these parents to abandon their baby in the woods (perhaps the only feasible way of ensuring she is not returned), even though the baby's death would be only a side effect. Clearly, we recognize that parents do have a responsibility to make sacrifices for their children, even if they have not voluntarily assumed such responsibilities, or given their consent to the personal relationship with the child.

The bodily rights argument implicitly supposes that we have a primordial right to construct a life simply as we please, and that others have claims on us only very minimally or through our (at least tacit) consent to a certain sort of relationship with them. On the contrary, we are by nature members of communities. Our moral goodness or character consists to a large extent (though not solely) in contributing to the communities of which we are members. We ought to act for our genuine good or flourishing (we take that as a basic ethical principle), but our flourishing involves being in communion with others. And communion with others of itself—even if we find ourselves united with others because of a physical or social relationship which precedes our consent—entails duties or responsibilities. Moreover, the contribution we are morally required to make to others will likely bring each of us some discomfort and pain. This is not to say that we should simply ignore our own good, for the sake of others. Rather, since what (and who) I am is in part constituted by various relationships with others, not all of which are initiated by my will, my genuine good includes the contributions I make to the relationships in which I participate. Thus, the life we constitute by our free choices should be in large part a life of mutual reciprocity with others.

For example, I may wish to cultivate my talent to write and so I may want to spend hours each day reading and writing. Or I may wish to develop my athletic abilities and so I may want to spend hours every day on the baseball field. But if I am a father of minor children, and have an adequate paying job working (say) in a coal mine, then my clear duty is to keep that job. Similarly, if one's girlfriend finds she is pregnant and one is the father, then one might also be morally required to continue one's work in the mine (or mill, factory, warehouse, etc.).

In other words, I have a duty to do something with my life that contributes to the good of the human community, but that general duty becomes specified by my particular situation. It becomes specified by the connection or closeness to me of those who are in need. We acquire special responsibilities toward people, not only by *consenting* to contracts or relationships with them, but also by having various types of union with them. So, we have special responsibilities to those people with whom we are closely united. For example, we have special responsibilities to our parents, and brothers and sisters, even though we did not choose them.

The physical unity or continuity of children to their parents is unique. The child is brought into being out of the bodily unity and bodies of the mother and the father. The mother and the father are in a certain sense prolonged or continued in their offspring. So, there is a natural unity of the mother with her child, and a natural unity of the father with his child. Since we have special responsibilities to those with whom we are closely united, it follows that we in fact do have a special responsibility to our children anterior to our having voluntarily assumed such responsibility or consented to the relationship.[2]

The second point is this: in the types of case we are considering, the harm caused (death) is much worse than the harms avoided (the difficulties in pregnancy). Pregnancy can involve severe impositions, but it is not nearly as bad as death—which is total and irreversible. One needn't make light of the burdens of pregnancy to acknowledge that the harm that is death is in a different category altogether.

The burdens of pregnancy include physical difficulties and the pain of labor, and can include significant financial costs, psychological burdens, and interference with autonomy and the pursuit of other important goals (McDonagh, 1996: ch. 5). These costs are not inconsiderable. Partly for that reason, we owe our mothers gratitude for carrying and giving birth to us. However, where pregnancy does not place a woman's life in jeopardy or threaten grave and lasting damage to her physical health, the harm done to other goods is not total. Moreover, most of the harms involved in pregnancy are not irreversible: pregnancy is a nine-month task—if the woman and man are not in a good position to raise the child, adoption is a possibility. So the difficulties of pregnancy, considered together, are in a different and lesser category than death. Death is not just worse in degree than the difficulties involved in pregnancy; it is worse in kind.

It has been argued, however, that pregnancy can involve a unique type of burden. It has been argued that the *intimacy* involved in pregnancy is such that if the woman must remain pregnant without her consent then there is inflicted on her a unique and serious harm. Just as sex with consent can be a desired experience but sex without consent is a violation of bodily integrity, so (the argument continues) pregnancy involves such a close physical intertwinement with the fetus that not to allow abortion is analogous to rape—it involves an enforced intimacy (Boonin, 2003: 84; Little, 1999: 300–3).

However, this argument is based on a false analogy. Where the pregnancy is unwanted, the baby's "occupying" the mother's womb may involve a harm; but the child is committing no injustice against her. The baby is not forcing himself or herself on the woman, but is simply growing and developing in a way quite natural to him or her. The baby is not performing any action that could in any way be construed as aimed at violating the mother.[3]

It is true that the fulfillment of the duty of a mother to her child (during gestation) is unique and in many cases does involve a great sacrifice. The argument we have presented, however, is that being a mother *does* generate a special responsibility, and that the sacrifice morally required of the mother is less burdensome than the harm that would be done to the child by expelling the child, causing his or her death, to escape that responsibility. Our argument equally entails responsibilities for the father of the child. His duty does not involve as direct a bodily relationship with the child as the mother's, but it may be equally or even more burdensome. In certain circumstances, his obligation to care for the child (and the child's mother), and especially his obligation to provide financial support, may severely limit his freedom and even require months or, indeed, years, of extremely burdensome physical labor. Historically, many men have rightly seen that their basic responsibility to their family (and country) has entailed risking, and in many cases, losing, their lives. Different people in different circumstances, with different talents, will have different responsibilities. It is no argument against any of these responsibilities to point out their distinctness.

So, the burden of carrying the baby, for all its distinctness, is significantly less than the harm the baby would suffer by being killed; the mother and father have a special responsibility to the child; it follows that intentional abortion (even in the few cases where the baby's death is an unintended but foreseen side effect) is unjust and therefore objectively immoral.

Notes

1. See, for example: Carlson (1994: chs. 2–4); Gilbert (2003: 183–220, 363–90); Larson (2001: chs. 1–2); Moore and Persaud (2003: chs. 1–6); Muller (1997: chs. 1–2); O'Rahilly and Mueller (2000: chs. 3–4).

2. David Boonin claims, in reply to this argument—in an earlier and less developed form, presented by Lee (1996: 122)—that it is not clear that it is impermissible for a woman to destroy what is a part of, or a continuation of, herself. He then says that to the extent the unborn human being is united to her in that way, "it would if anything seem that her act is *easier* to justify than if this claim were not true" (2003: 230). But Boonin fails to grasp the point of the argument (perhaps understandably since it was not expressed very clearly in the earlier work he is discussing). The unity of the child to the mother is the basis for this child being related to the woman in a different way from how other children are. We ought to pursue our own good *and the good of others with whom we are united in various ways.* If that is so, then the closer someone is united to us, the deeper and more extensive our responsibility to the person will be.

3. In some sense being bodily "occupied" when one does not wish to be *is* a harm; however, just as the child does not (as explained in the text), neither does the state inflict this harm on the woman, in circumstances in which the state prohibits abortion. By prohibiting abortion the state would only prevent the woman from performing an act (forcibly detaching the child from her) that would unjustly kill this developing child, who is an innocent party.

References

Boonin, David (2003). *A Defense of Abortion.* New York: Cambridge University Press.

Carlson, Bruce (1994). *Human Embryology and Developmental Biology.* St. Louis, MO: Mosby.

Gilbert, Scott (2003). *Developmental Biology,* 7th edn. Sunderland, MA: Sinnauer Associates.

Larson, William J. (2001). *Human Embryology,* 3rd edn. New York: Churchill Livingstone.

Lee, Patrick (1996). *Abortion and Unborn Human Life.* Washington, DC: Catholic University of America Press.

Little, Margaret Olivia (1999). "Abortion, intimacy, and the duty to gestate." *Ethical Theory and Moral Practice,* 2: 295–312.

McDonagh, Eileen (1996). *Breaking the Abortion Deadlock: From Choice to Consent.* New York: Oxford University Press.

Moore, Keith, and Persaud, T. V. N. (2003). *The Developing Human, Clinically Oriented Embryology,* 7th edn. New York: W. B. Saunders.

Muller, Werner A. (1997). *Developmental Biology.* New York: Springer Verlag.

O'Rahilly, Ronan, and Mueller, Fabiola (2000). *Human Embryology and Teratology,* 3rd edn. New York: John Wiley & Sons.

Thomson, Judith Jarvis (1971). "A defense of abortion." *Philosophy and Public Affairs,* 1: 47–66; reprinted, among other places, in Feinberg (1984, pp. 173–87).

Margaret Olivia Little 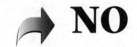 **NO**

The Morality of Abortion

Introduction

It is often noted that the public discussion of abortion's moral status is disappointingly crude. The positions staked out and the reasoning proffered seem to reflect little of the subtlety and nuance—not to mention ambivalence—that mark more private reflections on the subject. Despite attempts by various parties to find middle ground, the debate remains largely polarized—at its most dramatic, with extreme conservatives claiming abortion the moral equivalent of murder even as extreme liberals think it devoid of moral import.

To some extent, this polarization is due to the legal battle that continues to shadow moral discussions: admission of ethical nuance, it is feared, will play as concession on the deeply contested question of whether abortion should be a legally protected option for women. But to some extent, blame for the continued crudeness can be laid at the doorstep of moral theory itself.

For one thing, the ethical literature on abortion has focused its attention almost exclusively on the thinnest moral assessment—on whether and when abortion is "morally permissible." That question is, of course, a crucial one, its answer often desperately sought. But many of our deepest struggles with the morality of abortion concern much more textured questions about its placement on the scales of *decency, respectfulness,* and *responsibility.* It is one thing to decide that an abortion was permissible, quite another to decide that it was *honorable;* one thing to decide that an abortion was impermissible, quite another to decide that it was *monstrous.* It is these latter categories that determine what we might call the thick moral interpretation of the act—and, with it, the meaning the woman must live with, and the reactive attitudes such as disgust, forbearance, or admiration that she and others think the act deserves. A moral theory that moves too quickly or focuses too exclusively on moral permissibility won't address these crucial issues. . . .

To make progress on abortion's moral status, it thus turns out, requires us not just to arbitrate already familiar controversies in metaphysics and ethics, but to attend to the distinctive aspects of pregnancy that often stand at their margins. In the following, I want to argue that if we acknowledge gestation as an *intimacy,* motherhood as a *relationship,* and creation as a *process,* we will be in a far better position to appreciate the moral textures of abortion. I explore these textures, in the first half on stipulation that the fetus is a person, in the second half under supposition that early human life has an important value worthy of respect.

Fetal Personhood: From Wrongful Interference to Positive Responsibilities

If fetuses are persons, then abortion is surely an enormously serious matter: What is at stake is nothing less than the life of a creature with full moral standing. To say that the stakes are high, though, is not to say that moral analysis is obvious (which is why elsewhere in moral theory, conversation usually starts, not stops, once we realize people's lives are at issue). I think the most widely held objection to abortion is badly misguided; more importantly, it obscures the deeper ethical question at issue.

On the usual view, it is perfectly obvious what to say about abortion on supposition of fetal personhood: if fetuses are persons, then abortion is murder. Persons, after all, have a fundamental right to life, and abortion, it would seem, counts as its gross violation. On this view, we can assess the status of abortion quite cleanly. In particular, we needn't delve too deeply into the burdens that continued gestation might present for women—not because their lives don't matter or because we don't sympathize with their plight, but because we don't take hardship as justification for murder.

In fact, though, abortion's assimilation to murder will seem clear-cut only if we have already ignored key features of gestation. While certain metaphors depict gestation as passive carriage—as though the fetus were simply occupying a room until it is born—the truth is of course far different. One who is gestating is providing the fetus with sustenance—donating nourishment, creating blood, delivering oxygen, providing hormonal triggers for development—without which it could not live. For a fetus, to live *is* to be receiving aid. And whether the assistance is delivered by way of intentional activity (as when the woman eats or takes her prenatal vitamins) or by way of biological mechanism, assistance it plainly is. But this has crucial implications for abortion's alleged status as murder. To put it simply, the right to life, as Judith Thomson famously put it, does not include the right to have all assistance needed to maintain that life (Thomson, 1971). Ending gestation will, at early stages at least, certainly lead to the fetus's demise, but that does not mean that doing so would constitute murder. . . .

Even if the fetus is a person, then, abortion would not be murder. More broadly put, abortion, whatever its rights and wrongs, isn't a species of *wrongful interference*.

None of this, though, is to say that abortion under such supposition is therefore unproblematic. It is to argue, instead, that the crucial moral issue needs to be re-located. Wrongful interference is a central concern in morality, but it isn't the only one. We are also concerned with notions of *neglect, abandonment* and *disregard*. These are issues that involve abrogations of positive responsibilities to help others, not injunctions against interfering with them.

If fetuses are persons, the question we really need to decide is what positive responsibilities, if any, do pregnant women have to continue gestational assistance? This is a question that takes us into far richer, and far more interesting, territory than that occupied by discussions of murder.

One issue it raises is: what do pregnant women owe to the fetuses they carry as a matter of *general beneficence?* Philosophers, of course, familiarly divide over the ambitions of beneficence, generically construed; but abortion raises distinct difficulties of its own. On the one hand, the beneficence called for here is of a particularly urgent kind: the stakes are life and death, and the pregnant woman is the *only* one who can render the assistance needed. It's a rare (and, many of us will think, dreadful) moral theory that will think she faces no responsibilities to assist here: passing a drowning person for mere convenience when no one else is within shouting distance is a very good example of moral indecency. On the other hand, gestation is not just any activity. It involves sharing one's very body. It brings with it an emotional intertwinement that can reshape one's entire life. It brings another person into one's family. Being asked to gestate another person, that is, isn't like being asked to write a check to support an impoverished child; it's like being asked to adopt the child. Doing so is a caring, compassionate act; it is also an enormous undertaking that has reverberations for an entire lifetime. Deciding whether, and if so when, such action is obligatory rather than admirable is no light matter.

I don't think moral theory has begun to address the rich questions at issue here. When are intimate actions owed to generic others? How do we weigh the sacrifice morality requires of us when it is measured, not in terms of risk, but of intertwinement? What should we think of such obligations if the required acts would be performed under conditions of profound self-alienation? The *type* of issue paradigmatically represented by gestation—an assistance that combines life and death stakes with deep intimacy—is virtually nowhere discussed in ethical theory. (We aren't called upon in the usual course of events to save people's lives by, say, having sexual intercourse with them.) By ignoring these issues, mainstream moral theory has ended up deeply underselling the moral complexity of abortion.

Difficult as these questions are, though, it is actually a second issue, I suspect, that is responsible for much of the passion that surrounds abortion on supposition of fetal personhood. On reflection, many will say, the issues confronting the pregnant woman aren't about generic beneficence at all. The considerations she faces are not just those that would face someone uniquely well placed to serve as Good Samaritan to some stranger—as when one passes the drowning person: for the pregnant woman and fetus, crucially, aren't strangers. If the fetus is a person, many will say, it is *her child;* and for this reason she has special responsibilities to meet its needs. In the end, I believe, much of the animating concern with abortion is not about what we owe to generic others; it's about what parents owe their children.

But if it's parenthood that is carrying normative weight, then we need an ethics of parenthood—a theory of what makes someone a parent in this thickly normative sense and what the contours of its responsibilities really are. This should raise something of a warning flag. Philosophers, it must be said, have by and large done a rather poor job when it comes to parenthood—variously avoiding it, romanticizing it, or assimilating it to categories, like contractual relations, to which it stands in paradigmatic contrast. This general shortcoming is evident in discussions of abortion, where two remarkably unhelpful models dominate.

One position, advocated by Judith Thomson and some of the most recent treatments of abortion, is a classically liberal one. It agrees that special responsibilities attach to parenthood but argues that parenthood is thereby a status that is entered into only by consent. That consent is usually tacit, to be sure—taking the baby home from the hospital qualifies; nonetheless, special responsibilities to a child accrue only when one voluntarily assumes them.

Such a model is surely an odd one. The model yields the plausible view that the rape victim does not face the very same set of duties as many other pregnant women, but it does so by implying that a man who fathers a child during a one-night stand has no special responsibilities toward that child unless he decides he does. Perhaps most strikingly, such a view has no resources for acknowledging that there may be moral reasons why one *should* consent to the status. Those who sustain a biological connection may have a tendency to enter the role of parent, but on this scheme it's a mere psychological proclivity that rides atop nothing normative.

Another position is classically conservative. According to this view, the special responsibilities of parenthood are grounded in biological progenitorship. It is blood ties, to use the old-fashioned vernacular—"passing on one's genes," in more current translation—that makes one a parent and grounds heightened responsibilities. This view has its own blind spot. It has the resources for agreeing that a man who fathers a child from a one-night stand faces special responsibilities for the child whether he likes it or not, but none for distinguishing between the responsibilities of someone who has served as the special steward for a child—who has engaged for years in the *activity* of parenting—and the responsibilities of someone who bears literally no connection beyond a genetic or causal contribution to existence. On this view, a sperm donor faces all the responsibilities of a social father.

What both positions have in common is the supposition that parenthood is an all or nothing affair. Applied to pregnancy, the gestating woman either owes everything we imagine we owe to the children we love and rear or she owes nothing beyond general beneficence unless she decides she does. But parenthood—like all familial relations—is surely a more complicated moral notion than this. Parenthood, and its attendant responsibilities, admit of *layers*. It has a crucial existence as a social *role*—something with institutionally defined entrances, exits, and expectations that can attach to us quite independently of what our self-conceptions might say. It also has a crucial existence as a *relationship*—an emotional connection, a shared history, an intertwinement of lives. It is because of that intertwinement that parents' motivation to sacrifice is so often immediate. But it is also because of that relationship that even especially ambitious sacrifices are legitimately expected, and why failure to undertake them would be so problematic: absent unusual circumstances, it becomes a betrayal of the relationship itself. In short, parenthood is not monolithic: some of the responsibilities we paradigmatically associate as parental attach, not to the role, but to the relationship that so often accompanies it.

These layers matter especially when we get to gestation, for the pregnant woman stands precisely at their intersection. If a fetus is a person, then there is surely an important sense in which she is its mother: to regard her as just a passing stranger uniquely able to help it would grossly distort the situation. But she is not yet a mother most thickly described—a mother in standing relationship with a child, with the responsibilities born of shared history and the enterprise of caretaking.

These demarcations are integral, I think, to understanding the distinctive sorts of conflicts that pregnancy can represent—including, most notably, the conflicts it can bring *within* the mantle of motherhood. Women sometimes decide to abort even though they regard the fetus they carry as their child, because they realize, grimly, that bringing this child into the world will leave too little room to care adequately for the children they are already raising. This is a conflict we cannot even name, much less arbitrate, on standard views—if the fetus is her child, how could she possibly choose to sacrifice its life unless the stakes are literally equivalent for the others? But this is to ignore the layers of parenthood. She occupies the *role* of mother to the fetus, but with the other children, she is, by dint of time, interaction, and intertwinement, in a *relationship* of motherhood. The fetus is her baby, then—not just some passing stranger she alone can help—which is why this conflict brings the kind of agony it does. But if it is her child in the role sense only, she does not yet owe all that she owes to her other children. Depending on the circumstances, other family members with whom she is already in relationship may, tragically, come first.

None of this is to make light to the responsibilities pregnant women face on supposition of fetal personhood. If fetuses are persons, such responsibilities are surely profound. It is, rather, to insist that they admit of layer and degree, and that these distinctions, while delicate, are crucial to capturing the *types* of tragedy—and the types of moral compromise—abortion can here represent.

The Sanctity of Life: Respect Revisited

. . . For many women who contemplate abortion, the desire to end pregnancy is not, or not centrally, a desire to avoid the nine months of pregnancy; it is to avoid what lies on the far side of those months—namely, motherhood. If gestation were simply a matter of rendering, say, somewhat risky assistance to help a burgeoning human life they've come across—if they could somehow render that assistance without thereby adding a member to their family—the decision faced would be a far different one. But gestation doesn't just allow cells to become a person; it turns one into a mother.

One of the most common reasons women give for wanting to abort is that they do not want to become a mother—now, ever, again, with this partner, or no reliable partner, with these few resources, or these many that are now, after so many years of mothering, slated finally to another cause. Nor does adoption represent a universal solution. To give up a child would be for some a life-long trauma; others occupy fortunate circumstances that would, by their own lights, make it unjustified to give over a child for others to rear. Or again—and most frequently—she doesn't want to raise a child just now but knows that if she *does* carry the pregnancy to term, she won't *want* to give up the child for adoption. Gestation, she knows, is likely to reshape her heart and soul, transforming her into a mother emotionally, not just officially; and it is precisely that transformation she does not want to undergo. It is because continuing pregnancy brings with it this new identity and, likely, relationship, then, that many feel it legitimate to decline.

But pregnancy's connection to motherhood also enters the phenomenology of abortion in just the opposite direction. For some women, that it would be her child is precisely why she feels she must continue the pregnancy—even if motherhood is not what she desired. To be pregnant is to have one's potential child knocking at one's door; to abort is to turn one's back on it, a decision, many women say, that would haunt them forever. On this view, the desire to avoid motherhood, so compelling as a reason to contracept, is uneasy grounds to abort: for once an embryo is on the scene, it isn't about rejecting motherhood, it's about rejecting one's *child*. Not literally, of course, since there is no child yet extant to stand as the object of rejection. But the stance one should take to pregnancy, sought or not, is one of *acceptance:* when a potential family member is knocking at the door, one should move over, make room, and welcome her in.

These two intuitive stances represent just profoundly different ways of gestalting the situation of ending pregnancy. On the first view, abortion is closer to contraception—hardly equivalent, because it means the demise of something of value. But the desire to avoid the enterprise and identity of motherhood is an understandable and honorable basis for deciding to end a pregnancy. Given that there is no child yet on the scene, one does not owe special openness to the relationship that stands at the end of pregnancy's trajectory. On the second view, abortion is closer to exiting a parental relationship—hardly equivalent, for one of the key relata is not yet fully present. But one's decision about whether to continue the pregnancy already feels specially constrained: that one would be related to the resulting person exerts now some moral force. It would take especially grave reasons to refuse assistance here, for the norms of parenthood already have a toehold. Assessing the moral status of abortion, it turns out, then, is not just about assessing the contours of generic respect owed to burgeoning human life, it's about assessing the salience of *impending relationship*. And this is an issue that functions in different ways for different women—and, sometimes, in one and the same woman.

In my own view, until the fetus is a person, we should recognize a moral prerogative to decline parenthood and end the pregnancy. Not because motherhood is necessarily a burden (though it can be); but because it so thoroughly changes what we might call one's fundamental practical identity. The enterprise of mothering restructures the self—changing the shape of one's heart, the primary commitments by which one lives one's life, the terms by which one judges one's life a success or a failure. If the enterprise is eschewed and one decides to give the child over to another, the identity of mother still changes the normative facts that are true of one, as there is now someone by whom one does well or poorly. And either way—whether one rears the child or lets it go—to continue a pregnancy means that a piece of one's heart, as the saying goes, will forever walk outside one's body. As profound as the respect we should have for burgeoning human life, we should acknowledge moral prerogatives over identity-constituting commitments and enterprises as profound as motherhood.

But I also don't think this is the whole of the moral story. If women find themselves with different ways of gestalting the prospective relationship involved in pregnancy, it is in part because they have different identities, commitments, and ideals that such a prospect intersects with—commitments which, while permissibly idiosyncratic, are morally authoritative for *them*. If a woman feels already duty-bound by the norms of parenthood to nurture this creature, it may be for the very good reason that, in an important personal sense, she already *is* its mother. She finds herself—perhaps to her surprise, happy or otherwise—with a maternal commitment to this creature. As philosophers forget but women and men have long known, something can be your child even if it is not yet a person. But taking on the identity of mother towards something just *is* to take on certain imperatives about its well-being as categorical. Her job is thus clear—it's to help this creature reach its fullest potential. For other women, the identity is still something that can be assessed—tried on, perhaps accepted, but perhaps declined: in which case respect is owed, but is saved, or confirmed, for others—other relationships, other projects, other passions.

And again, if a woman feels she owes a stance of welcome to burgeoning human life that comes her way, it may be, not because she thinks such a stance authoritative for all, but because of the virtues around which her practical identity is now oriented: receptivity to life's agenda, for instance, or responsiveness to that which is most vulnerable. For another woman, the executive virtues to be exercised tug in just the other direction: loyalty to treasured life plans, a commitment that it be she, not the chances of biology, that should determine her life's course, bolstering self-direction after a life too long ruled by serendipity and fate.

Deciding when it is morally decent to end a pregnancy, it turns out, is an admixture of settling impersonally or universally authoritative moral requirements, and of discovering and arbitrating—sometimes after agonizing deliberation, sometimes in a decision no less deep for its immediacy—one's own commitments, identity, and defining virtues.

A similarly complex story appears when we turn to the second theme. Another thread that appears in many women's stories in the face of unsought pregnancy is respect for the weighty responsibility involved in creating human life. Once again, it is a theme that pulls and tugs in different directions.

In its most familiar direction, it shows up in many stories of why an unsought pregnancy is continued. Many people believe that one's responsibility to nurture new life is importantly amplified if one is responsible for bringing about its existence in the first place. Just what it takes to count as responsible here is a point on which individuals diverge (whether voluntary but contracepted intercourse is different from intercourse without use of birth control, and again from intentionally deciding to become pregnant at the IVF clinic). But triggering the relevant standard of responsibility for creation, it is felt, brings with it a heightened responsibility to nurture: it is disrespectful to create human life only to allow it to wither. Put more rigorously, one who is responsible for bringing about a creature that has intrinsic value in virtue of its potential to become a person has a special responsibility to enable it to reach that end state.

But the idea of respect for creation is also, if less frequently acknowledged, sometimes the reason why women are moved to *end* pregnancies. As Barbara Katz Rothman (1985) puts it, decisions to abort often represent, not a decision to destroy, but a refusal to create. Many people have deeply felt convictions about the circumstances under which they feel it right for them to bring a child into the world—can it be brought into a decent world, an intact family, a society that can minimally respect its agency? These considerations may persist even after conception has taken place; for while the *embryo* has already been created, a person has not. Some women decide to abort, that is, not because they do not *want* the resulting child—indeed, they may yearn for nothing more, and desperately wish that their circumstances were otherwise— but because they do not think bringing a child into the world the right thing for them to do.

These are abortions marked by moral language. A woman wants to abort because she knows she couldn't give up a child for adoption but feels she couldn't give the child the sort of life, or be the sort of parent, she thinks a child *deserves;* a woman who would have to give up the child thinks it would be *unfair* to bring a child into existence already burdened by rejection, however well grounded its reasons; a woman living in a country marked by poverty and gender apartheid wants to abort because she decides it would be *wrong* for her to bear a daughter whose life, like hers, would be filled with so much injustice and hardship.

Some have thought that such decisions betray a simple fallacy: unless the child's life were literally going to be worse than non-existence, how can one abort out of concern for the future child? But the worry here isn't that one would be imposing a *harm* on the child by bringing it into existence (as though children who are in the situations mentioned have lives that aren't worth living). The claim is that bringing about a person's life in these circumstances would do violence to her ideals of creating and parenthood. She does not want to bring into existence a daughter she cannot love and care for, she does not want to bring into existence a person whose life will be marked by disrespect or rejection.

Nor does the claim imply judgment on women who *do* continue pregnancies in similar circumstances—as though there were here an obligation to abort. For the norms in question, once again, need not be impersonally authoritative moral chums. Like ideals of good parenting, they mark out considerations all should be sensitive to, perhaps, but equally reasonable people may adhere to different variations and weightings. Still, they are normative for those who do have them; far from expressing mere matters of taste, the ideals one does accept carry an important kind of categoricity, issuing imperatives whose authority is not reducible to mere desire. These are, at root, issues about *integrity,* and the importance of maintaining integrity over one's participation in this enterprise precisely because it is so normatively weighty.

What is usually emphasized in the morality of abortion is the ethics of destruction; but there is a balancing ethics of creation. And for many people, conflict about abortion is a conflict *within* that ethics. On the one had, we now have on hand an entity that has a measure of sanctity: that it has begun is reason to help it continue—perhaps especially if one had a role in its procreation—which is why even early abortion is not normatively equivalent to contraception. On the other hand, not to end a pregnancy *is* to do something else, namely, to continue creating a person, and for some women, pregnancy strikes in circumstances in which they cannot countenance that enterprise. For some, the sanctity of developing human life will be strong enough to tip the balance towards continuing the pregnancy; for others, their norms of respectful creation will hold sway. For those who believe that the norms governing creation of a person are mild relative to the normative telos of embryonic life, being a responsible creator means continuing to gestate, and doing the best one can to bring about the conditions under which that creation will be more respectful. For others, though, the normativity of fetal telos is mild and their standards of respectful creation high, and the lesson goes in just the other direction: it is a sign of respect not to continue creating when certain background conditions, such as a loving family or adequate resources, are not in place.

However one thinks these issues settle out, they will not be resolved by austere contemplation of the value of human life. They require wrestling with the rich meanings of creation, responsibility, and kinship. And these issues, I have suggested, are just as much issues about one's integrity as they are about what is impersonally obligatory. On many treatments of abortion, considerations about whether or not to continue a pregnancy are exhausted by preferences, on the one hand, and universally authoritative moral demands, on the other; but some of the most important terrain lies in between.

References

Rothman, B. K. (1989). *Recreating motherhood: ideology and technology in a patriarchal society.* New York: Norton.

Thomson, J. J. (1971). A defense of abortion. *Philosophy and Public Affairs, 1,* 47–66.

POSTSCRIPT

Is Abortion Immoral?

According to the Centers for Disease Control and Prevention, more than half of all abortions in the United States are performed during the first eight weeks of pregnancy, and 88 percent before the twelfth week. Although uncommon, abortions performed in the second trimester of pregnancy are very controversial. Most often the reasons are fetal abnormalities, illness in the mother, or late diagnosis of pregnancy in a teenager. The procedure, which involves delivering a dead but intact fetus, is particularly troubling. The technical term is "intact dilatation and extraction" (D&X), but the more commonly used (and emotionally loaded) term is "partial-birth abortion."

In June 2000, the U.S. Supreme Court struck down a Nebraska law making it a crime to perform a partial-birth abortion. The five-to-four vote was the first abortion rights ruling in 8 years. Congress twice passed a bill banning partial-birth abortions, and President Bill Clinton twice vetoed it. President George W. Bush, however, signed the Partial-Birth Abortion Ban Act of 2003. In June 2004, a federal judge in San Francisco struck down the bill, ruling that the law jeopardizes other legal forms of abortion and threatens the health of women. The federal government appealed, and the case of *Gonzales v. Carhart* went to the U.S. Supreme Court in 2006.

In April 2007, by a five-to-four majority, the U.S. Supreme Court upheld the federal ban, which is limited to a particular, rarely used procedure. Lawrence O. Gostin criticizes the ruling on grounds that it interferes with clinical freedom, trust in the judiciary, and the autonomy of women ("Abortion Politics," *Journal of the American Medical Association*, October 3, 2007). For the Court opinion, with concurrence and dissents, see http://www.law.cornell .edu/supct/html/05-380.ZO.html. In October 2008, the Court declined to review a New Jersey court's decision in *Acuna v. Turkish* that state law did not require a physician to inform a woman considering a first-trimester abortion that it would result in killing an "existing human being."

While most attention focuses on federal challenges to *Roe v. Wade*, state legislatures have been very active in this arena. See http://www.stateline.org for information on abortion regulations in specific states.

For a history of the political and ethical issues surrounding abortion in the United States, see Eva R. Rubin, *The Abortion Controversy: A Documentary History* (Greenwood, 1994). See also Robert M. Baird and Stuart E. Rosenbaum, *The Ethics of Abortion: Pro-Life vs. Pro-Choice*, 3rd ed. (Prometheus Books, 2001).

ISSUE 8

Should a Pregnant Woman Be Punished for Exposing Her Fetus to Risk?

YES: Jean Toal, from Majority Opinion, *Cornelia Whitner, Respondent, v. State of South Carolina, Petitioner* (July 15, 1997)

NO: Lynn M. Paltrow, from "Punishment and Prejudice: Judging Drug-Using Pregnant Women," in Julia E. Hanigsberg and Sara Ruddick, eds., *Mother Troubles: Rethinking Contemporary Maternal Dilemmas* (Beacon Press, 1999)

ISSUE SUMMARY

YES: Jean Toal states the Majority Opinion in a case involving a pregnant woman's use of crack cocaine, the Supreme Court of South Carolina ruled that a state legislature may impose additional criminal penalties on pregnant drug-using women without violating their constitutional right of privacy.

NO: Attorney Lynn M. Paltrow argues that treating drug-using pregnant women as criminals targets poor, African American women while ignoring other drug usage and fails to provide the resources to assist them in recovery.

At first glance, Cornelia Whitner and Bobbi McCaughey have absolutely nothing in common. Cornelia Whitner gave birth to a baby after using crack cocaine in the last trimester of pregnancy. She was arrested and convicted of child neglect. Bobbi McCaughey gave birth to seven babies in November 1997 to public acclaim and an avalanche of gifts and community support. Yet she too placed her babies at risk, simply by the use of fertility drugs and her decision to continue the multiple pregnancy. Through laws and public attitudes, society views the risks taken by Whitner and McCaughey very differently and punishes or rewards women accordingly.

In 1989, fueled by the specter of an epidemic of drug use resulting in the birth of thousands of "crack babies," the Medical University of South Carolina established a program that required drug-using pregnant women to seek treatment and prenatal care or face criminal prosecution. This program applied only to patients attending the university's obstetric clinic, primarily poor black women, and not to private patients. Patients enrolled in the clinic saw a video and were given written information about the harmful effects of substance abuse during pregnancy. The information warned that the Charleston, South Carolina, police, the court system, and child protective services might become involved if illegal drug use were detected.

Women who met certain criteria were required to undergo periodic urine screening for drugs. A patient who had a positive urine test or who failed to keep scheduled appointments for therapy or prenatal care could be arrested and placed in custody. If a woman delivered a baby who tested positive for drugs, she would be arrested immediately after her medical release and her newborn taken into protective custody. If the drug use was detected within the first 27 weeks of gestation, the patient was charged with possession of an illegal substance; after that date, the charge was possession and distribution of an illegal substance to a minor. If the drug use were detected during delivery, the woman would be charged with unlawful neglect of a child.

This stringent policy was developed as a result of clinicians' concern about the harmful effects of drug use on fetal development and prosecutors' desires to take a strong public stand condemning drug use. Although the stated goal was to get women into treatment, there were few places that women could receive treatment and the necessary support, such as transportation and child care. At the time there was no women-only residential treatment center for substance-abusing pregnant women anywhere in the state.

The program ended because the federal Office of Protection from Research Risks determined that it constituted human experimentation conducted without required institutional review board approval. This determination was based on a published report comparing the outcomes before and after the program. The university's approval as a site that could receive federal funds was placed in jeopardy.

By the time the policy was discontinued in September 1994 as the result of a settlement with the Civil Rights Division of the federal Department of Health and Human Services, 42 pregnant women had been arrested. One of those women was Cornelia Whitner, whose baby was born with cocaine metabolites in his system. Whitner admitted to using crack cocaine during her pregnancy. Charged with criminal child neglect, she pled guilty and was sentenced to eight years in prison. She appealed the decision on the grounds that the law covered children, not fetuses, and her case went to the Supreme Court of South Carolina.

The court's majority decision, written by Justice Jean Toal, found that the state's statute includes a fetus within its definition of "child" and ruled that the state was not violating Whitner's constitutional right of privacy by punishing her for endangering her child through an already illegal activity. This ruling was appealed to the U.S. Supreme Court. Lynn Paltrow believes that criminalization of drug use is a punitive response that denies the humanity of the women who are denied treatment and support for recovering from their addiction.

YES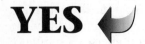

Jean Toal

Majority Opinion

Whitner v. South Carolina . . . ,

This case concerns the scope of the child abuse and endangerment statute in the South Carolina Children's Code. We hold the word "child" as used in that statute includes viable fetuses.

Facts

On April 20, 1992, Cornelia Whitner (Whitner) pled guilty to criminal child neglect, S.C.Code Ann. § 20-7-50 (1985), for causing her baby to be born with cocaine metabolites in its system by reason of Whitner's ingestion of crack cocaine during the third trimester of her pregnancy. The circuit court judge sentenced Whitner to eight years in prison. Whitner did not appeal her conviction.

Thereafter, Whitner filed a petition for Post Conviction Relief (PCR), pleading the circuit court's lack of subject matter jurisdiction to accept her guilty plea as well as ineffective assistance of counsel. Her claim of ineffective assistance of counsel was based upon her lawyer's failure to advise her the statute under which she was being prosecuted might not apply to prenatal drug use. The petition was granted on both grounds. The State appeals.

Law/Analysis

. . . South Carolina law has long recognized that viable fetuses are persons holding certain legal rights and privileges. In 1960, this Court decided Hall v. Murphy, 236 S.C. 257, 113 S.E.2d 790 (1960). That case concerned the application of South Carolina's wrongful death statute to an infant who died four hours after her birth as a result of injuries sustained prenatally during viability. The Appellants argued that a viable fetus was not a person within the purview of the wrongful death statute, because, inter alia, a fetus is thought to have no separate being apart from the mother.

We found such a reason for exclusion from recovery "unsound, illogical and unjust," and concluded there was "no medical or other basis" for the "assumed identity" of mother and viable unborn child. In light of that conclusion, this Court unanimously held: "We have no difficulty in concluding that a fetus having reached that period of prenatal maturity where it is capable of independent life apart from its mother is a person."

Four years later, in Fowler v. Woodward, 244 S.C. 608, 138 S.E.2d 42 (1964), we interpreted Hall as supporting a finding that a viable fetus injured

154

while still in the womb need not be born alive for another to maintain an action for the wrongful death of the fetus.

> Since a viable child is a person before separation from the body of its mother and since prenatal injuries tortiously inflicted on such a child are actionable, it is apparent that the complaint alleges such an "act, neglect or default" by the defendant, to the injury of the child. . . .
>
> Once the concept of the unborn, viable child as a person is accepted, we have no difficulty in holding that a cause of action for tortious injury to such a child arises immediately upon the infliction of the injury. . . .

More recently, [in State v. Horne,] we held the word "person" as used in a criminal statute includes viable fetuses. . . . The defendant in that case stabbed his wife, who was nine months' pregnant, in the neck, arms, and abdomen. Although doctors performed an emergency caesarean section to deliver the child, the child died while still in the womb. The defendant was convicted of voluntary manslaughter and appealed his conviction on the ground South Carolina did not recognize the crime of feticide.

This Court disagreed. In a unanimous decision, we held it would be "grossly inconsistent . . . to construe a viable fetus as a 'person' for the purposes of imposing civil liability while refusing to give it a similar classification in the criminal context." Accordingly, the Court recognized the crime of feticide with respect to viable fetuses.

Similarly, we do not see any rational basis for finding a viable fetus is not a "person" in the present context. Indeed, it would be absurd to recognize the viable fetus as a person for purposes of homicide laws and wrongful death statutes but not for purposes of statutes proscribing child abuse. Our holding in Hall that a viable fetus is a person rested primarily on the plain meaning of the word "person" in light of existing medical knowledge concerning fetal development. We do not believe that the plain and ordinary meaning of the word "person" has changed in any way that would now deny viable fetuses status as persons.

The policies enunciated in the Children's Code also support our plain meaning reading of "person." S.C. Code Ann. § 20-7-20(C) (1985), which describes South Carolina's policy concerning children, expressly states: "It shall be the policy of this State to concentrate on the prevention of children's problems as the most important strategy which can be planned and implemented on behalf of children and their families." . . . The abuse or neglect of a child at any time during childhood can exact a profound toll on the child herself as well as on society as a whole. However, the consequences of abuse or neglect which takes place after birth often pale in comparison to those resulting from abuse suffered by the viable fetus before birth. This policy of prevention supports a reading of the word "person" to include viable fetuses. Furthermore, the scope of the Children's Code is quite broad. It applies "to all children who have need of services." . . . When coupled with the comprehensive remedial purposes of the Code, this language supports the inference that the legislature intended to include viable fetuses within the scope of the Code's protection.

Whitner advances several arguments against an interpretation of "person" as used in the Children's Code to include viable fetuses. We shall address each of Whitner's major arguments in turn.

Whitner's first argument concerns the number of bills introduced in the South Carolina General Assembly in the past five years addressing substance abuse by pregnant women. Some of these bills would have criminalized substance abuse by pregnant women; others would have addressed the issue through mandatory reporting, treatment, or intervention by social service agencies. Whitner suggests that the introduction of several bills touching the specific issue at hand evinces a belief by legislators that prior legislation had not addressed the issue. Whitner argues the introduction of the bills proves that section 20-7-50 was not intended to encompass abuse or neglect of a viable fetus.

We disagree with Whitner's conclusion about the significance of the proposed legislation. Generally, the legislature's subsequent acts "cast no light on the intent of the legislature which enacted the statute being construed." . . . Rather, this Court will look first to the language of the statute to discern legislative intent, because the language itself is the best guide to legislative intent. . . . Here, we see no reason to look beyond the statutory language. . . . Additionally, our existing case law strongly supports our conclusion about the meaning of the statute's language.

Whitner also argues an interpretation of the statute that includes viable fetuses would lead to absurd results obviously not intended by the legislature. Specifically, she claims if we interpret "child" to include viable fetuses, every action by a pregnant woman that endangers or is likely to endanger a fetus, whether otherwise legal or illegal, would constitute unlawful neglect under the statute. For example, a woman might be prosecuted under section 20-7-50 for smoking or drinking during pregnancy. Whitner asserts these "absurd" results could not have been intended by the legislature and, therefore, the statute should not be construed to include viable fetuses.

We disagree for a number of reasons. First, the same arguments against the statute can be made whether or not the child has been born. After the birth of a child, a parent can be prosecuted under section 20-7-50 for an action that is likely to endanger the child without regard to whether the action is illegal in itself. For example, a parent who drinks excessively could, under certain circumstances, be guilty of child neglect or endangerment even though the underlying act—consuming alcoholic beverages—is itself legal. Obviously, the legislature did not think it "absurd" to allow prosecution of parents for such otherwise legal acts when the acts actually or potentially endanger the "life, health or comfort" of the parents' born children. We see no reason such a result should be rendered absurd by the mere fact the child at issue is a viable fetus.

Moreover, we need not address this potential parade of horribles advanced by Whitner. In this case, which is the only case we are called upon to decide here, certain facts are clear. Whitner admits to having ingested crack cocaine during the third trimester of her pregnancy, which caused her child to be born with cocaine in its system. Although the precise effects of maternal crack use during pregnancy are somewhat unclear, it is well documented and within the realm of public knowledge that such use can cause serious harm to the viable unborn child. . . . There can be no question here Whitner endangered the life, health, and comfort of her child. We need not decide any cases other than the one before us.

We are well aware of the many decisions from other states' courts throughout the country holding maternal conduct before the birth of the child does not give rise to criminal prosecution under state child abuse/endangerment or drug distribution statutes. . . . Many of these cases were prosecuted under statutes forbidding delivery or distribution of illicit substances and depended on statutory construction of the terms "delivery" and "distribution." . . . Obviously, such cases are inapplicable to the present situation. The cases concerning child endangerment statutes or construing the terms "child" and "person" are also distinguishable, because the states in which these cases were decided have entirely different bodies of case law from South Carolina. . . .

Massachusetts, however, has a body of case law substantially similar to South Carolina's, yet a Massachusetts trial court [in Commonwealth v. Pellegrini,] has held that a mother pregnant with a viable fetus is not criminally liable for transmission of cocaine to the fetus. . . . Specifically, Massachusetts law allows wrongful death actions on behalf of viable fetuses injured in utero who are not subsequently born alive. Mone v. Greyhound Lines, Inc., 368 Mass. 354, 331 N.E.2d 916 (1975). Similarly, Massachusetts law permits homicide prosecutions of third parties who kill viable fetuses. See Commonwealth v. Cass, 392 Mass. 799, 467 **783 N.E.2d 1324 (1984) (ruling a viable fetus is a person for purposes of vehicular homicide statute); Commonwealth v. Lawrence, 404 Mass. 378, 536 N.E.2d 571 (1989) (viable fetus is a person for purposes of common law crime of murder). Because of the similarity of the case law in Massachusetts to ours, the Pellegrini decision merits examination.

In Pellegrini, the Massachusetts Superior Court found that state's distribution statute does not apply to the distribution of an illegal substance to a viable fetus. The statute at issue forbade distribution of cocaine to persons under the age of eighteen. Rather than construing the word "distribution," however, the superior court found that a viable fetus is not a "person under the age of eighteen" within the meaning of the statute. In so finding, the court had to distinguish [Commonwealth v.] Lawrence and [Commonwealth v.] Cass, both of which held viable fetuses are "persons" for purposes of criminal laws in Massachusetts.

The Massachusetts trial court found Lawrence and Cass "accord legal rights to the unborn only where the mother's or parents' interest in the potentiality of life, not the state's interest, are sought to be vindicated." In other words, a viable fetus should only be accorded the rights of a person for the sake of its mother or both its parents. Under this rationale, the viable fetus lacks rights of its own that deserve vindication. Whitner suggests we should interpret our decisions in Hall, Fowler, and Horne to accord rights to the viable fetus only when doing so protects the special parent-child relationship rather than any individual rights of the fetus or any State interest in potential life. We do not think Hall, Fowler, and Horne can be interpreted so narrowly.

If the Pellegrini decision accurately characterizes the rationale underlying Mone, Lawrence, and Cass, then the reasoning of those cases differs substantially from our reasoning in Hall, Fowler, and Horne. First, Hall, Fowler, and Horne were decided primarily on the basis of the meaning of "person" as understood in the light of existing medical knowledge, rather than based on any policy of protecting the relationship between mother and child. As a homicide case, Horne also rested on the State's—not the mother's—interest in vindicating the life of the viable fetus. Moreover, the United States Supreme Court has repeatedly held that the states have a compelling interest in the life of a viable fetus. . . . If, as Whitner suggests we should, we read Horne only as a vindication of the mother's interest in the life of her unborn child, there would be no basis for prosecuting a mother who kills her viable fetus by stabbing it, by shooting it, or by other such means, yet a third party could be prosecuted for the very same acts. We decline to read Horne in a way that insulates the mother from all culpability for harm to her viable child. Because the rationale underlying our body of law—protection of the viable fetus—is radically different from that underlying the law of Massachusetts, we decline to follow the decision of the Massachusetts Superior Court in Pellegrini. . . .

Right to Privacy

Whitner argues that prosecuting her for using crack cocaine after her fetus attains viability unconstitutionally burdens her right of privacy, or, more specifically, her right to carry her pregnancy to term. We disagree.

Whitner argues that section 20-7-50 burdens her right of privacy, a right long recognized by the United States Supreme Court. . . . She cites Cleveland Board of Education v. LaFleur, 414 U.S. 632, 94 S.Ct. 791, 39 L.Ed.2d 52 (1974), as standing for the proposition that the Constitution protects women from measures penalizing them for choosing to carry their pregnancies to term.

In LaFleur, two junior high school teachers challenged their school systems' maternity leave policies. The policies required "every pregnant school teacher to take maternity leave without pay, beginning [four or] five months before the expected birth of her child." A teacher on maternity leave could not return to work "until the beginning of the next regular school semester which follows the date when her child attains the age of three months." The two teachers, both of whom had become pregnant and were required against their wills to comply with the school system's policies, argued that the policies were unconstitutional.

The United States Supreme Court agreed. It found that "[b]y acting to penalize the pregnant teacher for deciding to bear a child, overly restrictive maternity leave regulations can constitute a heavy burden on the exercise of these protected freedoms." The Court then scrutinized the policies to determine whether "the interests advanced in support of" the policy could "justify the particular procedures [the School Boards] ha[d] adopted." Although it found that the purported justification for the policy—continuity of instruction—was a "significant and legitimate educational goal," the Court concluded that the "absolute requirement[s] of termination at the end of the fourth or fifth month of pregnancy" was not a rational means for achieving continuity of instruction and that such a requirement "may serve to hinder attainment of the very continuity objectives that they are purportedly designed to promote." Finding no rational relationship between the purpose of the maternity leave policy and the means crafted to achieve that end, the Court concluded the policy violated the Due Process Clause of the Fourteenth Amendment.

Whitner argues that the alleged violation here is far more egregious than that in LaFleur. She first suggests that imprisonment is a far greater burden on her exercise of her freedom to carry the fetus to term than was the unpaid maternity leave in LaFleur. Although she is, of course, correct that imprisonment is more severe than unpaid maternity leave, Whitner misapprehends the fundamentally different nature of her own interests and those of the government in this case as compared to those at issue in LaFleur.

First, the State's interest in protecting the life and health of the viable fetus is not merely legitimate. It is compelling. . . .

Even more importantly, however, we do not think any fundamental right of Whitner's—or any right at all, for that matter—is implicated under the present scenario. It strains belief for Whitner to argue that using crack cocaine during pregnancy is encompassed within the constitutionally recognized right of privacy. Use of crack cocaine is illegal, period. No one here argues that laws criminalizing the use of crack cocaine are themselves unconstitutional. If the State wishes to impose additional criminal penalties on pregnant women who engage in this already illegal conduct because of the effect the conduct has on the viable fetus, it may do so. We do not see how the fact of pregnancy elevates the use of crack cocaine to the lofty status of a fundamental right.

Moreover, as a practical matter, we do not see how our interpretation of section 20-7-50 imposes a burden on Whitner's right to carry her child to term. In LaFleur, the Supreme Court found that the mandatory maternity leave policies burdened women's rights to carry their pregnancies to term because the policies prevented pregnant teachers from exercising a freedom they would have enjoyed but for their pregnancies. In contrast, during her pregnancy after the fetus attained viability, Whitner enjoyed the same freedom to use cocaine that she enjoyed earlier in and predating her pregnancy—none whatsoever. Simply put, South Carolina's child abuse and endangerment statute as applied to this case does not restrict Whitner's freedom in any way that it was not already restricted. The State's imposition of an additional penalty when a pregnant woman with a viable fetus engages in the already proscribed behavior does not burden a woman's right to carry her pregnancy to term; rather, the additional penalty simply recognizes that a third party (the viable fetus or newborn child) is harmed by the behavior.

Section 20-7-50 does not burden Whitner's right to carry her pregnancy to term or any other privacy right. Accordingly, we find no violation of the Due Process Clause of the Fourteenth Amendment.

Lynn M. Paltrow 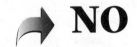 **NO**

Punishment and Prejudice: Judging Drug-Using Pregnant Women

The Villain Cocaine

In the late 1980s and into the 1990s newspapers, magazines, and television were full of stories documenting the devastating effects of cocaine and predicting a lost generation irredeemably damaged by the effects of their mothers' cocaine use. For example, in 1991 *Time* magazine ran a cover story on the subject.[1] Bold yellow letters read "Crack Kids" followed by the headline: "Their mothers used drugs, and now it's the children who suffer." The face of a tearful child filled the page beneath the words. . . .

The same year the *New York Times* ran a front page story entitled "Born on Crack and Coping with Kindergarten."[2] The story is accompanied by a photograph of a school teacher surrounded by young children. Underneath the caption reads: "I can't say for sure it's crack, said Ina R. Weisberg, a kindergarten teacher at P.S. 48 in the Bronx, but I can say that in all my years of teaching I've never seen so many functioning at low levels."

Throughout these years medical and popular journals, public school teachers and judges alike were willing to assume that if a child had a health or emotional problem and he or she had been exposed prenatally to cocaine, then cocaine and cocaine alone was the cause of the perceived medical or emotional problem. Rather than wait for careful research and evaluation of the drug's effect there was, as several researchers later criticized, a "rush to judgment" that blamed cocaine for a host of problems that the research simply has not borne out.[3]

Indeed, an article in the medical journal *Lancet* in 1989 found that scientific studies that concluded that exposure to cocaine prenatally had adverse effects on the fetus had a significantly higher chance of being published than more careful research finding no adverse effects.[4] The published articles, delineating the harmful effects on infants prenatally exposed to cocaine, reported brain damage, genito-urinary malformations, and fetal demise as just a few of the dire results of a pregnant woman's cocaine use. Infants that survived the exposure were described as inconsolable, unable to make eye contact, emitting a strange high-pitched piercing wail, rigid and jittery. These early studies, however, had numerous methodologic flaws that made generalization from them completely inappropriate. For example, these studies were based on individual case reports or on very small samples of women who used more than one drug. Researchers often failed to control for the other drugs and problems the mother might have, and/or failed to follow up on the child's health.[5] The articles describing these studies were nevertheless relied upon to show that cocaine alone was the cause of an array of severe and costly health problems.

Like alcohol and cigarettes, using cocaine during pregnancy can pose risks to the woman and the fetus. More carefully controlled studies, however, are finding that cocaine is not uniquely or even inevitably harmful. For example, unlike the devastating and permanent effects of fetal alcohol syndrome, which causes permanent mental retardation, cocaine seems to act more like cigarettes and marijuana, increasing certain risks like low birth weight but only as one contributing factor and only in some pregnancies.[6] Epidemiological studies find that statistically speaking many more children are at risk of harm from prenatal exposure to cigarettes and alcohol. In fact, one recent publication on women and substance abuse has created the label "Fetal Tobacco Syndrome" to draw attention to the extraordinarily high miscarriage and morbidity rates associated with prenatal exposure to cigarette smoke.[7]

By the late 1980s it was already becoming clear to researchers in the field that the labels "crack babies" and "crack kids" were dangerous and counter-productive.[8] If one read far enough in the *Time* article—past the pictures of premature infants and deranged children—the story reported that

> [a]n increasing number of medical experts, however, vehemently chal-
> lenge the notion that most crack kids are doomed. In fact, they detest
> the term crack kids, charging that it unfairly brands the children and
> puts them all into a single dismal category. From this point of view,
> crack has become a convenient explanation for problems that are
> mainly caused by a bad environment. When a kindergartner from a
> broken home in the impoverished neighborhood misbehaves or seems
> slow, teachers may wrongly assume that crack is the chief reason, when
> other factors, like poor nutrition, are far more important.

Even the *New York Times* article about crack-exposed children in kinder-garten eventually revealed that researchers "after extensive interviews [found] the problems in many cases were traced not to drug exposure but to some other traumatic event, death in the family, homelessness, or abuse, for example."[9] And despite the fact that school administrators "rarely know who the children are who have been exposed to crack . . . and the effects of crack are difficult to diag-nose because they may mirror and be mixed up with symptoms of malnutri-tion, low birth-weight, lead poisoning, child abuse and many other ills that frequently afflict poor children," the article resorts to crack as the only reasonable explanation for an otherwise seemingly inexplicable phenomenon. . . .

The Public Responds

The public response to the media and medical journal reports was largely one of outrage. The harshest reaction was the call for the arrest of the preg-nant women and new mothers who used drugs. Numerous states considered legislation to make it a crime for a woman to be pregnant and addicted.[10] Although not a single state legislature passed a new law creating the crime of fetal abuse, individual prosecutors in more than thirty states arrested women whose infants tested positive for cocaine, heroin, or alcohol. Many of these women were arrested for child abuse, newly interpreted as "fetal" abuse. Others, like Jennifer Johnson in Florida, were charged with delivery of drugs to a minor.[11] In that case, the prosecutor argued that the drug delivery occurred through the umbilical cord after the baby was born but before the umbilical cord was cut. Still other women were charged with assault with a deadly weapon (the weapon being cocaine), or feticide (if the woman suffered a miscarriage), or homicide (if the infant, once born, died). Some women were charged with contributing to the delinquency of a minor.

While arrests were almost always the result of the action of an individual prosecutor, in the state of South Carolina there was unprecedented coordination between health care providers, the prosecutor's office, and the police.

In 1989, the city of Charleston, South Carolina, established a collaborative effort among the police department, the prosecutor's office, and a state hospital, the Medical University of South Carolina (MUSC), to punish pregnant women and new mothers who tested positive for cocaine. Under the policy, the hospital tested certain pregnant women for the presence of cocaine. Women were tested for the presence of cocaine to further criminal investigations, but the women never consented to these searches and search warrants were never obtained.

While the hospital refused to create a drug treatment program designed to meet the needs of pregnant addicts, or to put even a single trained drug counselor on its obstetrics staff, it did create a program for drug-testing certain patients, their in-hospital arrest, and removal to jail (where there was neither drug treatment nor prenatal care); the ongoing provision of medical information to the police and prosecutor's office; and tracking for purposes of ensuring their arrest. Some women were taken to jail while still bleeding from having given birth. They were handcuffed and shackled while hospital staff watched with approval. All but one of the women arrested were African American. The program itself had been designed by and entrusted to a white nurse who admitted that she believed that the "mixing of races was against God's will."[12] She noted in the medical records of the one white woman arrested that she lived "with her boyfriend who is a Negro."[13] . . .

Who Are These Mothers?

As a report from the Southern Regional Project on Infant Mortality observed:

> Newspaper reports in the 1980s sensationalized the use of crack cocaine and created a new picture of the "typical" female addict; young, poor, black, urban, on welfare, the mother of many children and addicted to crack. In interviewing nearly 200 women for this study, a very different picture of the "typical" chemically dependent woman emerges. She is most likely white, divorced or never married, age 31, a high school graduate, on public assistance, the mother of two or three children, and

addicted to alcohol and one other drug. It is clear from the women we interviewed that substance abuse among women is not a problem confined to those who are poor, black, or urban, but crosses racial, class, economic and geographic boundaries.[14]

African American women have been disproportionately targeted for arrest and punishment, not because they use more drugs or are worse mothers, but because, as Dorothy Roberts explains, "[t]hey are the least likely to obtain adequate prenatal care, the most vulnerable to government monitoring, and the least able to conform to the white middle-class standard of motherhood. They are therefore the primary targets of government control."[15]

Beyond the stock images and prejudicial stereotypes, the media has given the public little opportunity to meet or get to know the pregnant women on drugs. If we never learn who they are it is inevitable that their drug use will seem inexplicably selfish and irresponsible. Yet, if we could meet them and learn their history, we might be able to begin to understand them and the problems that need to be addressed.

Let me give an example. In the popular television show *NYPD Blue* we get to know the irascible Detective Sipowicz. While he is neither handsome nor charming, we come to care for him. We learn that he is an alcoholic who is able to stop drinking and improve his life. When he has a massive relapse and behaves outrageously, effectively abandoning his new wife and their newborn son, committing crimes of violence and countless violations of his responsibilities as a police officer, we nevertheless want to forgive him and give him another chance.

We are able to sympathize, at least in part because we have been given the information about why he has relapsed. His first son, whom he has finally reconnected with, is murdered, and Sipowicz, who can't handle it emotionally, turns back to the numbing, relief-giving effects of alcohol.

Sipowicz, in the end, is supported by his police colleagues who cover up for him and give him yet another chance. By contrast, when the same program did an episode involving a heroin-addicted pregnant woman, whose drug habit leads her two older sons to a life of crime, we never get to know why she has turned to drugs. We do not know as we did with Sipowicz what could have driven her to this behavior. The viewer can only assume that her drug use is purely selfish, stemming from a thoughtless hedonism. Thus, she is not entitled to understanding, sympathy, or the many second chances Sipowicz's character routinely gets.

But like Sipowicz, pregnant women who use drugs also have histories and complex lives that affect their behavior and their chances of recovery. We know that substance abuse in pregnancy is highly correlated with a history of violent sexual abuse.[16] In one study 70 percent of the pregnant addicted women were found to be in violent battering relationships. A hugely disproportionate number, compared to a control group, were raped as children. Drugs appear to be used as a means to numb the pain of a violent childhood and adulthood. Like Vietnam veterans who self-medicated with drugs for their post-traumatic stress disorders, at least some pregnant women also use drugs to numb the pain of violent and traumatic life experiences.[17]

Are their difficult childhoods or their experiences with violence an excuse for drug use? No. But the information begins to provide some idea of root causes that might need to be taken into consideration when trying to imagine the appropriate societal reaction. Will the threat of jail remove the trauma and pain that in many instances prompted the drug use and stands in the way of recovery? It is not that a woman who uses drugs is not responsible, but rather that we have to hold her responsible in a context that takes into account the obstacles, internal and external, that stand in the way of recovery. . . .

All pregnant women, not just poor ones, are routinely denied access to the limited drug treatment that exists in this country. In a landmark study in 1990, Dr. Wendy Chavkin surveyed drug treatment programs in New York City. She found that 54 percent flat out refused to take pregnant women.[18] Sixty-seven percent refused to take women who relied on Medicaid for payment, and 84 percent refused to take crack-addicted pregnant women.

One hospital in New York was sued for excluding women from drug treatment. The program argued that its exclusion of all women was justified and no different from its medical judgment to exclude all psychotics.[19] While New York State courts found that such exclusion violated state law, this did not automatically increase needed services. . . .

Other barriers also exist. [In the case of Jennifer Johnson, a pregnant Florida woman,] Judge Eaton ruled that "the defendant also made a choice to become pregnant and to allow those pregnancies to come to term." The prosecutor argued that "[w]hen she delivered that baby she broke the law." By saying this, the judge makes clear that it was having a child that was against the law. If Ms. Johnson had had an abortion she would not have been arrested—even for possessing drugs.[20] But this statement not only reveals a willingness to punish certain women for becoming mothers, it also reflects a host of widely held beliefs and assumptions about access to reproductive health services for women.

For example, implicit in this statement is the assumption that Ms. Johnson had sex and became pregnant voluntarily. Given the pervasiveness of rape in our society, assuming voluntary sexual relations may not be justified. Perhaps, though, the judge, like many others, simply thought that addicts have no business becoming pregnant in the first place. A South Carolina judge put it bluntly: "I'm sick and tired of these girls having these bastard babies on crack cocaine." Apparently concerned about his candor, he later explained: "They say you're not supposed to call them that but that's what they are . . . when I was a little boy, that's what they called them."[21]

On call-in radio talk shows someone inevitably asks why these mothers can't just be sterilized or injected with Depo Provera until they can overcome their drug problems and, while they are at it, their low socioeconomic status. The consistency of this view should not be surprising given our country's history of eugenics and sterilization abuse. Indeed, the U.S. Supreme Court has declared sterilization of men unconstitutional, but has never overturned its decision upholding the sterilization of women perceived to be a threat to society.[22]

The suggestion of sterilization, however, is particularly attractive if there is no explanation about why a pregnant woman with a drug problem would want to become pregnant or to have a child in the first place. But drug-using pregnant women become pregnant and carry to term for the same range of reasons all women do. Because contraception failed. Because they fell in love again and hoped this time they could make their family work. Because they are "prolife" and would never have an abortion. Because when they found out the beloved father of the baby was really already married, they thought it was too late to get a legal abortion. Because they do not know what their options might be. Because they have been abused and battered for so long they no longer believe they can really control any aspect of their lives including their reproductive lives. Because they wanted a child. Because their neighbors and friends, despite their drug use, had healthy babies and they believed theirs would be healthy too.

The threat of sterilization is just another punitive response that denies the humanity of the women themselves. Although Judge Eaton did not propose sterilization as part of the sentence he imposed on Ms. Johnson, as some judges in related cases have,[23] he undoubtedly assumed that Ms. Johnson could decide, once pregnant, whether or not to continue that pregnancy to term. Since 1976, however, the United States government has refused to pay for poor women's abortions and few states have picked up the costs.[24] In Florida, like most other states, the "choice" Judge Eaton spoke of does not exist for low-income women. . . .

Lack of access to abortion services is only one of the many barriers that exist for a drug-addicted pregnant woman who attempts to make responsible "choices." There are many other barriers that make it extremely difficult for pregnant women on drugs to get the kind of help and support they need. Access to services for drug-addicted women who are physically abused is also limited. For example, many battered women's shelters are set up to deal with women who have experienced violence, but are not equipped to support a woman who has become addicted to drugs as a way to numb the pain of the abuse.[25] Other barriers include lack of housing, employment, and access to prenatal care. As one of the few news stories to discuss these women's dilemmas explains:

> Soon after she learned she was pregnant, [Kimberly] Hardy [who was eventually prosecuted for delivery of drugs to a minor], convinced she had to get away from her crowd of crack users as well as her crumbling relationship with her [boyfriend] Ronald, took the kids home to Mississippi for the duration of her pregnancy. But by moving, she lost her welfare benefits, including Medicaid. Unable to pay for clinic visits, she had to go without prenatal care.[26]

And what about the men in their lives? Their contributions to the problem, physiologically and socially, are ignored or deliberately erased. Rarely in the media do we know what has happened to the potential fathers. Their drug use, abandonment, and battering somehow miraculously disappear from view.

Nevertheless, men often do play a significant role. For example, in California Pamela Rae Stewart was arrested after her newborn died. One of her alleged crimes contributing to the child's ultimate demise was having sex with her husband on the morning of the day of the delivery. Her husband, with whom she had had intercourse, was never arrested for fetal abuse. Indeed, the prosecutor's court papers argued that Ms. Stewart had "subjected herself to the rigors of intercourse," thereby totally nullifying the man's involvement or culpability.[27]

Prosecutors in South Carolina have also managed to ignore male culpability, even when it is the father who is supplying the pregnant woman with cocaine or other potentially harmful substances. Many women arrested in this state were not identified as substance addicted until after they had given birth, a point at which their drug use could not even arguably have a biological impact on the baby. Prosecutors argued that arrest was still justified because evidence of a woman's drug use during pregnancy is predictive of an inability to parent effectively. But fathers identified as drug users are not automatically presumed to be incapable of parenting. Indeed, when a man who happens to be a father is arrested for drunk driving, a crime that entails a serious lack of judgment and the use of a drug, he is not automatically presumed to be incapable of parenting and reported to the child welfare authorities. Prosecutors nevertheless rely on biological differences between mothers and fathers, arguing that a man's drug use could not have hurt the developing baby in the first place. However, studies indicate that male drug use can affect birth outcome: Studies on male alcohol use have demonstrated a relationship between male drinking and low birth weight in their children and a study of cocaine and men suggests that male drug use can also affect birth outcome.[28]

We continue to live in a society with double standards and extremely different expectations for men and women. Drug use by men is still glorified, while drug use by women is shameful, and by pregnant women a crime. This could not have been better demonstrated than by an advertising campaign by Absolut vodka. On Father's Day, as a promotional gimmick, Absolut sent 250,000 free ties to recipients of the *New York Times* Sunday edition. Scores of little sperm in the shape of Absolut vodka bottles swim happily on the tie's blue background. So while many call for arrest when a pregnant woman uses drugs or alcohol, fathers who drink are celebrated and, in effect, urged to "tie one on."

Of course, none of these arguments is made to suggest that women are not responsible for their actions or that they are unable to make choices that reflect free will. Rather, it is to say that popular expectations of what acting responsibly looks like and notions of "choice" have to be modified by an understanding of addiction as a chronic relapsing disease, of the degree to which our country has abandoned programs for poor women and children, and of the time, strength, and courage it takes for a drug-addicted woman to confront her history of drug use, violence, and abandonment. Compassion and significantly more access to coordinated and appropriate services will not guarantee that all of our mothers and children are healthy. But medical experts and both children's and women's rights advocates agree that such an approach is far more likely to improve health than are punishment and blame. . . .

The problem with treating the fetus as a person is that women will not simply continue to be less than equal, they will become nonpersons under the law. [To oppose the recognition of fetal personhood as a matter of law is not to deny the value and importance of potential life as a matter of religious belief, emotional conviction, or personal experience. Rather, by opposing such a new legal construct, we can avoid devastating consequences to women's health, prenatal health care, and women's hope for legal equality.—L.P.] No matter how much value we place on a fetus's potential life, it is still inside the woman's body. To pretend that the pregnant woman is separate is to reduce her to nothing more than, as one radio talk show host asserted, a "delivery system" for drugs to the fetus.

Notes

1. *Time Magazine* (13 May 1991).

2. Suzanne Dale, "Born on Crack and Coping with Kindergarten," *New York Times* (7 February 1991), A1.

3. Linda C. Mayes, R. H. Granger, M. H. Bornstein, and B. Zuckerman, "The Problem of Cocaine Exposure, A Rush to Judgment," *Journal of the American Medical Association* 267 (1992): 406.

4. Gideon Koren, Karen Graham, Heather Shear, and Tom Einarson, "Bias Against the Null Hypothesis: The Reproductive Hazards of Cocaine," *Lancet* (1989): 1, 1440–1442.

5. Mayes, "The Problem of Cocaine Exposure"; B. Lutiger, K. Graham, T. R. Einarson, and G. Koren, "Relationship Between Gestational Cocaine Use and Pregnancy Outcome: A Meta-Analysis," *Teratology* (1991): 44, 405–414.

6. Barry Zuckerman et al., "Effect of Maternal Marijuana and Cocaine Use on Fetal Growth," *New England Journal of Medicine* 320, no. 12 (23 March 1990): 762–768; Deborah A. Frank and Barry S. Zuckerman, "Children Exposed to Cocaine Prenatally: Pieces of the Puzzle," *Neurotoxicology and Teratology* 15 (1993): 298–300; Deborah A. Frank, Karen Breshahn, and Barry Zuckerman, "Maternal Cocaine Use: Impact on Child Health and Development," *Advances in Pediatrics* 40 (1993): 65–99.

7. Center on Addiction and Substance Abuse at Columbia University, *Substance Abuse and the American Woman* (1997); Joseph R. DiFranza and Robert A. Lew, "Effect of Maternal Cigarette Smoking on Pregnancy Complications and Sudden Death Syndrome," *Journal of Family Practice* 40 (1995): 385. Cigarette smoking has been linked to as many as 141,000 miscarriages and 4,800 deaths resulting from perinatal disorders, as well as 2,200 deaths from sudden infant death syndrome, nationwide.

8. American Academy of Pediatrics, Committee on Substance Abuse. Drug Exposed Infants, *Pediatrics* 86 (1990): 639.

9. Dale, "Born on Crack."

10. Allison Marshall, 1992, 1993, 1994 Legislative Update, in *National Association for Families and Addiction Research and Education Update* (Chicago, 1993, 1994, 1995).

11. *Johnson v. State*, 602 So.2d 1288 (Fla. 1992).

12. Brown Trial Transcript, *Ferguson et al. v. City of Charleston et al.*, U.S. District Court for the District of South Carolina, Charleston Division, C/A No. 2:93-2624-1 at 5:18–21 (Dec. 10, 1996).

13. Plaintiffs' Exhibit 119, *Ferguson et al. v. City of Charleston et al.*, U.S. District Court for the District of South Carolina, Charleston Division, C/A No. 2:93-2624-1.

14. Shelley Geshan, "A Step Toward Recovery, Improving Access to Substance Abuse Treatment for Pregnant and Parenting Women," *Southern Regional Project on Infant Mortality* (1993): 1.

15. Dorothy Roberts, "Punishing Drug Addicts Who Have Babies: Women of Color, Equality, and the Right of Privacy," *Harvard Law Review* 104, no. 7 (1991): 1419, 1422.

16. Dianne O. Regan, Saundra M. Ehrlich, and Loretta P. Finnegan, "Infants of Drug Addicts: At Risk for Child Abuse, Neglect, and Placement in Foster Care," *Neurotoxicology and Teratology* 9 (1987): 315–319.

17. Sheigla Murphy and Marsha Rosenbaum, *Pregnant Women on Drugs: Combating Stereotypes and Stigma* (New Brunswick, N.J.: Rutgers University Press, 1999).

18. Wendy Chavkin, "Drug Addiction and Pregnancy: Policy Crossroads," *American Journal of Public Health* 80, no. 4 (April 1990): 483–487.

19. *Elaine W. v. Joint Diseases North General Hospital Inc.*, 613 N.E.2d 523 (N.Y. 1993).

20. Lynn M. Paltrow, "When Becoming Pregnant Is a Crime," *Criminal Justice Ethics* 9, no. 1 (Winter–Spring 1990): 41–47.

21. *State v. Crawley*, Transcript of Record (Ct. Gen. Sess. Anderson Cnty., S.C., Oct. 17, 1994).

22. *Skinner v. Oklahoma*, 316 U.S. 535 (1942); *Buck v. Bell*, 274 U.S. 200 (1927); Stephen J. Gould, "Carrie Buck's Daughter," *Natural History* (July 1984).

23. *People v. Johnson*, No. 29390 (Cal.Super.Ct. Jan. 2, 1991).

24. *Harris v. McRae*, 448 U.S. 297 (1980).

25. Amy Hill, "Applying Harm Reduction to Services for Substance Using Women in Violent Relationships," *Harm Reduction Coalition* 6 (Spring 1998): 7–8.

26. Jan Hoffman, "Pregnant, Addicted and Guilty?" *New York Times Magazine* (19 August 1990): 53.

27. Shelly Geshan, "A Step Toward Recovery, Improving Access to Substance Abuse Treatment for Pregnant and Parenting Women" Southern Regional Project on Infant Mortality (1993): 1.

28. Dorothy Roberts, "Punishing Drug Addicts who have Babies: Women of Color, Equality, and the Right of Privacy," Harvard Law Review 104, no. 7, (1991): 1419, 1422.

POSTSCRIPT

Should a Pregnant Woman Be Punished for Exposing Her Fetus to Risk?

In March 2001, the U.S. Supreme Court ruled in the case of *Ferguson v. City of Charleston* (121 S.C. 1281) that the Medical University of South Carolina's policy was unconstitutional. In a six-to-three decision, the Court reversed the decision of the lower Fourth Circuit Court of Appeals and sent the case back to the circuit court for a factual determination of whether the women had actually consented to the search that led to their arrest and imprisonment. The circuit court had ruled that the searches were reasonable under the Fourth Amendment to the Constitution (which prohibits "unreasonable" searches) because of the "special need" to protect women and children from the consequences of cocaine use in pregnant women.

The Supreme Court, however, rejected this claim, arguing that it did not meet the same standard as, for example, the purpose of testing railway workers, customs employees, and high school athletes. Because the Court's decision rested on an interpretation of the Fourth Amendment, it did not settle the public policy and ethical challenges that remain concerning drug use and pregnant women.

For more on this decision, see George Annas, "Testing Poor Pregnant Women for Cocaine: Physicians as Police Investigators," *The New England Journal of Medicine* (May 31, 2001) and Lawrence O. Gostin, "The Rights of Pregnant Women: The Supreme Court and Drug Use," *Hastings Center Report* (September–October, 2001).

In May 2008, the South Carolina Supreme Court overturned the 2001 conviction of Regina McKnight, who had been convicted of homicide because her stillborn child tested positive for cocaine. She will get a new trial, based on her inadequate defense, including a failure to introduce the baby's autopsy results in the trial and medical evidence challenging the prosecution. According to National Advocates for Pregnant Women, an advocacy organization, South Carolina leads the country in prosecutions of pregnant women for child abuse and neglect.

In New Mexico in May 2007, the Supreme Court struck down a law expanding the state's criminal child abuse law to drug-using pregnant women and fetuses. Courts in more than 20 other states have ruled similarly on this issue.

See also Drew Humphries, *Crack Mothers: Pregnancy, Drugs, and the Media* (Ohio State University Press, 1999).

Internet References . . .

Society for Adolescent Medicine

The Society for Adolescent Medicine is composed of professionals committed to improving the physical and psychosocial health of adolescents. This Web site provides many resources on the topic of adolescent health.

http://www.adolescenthealth.org

Center for Adolescent Health and the Law

This site has extensive material about minors' right to consent to medical treatment and access to health care.

http://www.cahl.org

National Disability Rights Network

This is an organization made up of agencies that work to protect and advocate for individuals with disabilities.

http://www.napas.org/index.htm

Children, Adolescents, and Bioethics

*C*hildren *are often the subjects of controversies in biomedical ethics. Too young to make fully autonomous decisions, vulnerable to the pressures and interests of adults (including parents and health care providers), children are nonetheless persons in their own right with clear interests and a need for guidance and protection. Unless proven otherwise, parents are presumed to be the primary decision makers for their children. The common belief is that parents know and love their children, have a family history of values and choices, and can make informed choices about the best interests of their children. Yet this ideal does not always hold true, and in many cases what parents find acceptable, physicians or public health officials see as medical negligence. This section presents some of the most vexing dilemmas in medical ethics.*

- Should Adolescents Be Allowed to Make Their Own Life-and-Death Decisions?

- Is It Ethical to Use Steroids and Surgery to Stunt Disabled Children's Growth?

- Should Vaccination for HPV Be Mandated for Teenage Girls?

ISSUE 9

Should Adolescents Be Allowed to Make Their Own Life-and-Death Decisions?

YES: Robert F. Weir and Charles Peters, from "Affirming the Decisions Adolescents Make About Life and Death," *Hastings Center Report* (November–December 1997)

NO: Lainie Friedman Ross, from "Health Care Decisionmaking by Children: Is It in Their Best Interest?" *Hastings Center Report* (November–December 1997)

ISSUE SUMMARY

YES: Ethicist Robert F. Weir and pediatrician Charles Peters assert that adolescents with normal cognitive and developmental skills have the capacity to make decisions about their own health care. Advance directives, if used appropriately, can give older pediatric patients a voice in their care.

NO: Pediatrician Lainie Friedman Ross counters that parents should be responsible for making their child's health care decisions. Children need to develop virtues, such as self-control, that will enhance their long-term, not just immediate, autonomy.

$\mathbf{A}$ patient is brought to the emergency room after an accident. The physicians believe that he will die if he does not receive a blood transfusion, but the patient says that he is a Jehovah's Witness and will not accept blood. A cancer patient has undergone months of debilitating therapy with discouraging results; she says that she does not want any more treatment. These patients have the right to refuse treatment because they are adults. What if they were 15 or 16 years old? Would they have the same rights or could their wishes be overruled?

If there is one Golden Rule of contemporary bioethics, it is that competent adults are legally and ethically empowered to make health care decisions for themselves. Competent in this context means able to understand the choices and the consequences of decisions made. People base these decisions on values and preferences, personal experiences, religious beliefs, the availability of alternatives, level of pain and suffering, economic consequences, or any combination of these and other factors.

Except in unusual situations, parents are presumed to be in the best position to make these decisions for their children. Children, especially young children, are assumed to have neither the cognitive skills nor the mature judgment to make complex choices that may have far-reaching health consequences. Parents share the consequences of the decision so they make it with the best interests of their children and themselves in mind.

But adolescents are neither children nor fully mature adults. Where do they fit in this scheme? There are differences of opinion of how to define adolescence. Depending on the definition, adolescence may begin as young as 10 and end as late as 21. Legally the age of 18 defines the end of adolescence. However, that may not be an appropriate boundary for health care decision making. Those who support the idea that young people of a certain age should make their own health care decisions tend to call them "adolescents"; those who are critical of this view tend to call them "children" or "minors." In general adolescents have achieved a degree of emotional and intellectual maturity that surpasses that of young children. Still, they may be unable to appreciate long-term consequences of their actions.

In making health care decisions for children and adolescents, an alliance among the patient, parents, and physicians sometimes develops. Together they choose among alternative plans for treatment or, in the case of terminal illness, palliative care instead of aggressive treatment. However, parents, adolescents, and physicians do not always agree.

The selections that follow present two opposing views on whether adolescents should make their own life-and-death decisions. Robert F. Weir and Charles Peters argue for adolescent capacity and autonomy. They summarize an expanding body of professional literature to indicate that, with a few exceptions, adolescents are capable of making major health decisions and giving informed consent. Lainie Friedman Ross argues against the 1995 American Academy of Pediatrics recommendations that give children a greater voice in their care. She contends that it is the parents' right and responsibility to make decisions that enhance their children's long-term autonomy.

YES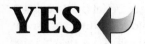

**Robert F. Weir and
Charles Peters**

Affirming the Decisions Adolescents Make About Life and Death

Some Illustrative Cases

Scott Rose was a talented adolescent who loved poetry, music, writing, and acting. Unfortunately, he had Nezelof syndrome, a cellular immunodeficiency disease similar to the condition of the famous "bubble boy" in Houston. Scott refused to remain in a similar enclosure, preferring to live as normal a life as his condition permitted. At the age of fourteen, with his lungs deteriorating and his suffering increasing, Scott decided that he could accept no more life-sustaining treatment. Against his physician's wishes but with tacit approval from his family, Scott died by disconnecting himself from the ventilator that was keeping him alive in a community hospital in Oklahoma.

C.G. was a fifteen-year-old with end-stage cystic fibrosis. During the last year of his life, he was hospitalized four times in a critical care unit for pneumonia and respiratory distress. He repeatedly expressed fear that his life would end in a slow, agonizing death. He realized that he was dying and stated that he did not want to "smother" or die on a ventilator. On his last admission, he experienced increasing respiratory distress and became disoriented as his carbon dioxide rose. However, his parents were adamant, insisting to the attending physician that "everything possible" be done to keep C.G. alive, including prolonged intubation and mechanical ventilation.

Benito Agrela was born with an enlarged liver and spleen. He received a liver transplant when he was eight years old, had a second liver transplant when he was fourteen, and then stopped taking his medication several months after the second transplant because he could not tolerate its side effects. When the Florida Department of Social Services discovered that he was not taking his antirejection medications, they forcibly removed him from his parents' home and admitted him to a transplant floor of a Miami hospital. After he refused further treatment, his case was taken to court; the circuit court judge spent several hours with Benito and his physicians, then ruled that Benito had a legal right to refuse the medications and return home. Before his death at the age of fifteen, Benito said: "I should have the right to make my own decision. I know the consequences, I know the problems."

M.C. was ten years old when she was diagnosed with acute lymphoblastic leukemia. During two years of chemotherapy, she maintained excellent grades,

From *Hastings Center Report*, November/December 1997. Copyright © 1997 by The Hastings Center. Reprinted by permission of the publisher and Robert Weir and Charles Peters.

joined a swim team, and demonstrated, according to her teachers, "a particularly mature and far-reaching perspective on her life." Then the leukemia relapsed. Following discussions with a health care team and her parents, she decided that a partially matched, related donor bone marrow transplant was her best chance for continued life. Before she received the transplant, at the age of thirteen, she told her parents and others that she did not want to "grow up to be a vegetable," did not want to be supported on "a lot of machines," and did not want to be a psychological or financial burden on the family. Two months after the transplant, she was diagnosed as having an Epstein Barr virus-associated lymphoproliferative disorder. Despite aggressive treatment efforts in a pediatric ICU, her condition did not improve. Four days later the ventilator sustaining her life was withdrawn, at the request of her family and in keeping with her previously expressed wishes.

B.C. was a sixteen-year-old adolescent who was diagnosed with cystic fibrosis shortly after birth. Over the years, both his medical condition and his relationship with his parents deteriorated. He watched several friends with cystic fibrosis die, and mentioned on several occasions that he did not want to be placed on a ventilator. Nevertheless, even as his pulmonary tests deteriorated rapidly, his parents refused to discuss death with him, or any decisions that might need to be made about limiting life-sustaining treatment, the possibility of do-not-resuscitate status, or his preferences about treatment options. When he was soon thereafter admitted, unresponsive, following an unsuccessful suicide attempt, his parents requested that no life-sustaining measures be employed. They forbade the medical staff from discussing this matter with B.C., even when he became sufficiently alert to communicate.

Our reason for presenting these cases is simple. Every day, in hospitals throughout this country, adolescent patients cope with chronic conditions, struggle to survive with life-threatening illnesses, and think about the burdens of continued existence compared with the prospect of death. Sometimes, as indicated by Scott Rose and Benito Agrela, these adolescent patients conclude that death is preferable to the suffering they are experiencing, decide to refuse further life-sustaining interventions, and carry out that decision in spite of opposition from physicians and/or parents. Other times, as in the case of M.C., parents and physicians carry out the decision to abate life-sustaining treatment, knowing it to be consistent with the adolescent patient's wishes. Yet other times, as in the cases of C.G. and B.C., parents request, and physicians carry out, a plan of care that has not been discussed with the adolescent patient and may be completely contrary to his or her expressed wishes.

Such cases reflect the considerable uncertainty that sometimes surrounds the medical management of these patients. Do most adolescents have the capacity to make major decisions about their lives and health, even when they are hospitalized? Do only *some* adolescents have this decisionmaking capacity and, if so, what kinds of lines need to be drawn in terms of adolescent decisional abilities? Do adolescents have the right not only to *assent,* but also to *consent*—and to refuse to consent—to recommended medical treatment or participation in research studies? . . .

Adolescents as Capable Decisionmakers

An expanding body of professional literature indicates that adolescents, with some exceptions, are capable of making major health decisions and giving informed consent, whether in a clinical or research setting. An increasing number of professionals in developmental psychology, pediatrics, biomedical ethics, and health law agree that a fundamental reorientation toward adolescents—in clinical medicine, in research settings, and in the law—is necessary to increase adult acceptance of the important decisions that many adolescents now seem capable of making for themselves.

Numerous studies can be cited to make the basic point. Almost twenty years ago, a comprehensive analysis of the literature in developmental psychology by Thomas Grisso and Linda Vierling indicated that "generally minors below the ages of 11–13 do not possess many of the cognitive capacities one would associate with the psychological elements of 'intelligent' consent."[1] By contrast, the authors stated that there "is little evidence that minors of age 15 and above as a group are any less competent to provide consent than are adults." On the basis of their literature analysis, they concluded that "minors are entitled to have some form of consent or dissent regarding the things that happen to them in the name of assessment, treatment, or other professional activities that have generally been determined unilaterally by adults in the minor's interest." Similar conclusions came from an empirical study reported by Lois Weithron and Susan Campbell.[2]

In the pediatric literature, Sanford Leikin surveyed the findings of developmental psychologists, mainly those of Jean Piaget, and applied them to the issue of minors' assent or dissent to medical treatment. He observed that while cognitive development cannot always be equated with chronological age, good evidence exists "that, by age 14 years, many minors attain the cognitive developmental stage associated with the psychological elements of rational consent." As to other adolescent ages, he concluded that "minors between 11 and 14 years of age appear to be in a transition period . . . [and] there appear to be no psychological grounds for the general assumption that minors 15 years of age or older cannot provide competent consent."[3]

In a subsequent publication Leikin addressed the question of how parents and physicians should respond to the decisions made by adolescents to withhold or withdraw life-sustaining treatment. In large part, he argued, it depends on the psychological development of the adolescent in question and that person's ability to make "authentic choices" guided by logical thought patterns, a physiologic understanding of illness, and a willingness to make decisions independent of authority figures (a willingness, he pointed out, not usually found in adolescents less than fourteen or fifteen years of age).[4] Other writers agree.[5] . . .

Legal Developments

Even if most adolescents between age fourteen and seventeen increasingly are regarded as having the capacity to make health decisions for themselves, and even if leading pediatric groups have for over twenty years called for an expansion of adolescent rights in health care settings, important questions about the law remain. . . .

Traditionally, state laws reflected the view that adolescents and other legal minors under the age of twenty-one were incapable of understanding, deliberating about, and making decisions regarding important health care choices. The power to make such decisions was vested in parents, legal guardians, or someone standing in *loco parentis* to a child. Any physician who might have provided nonemergency medical care to a legal minor without parental consent risked being charged with civil battery (performing treatment without consent), even if there was no charge of malpractice.[6]

Legal minors and personal health decisions.   During the past three decades, this view of legal minors has changed in a number of ways. One important change involves the age of majority. Until 1971, the standard age of majority was twenty-one, with a perennial debate focusing on the differences in age required for voting compared with the age required for being drafted into the military. That debate stopped with the passage of the 26th amendment to the Constitution in 1971, thereby permitting persons aged between eighteen and twenty to vote in federal elections. Most state legislatures subsequently lowered the age of majority to eighteen, thus granting legal adulthood to millions of persons who previously could not vote, make contractual obligations, or consent to medical treatment apart from their parents.[7]

Another change in the law involves the creation of exceptional legal categories for some adolescents to make personal health decisions. Two such categories are common among the states. Some adolescents, depending on the state, are legally recognized as *emancipated minors* on the basis of marriage, parenthood, military service, consent of parents (for example, adolescents who are "thrown away" by parents after family conflicts), judicial order of emancipation, or financial independence. Some state statutes (such as in Arizona, Idaho, Massachusetts, Montana, Nevada, North Carolina, Oregon, and Texas) specifically grant emancipated minors the right to consent to medical treatment.

Other adolescents are legally recognized in some jurisdictions as *mature minors* for the purpose of making health decisions because of their individual ability to understand the nature and purposes of recommended medical treatment. The "mature minor rule" recognizes that some adolescents are sufficiently mature to make their own decisions about recommended medical treatment and, when necessary, to go against their parents' views regarding the treatment. Physicians who carry out these decisions seem to run little legal risk, since there are no reported judicial decisions over the past twenty-five years in which parents have recovered damages for the medical treatment of an adolescent over the age of fifteen without parental consent.[8]

A third change in the law pertains to *minor treatment statutes* according to which states permit legal minors to consent to certain types of medical care. These statutes usually specify certain health problems for which legal minors can seek medical treatment without parental consent, precisely because the nature of the health problems is such that some adolescents would probably choose to go without medical treatment rather than seek their parents' consent for the treatment. Such statutes are typically limited to treatment for sexually transmitted diseases, pregnancy and pregnancy prevention (including abortion in some states, but not sterilization), alcohol and other drug abuse, and in some states, psychiatric problems.

Legal minors, end-of-life decisions, and state legislatures. Despite these changes, most state legislatures have not addressed the issue of treatment refusal by adolescents, especially in circumstances in which a refusal of life-sustaining treatment is likely to result in the adolescent's death. Thus, even though forty-seven states have living will statutes (the exceptions are Massachusetts, Michigan, and New York) and forty-eight states have surrogate decisionmaking statutes that include end-of-life decisions (the exceptions are Alabama and Alaska), the legislative statutes in thirty-eight states and the District of Columbia do not specifically address end-of-life decisions made by legal minors.[9]

Most state legislatures seem to think that adolescents either do not die in clinical settings, or are incapable of making informed consent or informed refusal decisions about treatment options, must be protected from their own lack of judgment, or simply should not be permitted to give legally binding advance directions regarding life-sustaining treatments and surrogate decisionmakers. If a given adolescent does not qualify for emancipation under state law, does not live in one of the three states (Alaska, Arkansas, and Mississippi) having a mature-minor statute, and is unable or unwilling for some reason to go through a judicial hearing to be designated a mature minor, he or she is left with only three options: (1) persuading parents and physicians to act according to the adolescent's expressed views on life-sustaining treatment, (2) persuading parents to execute an advance directive on the patient's behalf (in the seven states having this legal option), or (3) acquiescing to the views of legal adults (namely, parents and physicians) regarding the medical circumstances under which the remaining portion of life is to be lived. . . .

Advance Directives and Moral Persuasion

Most adolescents who want to participate in the decisionmaking process connected with their medical conditions, especially in regard to decisions about life-sustaining medical interventions, have chronic conditions that often deteriorate over time: certain kinds of cancer, cystic fibrosis, AIDS, complicated types of heart disease, and so on. Having experienced years of physical and psychological suffering, gone through multiple hospitalizations and numerous treatments, probably experienced depression, and probably observed the suffering and dying of several hospitalized friends with similar medical problems, these adolescent patients are frequently mature beyond their chronological years. They have had, at the very least, multiple opportunities to think about the inescapable suffering that characterizes their lives, the features of life that make it worth continuing, the benefits and burdens that accompany medical treatment, and the prospect of death. At least some of these adolescents want to give voice to their values, provide directions for parents, physicians, and nurses regarding end-of-life care, and be assured that their wishes and preferences will be respected and carried out should their medical conditions deteriorate to the point that they will no longer be able to communicate their deeply felt views.

How parents, physicians, nurses, and other health professionals respond to these adolescents' desires for control and self-determination at the end of life is vitally important. These adults, individually and collectively, may simply *choose not to* listen. Alternatively, parents, physicians, and other adults involved in these cases may think that these personal life-and-death decisions are *primarily matters of law,* quite apart from the wishes and preferences expressed by individual patients. If so, the attending physician will likely check with hospital legal counsel, who will report on relevant statutory and case law and give legal advice that, understandably, will be protective of the hospital's legal interests. . . .

There is a third alternative. Parents, physicians, and other adults involved in these cases may regard the thoughtful comments, the verbalized reflections on the meaning of life and death, and the communicated choices regarding treatment options by *at least some* (perhaps most) adolescents with life-threatening conditions as *efforts of moral persuasion,* quite apart from what the law may or may not say.[10] Parents may reluctantly conclude that their son or daughter has suffered enough, seen enough, and communicated enough to convince them that however much they may want their child to live, he or she has the moral right to make end-of-life decisions that, when carried out, will result in death. Physicians, nurses, and other health care professionals also may be convinced.

Advance directives can help meet this goal, especially if the use of such directives becomes an acceptable part of the informed consent process in pediatric medicine. Enabling at least some adolescent patients—patients with chronic, life-threatening conditions—to communicate their decisions about treatment options through oral or written advance directives would also provide a measure of legal protection for physicians. Pediatricians, family practice physicians, and other physicians having such cases would be more able to document the specific end-of-life treatment decisions made by these patients, the maturity and decisionmaking capacity of individual patients, and the conversations about consenting to or refusing life-sustaining treatment that had taken place with the patients and their parents.

References

1. Thomas Grisso and Linda Vierling, "Minors' Consent to Treatment: A Developmental Perspective," *Professional Psychology* 9 (August 1978): 412–427, at 420.

2. Lois A. Weithorn and Susan B. Campbell, "The Competency of Children and Adolescents to Make Informed Treatment Decisions," *Child Development* 53 (1982): 1589–98.

3. Sanford L. Leikin, "Minors' Assent or Dissent to Medical Treatment," *Journal of Pediatrics* 102 (1983): 173.

4. Sanford L. Leikin, "A Proposal Concerning Decisions to Forgo Life-Sustaining Treatment for Young People," *Journal of Pediatrics* 108 (1989): 17–22, at 20; Leikin, "The Role of Adolescents in Decisions Concerning Their Cancer Therapy," *Cancer Supplement* 71 (15 May 1993): 3342–46.

5. For example, C. E. Lewis, "A Comparison of Minors' and Adults' Pregnancy Decisions," *American Journal of Orthopsychiatry* 50 (1980): 446–53; Richard H. Nicholson, ed., *Medical Research with Children* (Oxford: Oxford University Press, 1986), p. 140–52; Angela Holder, *Legal Issues in Pediatrics and Adolescent Medicine,* 2d ed. (New Haven: Yale University Press, 1985), p. 133.

6. Sarah D. Cohn, "The Evolving Law of Adolescent Health Care," *Clinical Issues 2* (1991): 201–7, at 201; Angela R. Holder, "Disclosure and Consent Problems in Pediatrics," *Law, Medicine & Health Care* 16 (1988): 219–28; Steven M. Selbst, "Treating Minors Without Their Parents," *Pediatric Emergency Care* 1 (1985): 168–73.

7. Richard A. Leiter, ed., *National Survey of State Laws* (Detroit: Gale Research Inc., 1993), pp. 279–91.

8. Angela R. Holder, "Children and Adolescents: Their Right to Decide about Their Own Health Care," in *Children and Health Care: Moral and Social Issues,* ed. Loretta Kopelman and John C. Moskop (Boston: Kluwer Academic Publishers, 1989), p. 163.

9. Information from Choice in Dying, New York, 1995.

10. Robert F. Weir, "Advance Directives as Instruments of Moral Persuasion," in *Medicine Unbound,* ed. Robert H. Blank and Andrea L. Bonnicksen (New York: Columbia University Press, 1994), pp. 171–87.

Lainie Friedman Ross

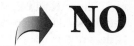 **NO**

Health Care Decisionmaking by Children

In pediatrics, the doctor-patient relationship traditionally has included three parties: the physician, the child, and his or her parents. Parents were not merely surrogate decisionmakers on the grounds of child incompetence, but rather, parents were believed to have both a right and a responsibility to partake in their child's medical decisions.[1] In this [selection] I will examine the evolving position regarding the role of the child in the decisionmaking process as advocated by the American Academy of Pediatrics (AAP). I will offer both moral and pragmatic arguments why I believe this position is misguided.

Recommendations of the American Academy of Pediatrics

In 1995, the AAP published its recommendations for the role of children in health care decisionmaking. The AAP recommended that the child's voice be given greater weight as the child matured. The AAP categorized children as (1) those who lack decisionmaking capacity; (2) those with a developing capacity; and (3) those who have decisionmaking capacity for health care decisions.[2]

For children who lack decisionmaking capacity, the AAP recommended that their parents should make decisions unless their decisions are abusive or neglectful. When children have developing decisionmaking capacity, the physician should seek parental permission and the child's assent. In many cases, the child's dissent should be binding, or at minimum, the physician should seek third-party mediation for parent-child disagreement. Although the child who dissents to life-saving care can be overruled, attempts should be made to persuade the child to assent for "coercion in diagnosis or treatment is a last resort." When children have decisionmaking capacity, the AAP concluded that the children should give informed consent for themselves and their parents should be viewed as consultants.

A major problem with the AAP recommendations is that it assumes decisionmaking capacity can be defined and measured, although the AAP offers no guidance as to what this definition is or how to test for it. Instead, the AAP recommends individual assessment of decisionmaking capacity in

From *Hastings Center Report*, November/December 1997, pp. 41–45. Copyright © 1997 by The Hastings Center. Reprinted by permission of the publisher and Lainie Friedman Ross.

each case. However, since there are no criteria on which to base maturity or decisionmaking capacity, the decision of whether to respect a child's decision is dependent upon the judgment of the particular pediatrician—a judgment he or she has no training to make.

My main concern with the AAP recommendations, however, is what should be done when parents and children disagree on health care decisions: according to the AAP, if there is parental-child disagreement and the child is judged to have decisionmaking authority, the child's decision should be binding. If the child has developing capacity, various mechanisms to resolve the conflict should be attempted. They propose:

> short term counseling or psychiatric consultation for patient and/or family, "case management" or similar multidisciplinary conference(s), and/or consultation with individuals trained in clinical ethics or a hospital based ethics committee. In rare cases of refractory disagreement, formal legal adjudication may be necessary.

I will ignore the difficulties in determining whether a minor has decisionmaking capacity and assume that some minors are competent to make at least some health care decisions. If autonomy is based solely on competency, then competent children should have decisionmaking autonomy in the health care setting. It is my view, however, that even if children are competent, there is a morally significant difference between competent minors and adults. Competency is a necessary but not a sufficient condition on which to base respect for a minor's health care decisionmaking autonomy.

Competency of Children

The psychological literature divides the process of giving informed consent into three components: the patient's consent is informed (made knowingly), is competent (made intelligently), and is voluntary.[3] Although a survey of the literature reveals scant empirical data, existing data suggest that most health care decisions made by adults and children do not fulfill these three components.[4] The data also suggest that adults and older children do not significantly differ in their consent skills.[5] If competency is the only criterion on which respect for autonomy in health care is based, then this difference in treatment cannot be justified.

No test has been developed that uniformly distinguishes all competent individuals from incompetent individuals. Given that competency is context-specific, it is doubtful whether such a test could be developed. And even if a nonculturally biased, objective test could be devised, individual testing of every potential patient would exact a high price in terms of efficiency, privacy, and respect for autonomy. Instead, adults have traditionally been presumed competent and children have been presumed incompetent. That is, respect for autonomy in health care uses both a threshold concept of competency and an age-standard.

To some extent the age-standard is arbitrary as there are individuals above the line (older than the legal age of emancipation) who are incompetent and individuals below the line (younger than the legal age of emancipation) who are competent. But the statutes are not capricious: in general, individuals above the line are more likely to be competent than individuals below it.

Autonomy of Children

One reason to limit the child's present-day autonomy is based on the argument that parents and other authorities need to promote the child's life-time autonomy. Given the value that is placed on self-determination, it makes sense to grant adults autonomy provided that they have some threshold level of competency. Respect is shown by respecting their present project pursuits. But respect for a threshold of competency in children places the emphasis on present-day autonomy rather than on a child's life-time autonomy. Children need a protected period in which to develop "enabling virtues"—habits, including the habit of self-control, which advance their life-time autonomy and opportunities. Although many adults would also benefit from developing their potentials and improving their skills and self-control, at some point (and it is reasonable to use the age of emancipation as the proper cut-off), the advantages of self-determination outweigh the benefits of further guidance and its potential to improve life-time autonomy.

A second reason to limit the child's present-day autonomy is the fact that the child's decisions are based on limited world experience and so her decisions are not part of a well-conceived life plan. Again, many adults have limited world experience, but children have a greater potential for improving their knowledge base and for improving their skills of critical reflection and self-control. . . . By protecting the child from his own impetuosity, his parents help him obtain the background knowledge of the world and the capacities that will allow him to make decisions that better promote his life plans. His parents' attempt to help him flourish may not be achieved, but that does not invalidate their attempt.

A third reason childhood competency should not necessarily entail respect for a child's autonomy is the significant role that intimate families play in our lives. Elsewhere, I have argued that when the family is intimate, parents should have wide discretion in pursuing family goals, goals which may compete and conflict with the goals of particular members.[6] In general, parental autonomy promotes the interests and goals of both children and parents. It serves the needs and interests of the child to have autonomous parents who will help him become an autonomous individual capable of devising and implementing his own life plan. It serves the adults' interest in having and raising a family according to their own vision of the good life. These interests do not abruptly cease when the child becomes competent. If anything, now parents have the opportunity to inculcate their beliefs through rational discourse, instead of through example, bribery, or force.

There are also pragmatic reasons to permit parents to override the present-day autonomy of competent children. First, one can argue for a determination of competency that allows unusually mature children to be emancipated. The problem, as I have already mentioned, is that no such test exists. Second, one can acknowledge that it is best if parents recognize their child's maturity and treat them accordingly, but deny that this justifies granting competent children legal emancipation. Many parents respect their mature child's decisions voluntarily. Laura Purdy remarks: "It is plausible to think that children's maturity is not completely unrelated to parental good sense."[7] Child liberationists may object because a voluntary approach only encourages parents to respect their children's autonomy, but it does not legally enforce it. However, the voluntary approach is more consistent with a policy to limit the state's role in intrafamilial decisions, which is important for the family's ability to flourish.

Health Care Rights in Context

A final argument against respecting the health care decisions of minors is based on placing the notion of health care rights in context. Most individuals who support health care decisionmaking for children view it as an exception and do not seek to emancipate children in other spheres. But why should a child who is competent to make major health care decisions not have the right to make other types of decisions? That is, if a fourteen-year-old is competent to make life-and-death decisions, then why can't this fourteen-year-old buy and smoke cigarettes? Participate in interscholastic football without his parents' consent? Or even drop out of school? . . .

What would it mean to endorse equal rights for children? It is a radical proposal with wide repercussions.[8] It would mean that children could make binding contracts, and that there would be the dissolution of child labor laws, mandatory education, statutory rape laws, and child neglect statutes. As such, it would give children rights for which they are ill-prepared and deny them the protection they need from predatory adults. It would leave children even more vulnerable than they presently are.

Endorsement of child liberation would make a child's membership in a family voluntary. For example, Howard Cohen argues that children should be allowed to change families, either because the child's parents are abusive, or because a neighbor or wealthy stranger offers him a better deal.[9] Such freedom ignores the important role that continuity and permanence play in the parent-child relationship—a significance the child may not yet appreciate.[10] . . .

The Family as the Locus of Decisionmaking

One of my major concerns with the AAP's recommendations is their willingness to involve third-parties in the decisionmaking process. My concern is that these decisions undermine the family. Physicians provide only for the child's transient medical needs; his parents provide for all of his needs and are responsible for raising the child in such a way that he becomes an autonomous responsible adult. Goldstein and colleagues at Yale University's Child Study Center expressed their concern that health care professionals sometimes forget where their professional responsibilities end, and described the harm that we do when we think we can replace parents.[11] By deciding that the child's decision should be respected over the parents' decision, physicians are replacing the parents' judgment that the decision should be overridden with their judgment that the child's decision should be respected. To do so makes this less an issue of respecting the child's autonomy, and more about deciding who knows what is best for the child. In general, parents are the better judge as they have a more vested interest in their child's well-being and are responsible for the day-to-day decisions of child-rearing. It behooves physicians to be humble as they are neither able nor willing to take over this daily function.

I do not mean to suggest that children, particularly mature children, should be ignored in the decisionmaking process. Diagnostic tests and treatment plans should be explained to children to help them understand what is being done to them and to garner, when possible, their cooperation. Parents should include their children in the decisionmaking process both to get their active support and to help them learn how to make such decisions. However, when there is parental-child disagreement, the child's decision should not be decisive nor should health care providers, as I have argued, seek third-party mediation. Rather, as I have already argued, there are both moral and pragmatic reasons why the parents should have final decisionmaking authority.

References

1. Allen Buchanan and Dan Brock, *Deciding for Others: The Ethics of Surrogate Decision Making* (New York: Cambridge University Press, 1989).
2. American Academy of Pediatrics, Committee on Bioethics, "Informed Consent, Parental Permission, and Assent in Pediatric Practice," *Pediatrics* 95 (1995): 314–17.
3. Thomas Grisso and Linda Vierling, "Minor's Consent to Treatment: A Developmental Perspective," *Professional Psychology* 9, no. 3 (1978): 412–27.
4. Paul S. Appelbaum, Charles W. Lidz, and Alan Meisel, *Informed Consent: Legal Theory and Clinical Practice* (New York: Oxford University Press, 1987); Stanley Milgram, *Obedience to Authority: An Experimental View* (New York: Harper and Row, 1974).
5. Grisso and Vierling, "Minor's Consent to Treatment."
6. Lainie Friedman Ross, *Health Care Decision Making for Children*, unpublished manuscript, 1996.
7. Laura M. Purdy, *In Their Best Interest? The Case Against Equal Rights for Children* (New York: Cornell University Press, 1992).
8. Richard Farson, "A Child's Bill of Rights," in *Justice: Selected Readings,* ed. Joel Feinberg and Hyman Gross (Belmont, Calif.: Dickenson Publishing Co. 1977).
9. Howard Cohen, *Equal Rights for Children* (Totowa, N.J.: Rowman and Littlefield, 1980); John Harris, "The Political Status of Children," in *Contemporary Political Philosophy,* ed. Keith Graham (Cambridge, Mass.: Cambridge University Press, 1982), pp. 35–55.
10. Joseph Goldstein, Anna Freud, and Albert J. Solnit, *Before the Best Interests of the Child* (New York: The Free Press, 1979).
11. Joseph Goldstein et al., *In the Best Interest of the Child* (New York: The Free Press, 1986).

POSTSCRIPT

Should Adolescents Be Allowed to Make Their Own Life-and-Death Decisions?

In August 2006, Starchild Abraham Cherrix, a 16-year-old Virginia adolescent with Hodgkin's disease, a form of cancer, was granted the right to pursue a course of Hoxsey therapy instead of chemotherapy. Hoxsey therapy is an alternative form of herbal therapy that is illegal in the United States but is available in Mexico. The case was settled out of court at the start of what was to be a two-day hearing. In this case, Starchild Abraham's parents supported his decision to forego the second round of chemotherapy that his doctors recommended.

As of June 2008, when Abraham turned 18, he was free of Hodgkin's disease and no longer had to report his blood test results to a court. "Abraham's law," passed in Virginia, gives teenagers and their parents the right to refuse doctor-recommended treatments for life-threatening ailments.

In Washington State, Dennis Lindberg, 14, died in November 2007, 3 weeks after a court granted his right to refuse blood transfusions for leukemia because of his Jehovah's Witness religious beliefs. His biological parents opposed the court's decision, but it was supported by his aunt, a Jehovah's Witness, and uncle, who had taken over his care because his birth parents were addicted to drugs. For a commentary opposing the court decision, see Rosamond Rhodes, "Death or Damnation: An Adolescent's Treatment Refusal," online at http://www.thehastingscenter.org/BioethicsForum.

Three earlier cases are discussed in Isabel Traugott and Ann Alpers, "In Their Own Hands: Adolescents' Refusals of Medical Treatment," *Archives of Pediatric and Adolescent Medicine* (September 1, 1997). Although published in 1985, *Legal Issues in Pediatrics and Adolescent Medicine* by Angela Roddey Holder (Yale University Press) is still a classic text. She supports the right of competent adolescents to make treatment decisions. Other documents supporting this position are the 1995 statement of the American Academy of Pediatrics (cited in the selection by Ross) and "Health Care Decision Making Guidelines for Minors" (Midwest Bioethics Center, 1995). Hillary Rodham Clinton also supports children's rights in several articles, including "Children's Rights: A Legal Perspective," *Children's Rights: Contemporary Perspectives,* edited by Patricia A. Vardin and Ilene N. Brody (Teachers College Press, 1979). Among those critical of the movement to grant children and adolescents more decision-making authority is Laura M. Purdy, *In Their Best Interests? The Case Against Equal Rights for Children* (Cornell University Press, 1992). In "Minor Rights and Wrongs," *Journal of Law, Medicine & Ethics* (Summer 1996), Michelle Oberman urges particular concern about cases in which adolescents refuse life-sustaining treatment.

In *The Adolescent "Alone": Decision Making in Health Care in the United States* (Cambridge University Press, 1999), Jeffrey Blustein, Nancy N. Dubler, and Carol Levine present a series of papers and case studies concerning adolescents who do not have a parent or surrogate in their lives to help them make health care decisions.

ISSUE 10

Is It Ethical to Use Steroids and Surgery to Stunt Disabled Children's Growth?

YES: **Sarah E. Shannon**, from "In Support of the Ashley Treatment," *Pediatric Nursing* (March/April 2007)

NO: **Teresa A. Savage**, from "In Opposition of the Ashley Treatment," *Pediatric Nursing* (March/April 2007)

ISSUE SUMMARY

YES: Nurse Sarah E. Shannon believes that ethically and legally parents have the right and duty to make decisions and to care for their family members who are unable to do so themselves and that we should not abandon parents of severely developmentally disabled children to the harsh social and economic realities that are barriers to good care.

NO: Nurse Teresa A. Savage believes that children like Ashley should have independent advocates, preferably persons with disabilities, to weigh the risks and benefits of proposed interventions.

Ashley (her real name) was born in 1997 with a severe brain impairment condition called static encephalopathy. She will never progress beyond the developmental level of an infant. At the age of 7, she was already showing signs of early puberty. Her parents wanted to keep her at home, but felt that as she grew older and bigger, and matured physically, it would be difficult to manage. They were concerned that the quality of life of the child they called their "pillow angel" would be diminished. In 2004, the parents and doctors at the Children's Hospital in Seattle devised a new treatment, which came to be called the "Ashley treatment."

This treatment included the administration of high-dose estrogen (sex steroid) therapy, which would stunt her growth; a hysterectomy (removal of her reproductive organs), which would prevent menstruation and make her infertile; and removal of her breast buds to prevent normal breast development. Before embarking on this treatment, the doctors consulted the hospitals' ethics committee, which met with the parents, Ashley herself, and her physicians. The committee agreed that the requests for estrogen therapy and hysterectomy were ethical in this case but should be considered in future patients only after review by an interdisciplinary panel.

This was not the first time the use of sex steroids has been proposed as a solution to perceived problems of children's growth patterns. In "Tall Girls: The Social Shaping of a Medical Therapy," Joyce M. Lee and Joel D. Howell describe the practice in the second half of the 20th century of prescribing estrogen therapy to otherwise healthy girls to keep them from growing too tall (*Archives of Pediatric and Adolescent Medicine,* October 2006). The definition of "too tall" was determined by societal beliefs about what it meant to be tall and female—not a good thing in those days.

As early as the 1940s, scientists observed that abnormal hormone levels influenced growth patterns both by prematurely closing long-bone growth plates (leading to short stature) and by keeping growth plates open over a prolonged time (leading to acromegaly, or extreme height). Through the 1950s and 1960s articles appeared in medical journals attesting to the success of estrogen therapy in preventing girls from growing too tall, a condition that made them "self-conscious" and "embarrassed."

Lee and Howell assert that in this period the most important career for women was that of homemaker and mother. If this was the ideal, girls who were very tall were less likely to find marriage partners because men were assumed to seek women shorter than them. As social norms changed toward the end of the twentieth century, scientific and medical interest in keeping girls from growing to their natural height diminished. And even among doctors who continued to treat girls, the expected height to which they might grow also increased. In 1956, a girl expected to reach 5'9" might be offered treatment, while by 1999 only girls who might grow to 6'2" would be in that category.

On the other hand, the use of growth hormone for very short but otherwise healthy boys has increased. The reasons are also socially determined. Tall men achieve more in society, it is believed, and have a greater choice of mates.

While Ashley's treatment raises somewhat different questions because she has an underlying medical condition, the social context and limited resources for caring for a severely disabled child are also relevant.

The following selections lay out the issues. Nurse Sarah E. Shannon believes that Ashley's parents' desire to care for her at home is their ethical and legal right, and that they should be able to make decisions in what they understand as Ashley's best interest. Nurse Teresa A. Savage argues that children like Ashley should have independent advocates to weigh the risks and benefits so that perceptions of "quality of life" from a disability perspective are included.

YES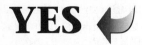

Sarah E. Shannon

In Support of the Ashley Treatment

The news about Ashley, a severely cognitively and developmentally delayed child whose parents chose to medically limit her physical size, grabbed the attention of all of us. What if this was my child? Would I want to make my child smaller so that she would always be able to be cared for in a home, by family members? Growth attenuation treatment for children such as Ashley challenges us to think beyond our initial reactions. Ashley has the developmental and cognitive capacity of a young infant (Gunther & Diekema, 2006). She cannot hold up her head, roll or otherwise change her body position. She moves her arms and legs but cannot sit unsupported. Ashley responds positively to music and is able to vocalize but cannot talk (Parents' blog, 2006). She is alert to her environment but it is not clear that she recognizes people, including her own family. Ashley cries to express her frustration or discomfort. Currently, she lives at home with her parents and two siblings and is cared for by extended family.

Ashley's parents chose to attenuate Ashley's growth – to make her smaller – through the use of high dose estrogen therapy. In addition, Ashley's parents requested, and her physicians agreed, to remove her uterus and breast buds (Gunther & Diekema; Parents' blog; 2006). These three choices were made for separate therapeutic reasons. Growth attenuation through high dose estrogen therapy hastens the normal impact of puberty on girls' height. With puberty, estrogen levels rise and growth plate maturation occurs (Gunther & Diekema, 2006). High dose estrogen therapy takes advantage of this normal effect by stimulating growth plate maturation to occur prematurely. Therapy usually lasts for several years and, while data in developmentally delayed young children is sparse, the major risks appear similar to those for birth control pills, including uterine bleeding, breast development, and a small increased risk of deep vein thrombosis (DVT). Once puberty begins or growth attenuation is achieved, estrogen is stopped. The younger the child, the greater will be the effect on height. Ashley's physicians predict that "treatment beginning in a 5-year-old boy of average height and weight might result in a reduction in final length of as much as 24 inches (60 cm) and in weight of more than 100 pounds (45 kg)." (Gunther & Diekema, 2006, p. 1015).

Reprinted from *Pediatric Nursing Journal,* vol. 33, no. 2, April 2007, pp. 175–178. Reprinted with permission of the publisher, Jannetti Publications, Inc., East Holly Avenue, Box 56, Pitman, NJ 08071-0056; (856) 256-2300; fax: (856) 589-7463; Web site: http://www.pediatricnursing.net; for a sample copy of the journal, please contact the publisher.

Hysterectomy raises the issue of sterilization and whether this procedure was done primarily for birth control. Ashley has the mental capacity of an infant however making any possibility of consensual sex or parenthood impossible. Conversely, there are several health benefits resulting from removal of the uterus. First, it allows the high dose estrogen therapy to be administered without progesterone, reducing the risk of DVT (Gunther & Diekema, 2006). Second, hysterectomy avoids future hormone therapy to control menses. Menses can be a significant source of discomfort and a hygiene challenge that can aggravate skin breakdown when mobility is already impaired. For these reasons, a significant number of disabled women receive depot medroxyprogesterone acetate (DepoProvera) to suppress menstrual bleeding. However recent research has found that this increases their fracture risk 2.4 times above disabled women not on this medication (Watson, Lentz, & Cain, 2006). Hence, hysterectomy is being reconsidered as a more appropriate treatment for long-term control of menses. Third, a hysterectomy removes the cervix, alleviating the need to do routine PAP smears for health maintenance. For a woman as profoundly disabled as Ashley, the personal invasion and discomfort of a routine PAP smear can be intolerable (Brakman & Amari-Vaught, 1999).

The third procedure was breast bud removal, done while Ashley was under anesthesia for the hysterectomy. Was this cosmetic? An effort on the part of Ashley's parents to keep her child-like? How could removal of her breasts possibly benefit Ashley? Ashley's maternal lineage includes large and often, fibrocystic breasts, a painful condition (Parents' blog, 2006). Due to her profound developmental disability, Ashley is unable to sit up without chest support such as a chest strap, which puts pressure on breast tissue. This is a potential source of skin breakdown and discomfort aggravated by large breasts. Breast bud removal is a relatively simple procedure to remove the small subcutaneous breast tissue while retaining the nipple and areola. It is true that if Ashley's breast size becomes problematic later, she could have breast reduction surgery done. However, this is a much more complicated, painful and risky procedure.

Ashley's parents believe that the two biggest challenges Ashley faces in life are discomfort and boredom (Parents' blog, 2006). Avoiding discomfort in persons such as Ashley is a complex goal involving the entire multidisciplinary team. Ashley is fortunate to not suffer from any chronic health problems. However, persons with profound limitations in mobility have a lifetime risk of increased skin breakdown, a major cause of discomfort and morbidity. This risk is increased through factors that include increased body weight, body morphology (such as large breasts), and poor nutritional status and is decreased through actions such as frequent repositioning, optimal hygiene, and good nutritional status. Having a smaller body size minimizes the potential for skin breakdown. A smaller size also increases the opportunity that caregivers can reposition a person more frequently and effectively. Ashley's parents have argued that having Ashley remain small affords other benefits to her. Her grandparents can physically continue to provide care for her. She can continue to use a stroller that she seems to prefer and allows her to be moved around the home to hear and watch family activities, as is often done with an infant. She will continue to fit into a standard bathtub. She will be able to be picked up and held on a parent's lap. She will be kept at home to be cared for within a family environment.

Yet should we change Ashley to fit the home, or change the home to fit Ashley? We could insure that caregivers who are large and strong be available to families to provide care for profoundly disabled persons. We could redesign homes to accommodate persons with disabilities so that their wheelchairs could fit through doorways, their bodies into bathtubs. Yet this utopian view of care would require a level of public financing that is currently unavailable. Americans currently tolerate having 46 million of their neighbors, co-workers, and the strangers they walk past on the sidewalk living without heath care insurance (Hoffman, 2007). Custodial care, such as Ashley needs, is not covered by even the most generous of health care plans. After a few weeks, care at home must be provided by non-paid family caregivers, or helpers paid out-of-pocket, or those paid for through long-term care insurance that the adult person obtained prior to the event, or paid for by public assistance through the Medicaid program after the person (and their spouse) have exhausted their personal finances (U.S. Department of Health and Human Services, 2007). For the elderly who require assistance with activities of daily living, for example after suffering a stroke, finding homecare is difficult. For disabled infants and children it may be nearly impossible. Catlin (2007) described the plight of parents who are trying to secure home health nursing for fragile children. Pediatric-trained caregivers willing to work for the low wages paid in home care settings are in short supply. Reimbursement is nearly non-existent. Equipment for pediatric patients is in short supply. Ashley does not live in a utopian world. By allowing parents of severely developmentally disabled children to have access to growth attenuation treatment, we do not abandon them to these harsh social and economic realities.

The last criticism to address is that Ashley's parents have attenuated her growth for their own convenience. We are disquieted by the thought that Ashley's parents might have decided to keep her small, a 'pillow angel' as they call her, without regard for her dignity or safety. Perhaps it is this last point that disturbs us most deeply. Yet in most healthcare settings, across all age groups, we are witnesses to family decision-making for loved ones who lack decision-making capacity: the distraught family in the intensive care setting making choices for a seriously ill or injured loved one, the exhausted family in mental health making choices for the acutely mentally ill person, the young parents in the NICU making choices for the babies who came too soon and too small. Families approach these decisions without medical training, often in crisis, and with multiple demands on their care giving and financial means. Ethically and legally, we invest in the family the right and duty to make decisions and to care for family members who are unable to do so themselves. Why? Because families do the best they can and it is better than we, as professionals, could do for them. Sometimes we are called upon to protect our patients in situations of abuse or neglect. But most often, we are asked to simply bear witness to the daily sacrifices and acts of love that constitute family caregiving and to humbly guide these families in their decision-making. Ashley's parents, physicians and the multidisciplinary ethics committee have allowed us to share, and judge, their thoughtful deliberations (Gunther & Diekema; Parents' blog; 2006). Each of us can learn from their decisions and benefit from their generosity. So ask yourself again, what if this were my child – who I loved dearly and desperately wanted to ensure would always be able to be cared for in a home setting, by family members? What would I do?

References

Brakman S.V., & Amari-Vaught E. (1999). *Resistance and refusal. Hastings Center Report, 29*(1), 22.

Catlin A.J. (2007). Home care for the high-risk neonate: success or failure depends on home health nurse funding and availability. *Home Healthcare Nurse, 25*(2), 1–5.

Gunther D.F., & Diekema D.S. (2006). Attenuating growth in children with profound developmental disability: A new approach to an old dilemma. *Archives of Pediatrics & Adolescent Medicine, 160*(10), 1013–1017.

Hoffman C.B. (2007). Simple truths about America's uninsured. *American Journal of Nursing, 107*(1), 40–3, 46–47.

Parents' Blog: Ashley's Mom and Dad. (2006). The "Ashley Treatment", toward a better quality of life for "Pillow Angels." . . .

U.S. Department of Health and Human Services, *Medicare: The Official U.S. Government Site for People with Medicare. Long-term Care.* . . .

Watson K.C., Lentz M.J., & Cain K.C. (2006). Associations between fracture incidence and use of depot medroxyprogesterone acetate and anti-epileptic drugs in women with developmental disabilities. *Womens Health Issues 16*(6), 346–52.

Teresa A. Savage 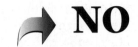 **NO**

In Opposition of the Ashley Treatment

Ashley, at age 6 years, had surgery to remove her uterus and breast buds and after recovering from surgery, was placed on high doses of estrogen for 3 years to permanently stunt her linear growth; her parents refer to the surgeries and hormonal medication as the "Ashley treatment." Her parents believed the surgery and medication would improve their daughter's quality of life by keeping her from reaching adult growth in height and weight. Ashley is permanently disabled from a static encephalopathy. She is reported to have the cognitive abilities arrested at a 3-month level. She is unable to move out of the position in which she is placed and prefers not to be in a sitting position but in a lying position. Her parents are devoted to their daughter and say that they made the decision for the "Ashley treatment" in order to keep her at home. They fear that if she grew an anticipated adult height of 5'6" and adult weight, they would be unable to move and carry her and include her in family gatherings.

Her parents described their reasoning in choosing the "Ashley treatment" in their blog (http://ashleytreatment.spaces.live.com/). Within their blog, there are certain assumptions that underlie their reasoning. I challenge these assumptions.

Assumption 1: Keeping Ashley small will improve her quality of life. Her parents listed "bedsores," "pneumonia," and "bladder infection" as reasons for keeping her small and therefore less likely to be "bedridden" and susceptible to those three complications of immobility.

In my experience in caring for premature infants, who are the smallest human beings ex utero, if you do not re-position them, they will get skin breakdown. If you do not use appropriate bedding, they will get skin breakdown. If you do not re-position them and perform pulmonary hygiene, they will get pneumonia. If you do not keep them adequately hydrated with appropriate nourishment, they are at risk for bladder infections. Size is less important as attention to positioning, bedding materials, pulmonary hygiene, nutrition, and elimination.

Ashley will still require total care and keeping her smaller will make it easier to provide her care. Keeping her small makes it physically easier to care for her, which will positively impact the quality of her life. If she was not kept

Reprinted from *Pediatric Nursing Journal*, vol. 33, no. 2, April 2007, pp. 175–178. Reprinted with permission of the publisher, Jannetti Publications, Inc., East Holly Avenue, Box 56, Pitman, NJ 08071-0056; (856) 256-2300; fax: (856) 589-7463; Web site: http://www.pediatricnursing.net; for a sample copy of the journal, please contact the publisher.

small, she could still have a "good" quality of life, but her care may require more effort. Caregiver effort is no minor factor in Ashley's quality of life; it is perhaps the most critical factor in her quality of life, so I don't think her parents should deny that it was a motivating factor in the decision to use high dose estrogen to stunt her growth.

Assumption 2: Ashley will never bear children so she doesn't need her uterus. It is anticipated that menstrual hygiene will pose a caregiver problem and she may have menstrual cramps.

Do the risks of a hysterectomy outweigh the potential for monthly cramps and bleeding? One might argue that she will be wearing diapers all her life, so what difference does it make if there is urine, stool, or blood in the diaper? She may have discomfort with her periods or she may not. Do the known and real risks of a hysterectomy outweigh the potential risks of her monthly periods?

If she does have skin problems associated with her menses, or she has discomfort that cannot be relieved with medication, she can be treated as any woman is treated—with hormonal therapy to relieve symptoms or to reduce or eliminate menstrual flow. If conservative therapy fails, she could have endometrial ablation or a hysterectomy. Why is it necessary to make this decision at age 6?

Some parents believe that a hysterectomy will protect their child from sexual abuse. A hysterectomy will protect against pregnancy but not molestation, rape, or sexually transmitted diseases.

Assumption 3: Ashley will have large breasts because there is a family history of large breasts, fibrocystic disease, and breast cancer. [It is unclear if she tested positive for the BRCA1/2 gene. If she has the gene, she's at a greater than average risk for ovarian cancer, so why weren't her ovaries removed too?] Therefore, she is better off having her breast buds removed.

Large breasts can be uncomfortable, although there are many women with large breasts who do not choose to have them removed or even reduced. Her parents worry that her breasts will create difficulties in strapping her into her adaptive seating. A penis and scrotum may present difficulties when positioning boys with the same type and degree of disability as Ashley's, but it has not been suggested that the penis and scrotum be removed because of ease in positioning. A boy with the same disability will not reproduce and can void through a shortened urethra, much like a girl's urethra, and surgery may require minimal cutting. So the same argument about justifying removal of the uterus and breasts could be made to remove a disabled boy's penis and scrotum, but that sounds more like mutilation.

Her parents' blog also maintained that large breasts could "invite" abuse. Parents of children with this level of disability worry about vulnerability to sexual molestation. No surgery or hormonal medicating can prevent molestation, and large breasts do not "invite" abuse. Opportunity and lack of supervision invite abuse. Only close supervision of anyone coming in contact with the vulnerable person can protect against abuse.

Assumption 4: High dose estrogen will cause the growth plates to close, thereby stopping linear growth and concomitant weight gain.

Are the long-term risks of high dose estrogen in a 6-year old girl known? Is it known whether or not the high dose estrogen will reduce growth to the degree that is desired? (Were the breast buds removed because of the possibility for breast cancer with high dose estrogens?) Again, it is disturbing to have healthy tissue removed in anticipation of a problem.

Assumption 5: Adults with a mental age of an infant are undignified.

Adults with profound intellectual disability often do not look like the rest of the population. Their features may be coarse; they may have open mouths, protruding tongues, and drooling. They are often the subject of ridicule by unkind, cruel people. Do the attitudes and behavior of uncouth people warrant surgery and hormonal medicating of the recipient of the bad behavior? The stigma toward people with disabilities has persisted despite community integration, mainstream education, independent living, and the Americans with Disabilities Act. The parents' view of dignity, keeping Ashley's appearance more consistent with her intellectual level, differs from the view of dignity from people in the disability communities. The parents quote a passage in their blog that says "The estrogen treatment is not what is grotesque. Rather, it is the prospect of having a full-grown and fertile woman endowed with a mind of a baby." It is regrettable if her parents capitulate to the stigma and believe growth attenuation is necessary to preserve their daughter's dignity.

Disability groups have responded to the "Ashley treatment" with a fervor. They view the choices these parents made as a failure of society to provide the support to people with disabilities and their families (American Association on Intellectual and Developmental Disabilities, 2007; Disability Rights Education & Defense Fund, 2007; Not Dead Yet, 2007; Dick Sobsey [parent of a child with a disability and Director of the John Dossetor Health Ethics Centre, University of Alberta], 2007; Feminists Response in Disability Activism, 2007; ADAPT Youth, 2007r; TASH, 2007). They criticize the medical establishment for offering drastic interventions with unknown long-term risks instead of advocating for social changes that would support Ashley and her family.

I have a colleague who talks about "holding families hostage to the revolution." It's unfair to malign this family who acted with medical endorsement in choosing interventions that many people in the disability community find repugnant. They were doing what they thought was best for Ashley and their family and were extremely brave in publicly sharing their experience. However, before the revolution is over, and to afford children like Ashley all the protections that a human being should have, due process should occur when interventions like the "Ashley treatment" is recommended. The child should have an independent advocate to weigh the risks and benefits of the proposed intervention. Preferably, the advocate should be a person with a disability who is better able to envision from a disability perspective what able-bodied parents can never know—what it is like to live with a disability. Albrecht and Devlieger (1999) describe the disability paradox where people with moderate to severe disabilities report a good or excellent quality of life. The parents' projection of Ashley's quality of life may be conflated with the projection of their own or their family's quality of life. They fear the effects of the "unending work" (to borrow from Corbin and Strauss, 1988) on their lives and, in turn, believe it will adversely affect Ashley's quality of life. It seems the vast majority of disability activists strongly oppose the "Ashley treatment." I wonder if her parents viewed it as the lesser of two evils.

References

ADAPT Youth. (2007). ADAPT Youth appalled at parents surgically keeping disabled daughter childlike. . . .

Albrecht, G. L., & Devlieger, P. J. (1999). The disability paradox: High quality of life against all odds. *Social Science & Medicine, 48,* 977–988.

American Association on Intellectual and Developmental Disabilities. (2007). Unjustifiable non-therapy: A response to Gunther & Diekema (2006), and to the issue of growth attenuation for young people on the basis of disability. . . .

Corbin, J., & Strauss, A. (1988). *Unending work and care: Managing chronic illness at home.* San Francisco: Jossey-Bass publishers.

Disability Rights Education and Defense Fund. (2007). Modify the system, not the person. . . .

Feminists Response in Disability Activism (FRIDA). (2007). FRIDA demands ethics and accountability from the AMA. . . .

Gunther, D. F., & Diekema, D. S. (2006). Attenuating growth in children with profound developmental disability: A new approach to an old dilemma. *Archives of Pediatric & Adolescent Medicine, 160,* 1013–1017.

Not Dead Yet. (2007). *Not Dead Yet statement on "Growth Attenuation" experimentation.* . . .

Sobsey, D. (2007). Growth attenuation and indirect-benefit rationale. *Ethics and Intellectual Disability: Newsletter of the Network on Ethics and Intellectual Disability, 10*(1), 1–2, 7–8.

TASH. (2007). Attenuating growth. . . .

Turnbull, R., Wehmeyer, M., Turnbull, A., & Stowe, M. (2007). *KU experts examine issues in surgery to halt girl's growth.* . . .

POSTSCRIPT

Is It Ethical to Use Steroids and Surgery to Stunt Disabled Children's Growth?

Ashley is now 14 years old and according to her parent's blog, http:// ashleytreatment.spaces.live.com/blog/, she is happy and doing well. (There are no entries after January 2010.) The blog contains pictures of Ashley and reports from other families with "pillow angels," most of whom support the treatment.

Daniel F. Gunther and Douglas A. Diekema, physicians involved in the case, describe their decision-making process in "Attenuating Growth in Children with Profound Developmental Disability: A New Approach to an Old Dilemma," *Archives of Pediatric and Adolescent Medicine,* October 2006.

Most of the commentaries on the "Ashley treatment" have acknowledged the parents' deep love for their child and their good intentions but have criticized the treatment on several grounds: unknown risks, the possibility of abuse in other cases; focus on the parent's convenience rather than benefit to Ashley; and failure to consider the rights of persons with disabilities. S. D. Edwards, a British philosopher, believes that the treatment sets a worrisome precedent that could be used to justify even more radical interventions ("The Ashley Treatment: A Step Too Far, or Not Far Enough?" *Journal of Medical Ethics,* May 2008). Heather T. Battles and Lenore Manderson emphasize the importance of medical anthropological research on the meanings of personhood and childhood disability, autonomy, and the ethics of body modification surgery ("The Ashley Treatment: Furthering the Anthopology of/on Disability," *Medical Anthropology,* vol. 27, no. 3, July 2008).

After weighing all the arguments, Peter A. Clark and Lauren Vasta conclude that "When solutions exist that allow individuals with severe brain impairments to be cared for without interfering with their natural developmental patterns, then these solutions should always take priority." They recommend that until more research is done, no other children be offered the Ashley treatment ("The Ashley Treatment: An Ethical Analysis," *The Internet Journal of Law, Healthcare and Ethics,* vol. 5, no. 1, 2007).

See also S. Matthew Liao, Julian Savulescu, and Mark Sheehan, "The Ashley Treatment: Best Interests, Convenience, and Parental Decision-Making," *Hastings Center Report,* March/April 2007.

Two articles in the January–February 2009 issue of *The Hastings Center Report* conclude, for different reasons, that the Ashley treatment can be ethically justified. Erik Parens believes that parents' wishes, as well as those of people with disabilities, should be respected but that their assumptions can be discussed to ensure that they are truly informed ("Respecting Children with Disabilities—and Their Parents"). Gregory J. Kaebnick uses the Ashley treatment to analyze the claim that it is "against nature" ("It's Against Nature"). N. Tan and I. Brassington look at the Ashley treatment from the viewpoint of professional responsibilities and find worrisome aspects ("Agency, Duties, and the 'Ashley Treatment,'" *Journal of Medical Ethics,* vol. 35, 2009).

ISSUE 11

Should Vaccination for HPV Be Mandated for Teenage Girls?

YES: Joseph E. Balog, from "The Moral Justification for a Compulsory Human Papillomavirus Vaccination Program," *American Journal of Public Health* (April 2009)

NO: Gail Javitt, Deena Berkowitz, and Lawrence O. Gostin, from "Assessing Mandatory HPV Vaccination: Who Should Call the Shots?" *The Journal of Law, Medicine and Ethics* (Summer 2008)

ISSUE SUMMARY

YES: Health science professor Joseph E. Balog believes that a principle-based approach to moral reasoning leads to the conclusion that compulsory HPV vaccinations for teenage girls can be justified on moral, scientific, and public health grounds.

NO: Law professors Gail Javitt and Lawrence O. Gostin and physician Deena Berkowitz believe that, given the limited data and experience, and the fact that HPV does not pose imminent and significant risk to others, mandating HPV vaccine is premature.

Human papillomavirus (HPV) is the most common sexually transmitted infection in the United States, with about 6.2 million individuals newly infected every year. Over a quarter (26.8 percent) of females aged 14–24 have an HPV infection, and among the age group 20–24, almost half (44.8 percent) are infected. There is no treatment, but the vast majority (90 percent) of the women clear the virus within 2 years.

HPV is linked to cancer of the cervix (the narrow end of the uterus, or womb), which is the second most common cancer among women globally. (Breast cancer is the first.) Each year around the world about 493,000 cases of cervical cancer are diagnosed, and 274,000 deaths from this disease are reported. Most of these cases are among young women in their child-bearing and child-rearing years. More than 80 percent of the cases occur in developing countries, and this percentage is rising. In the United States, the incidence of cervical cancer is low, but still significant; about 11,000 new cases occur every year, leading to 3,700 deaths. The risk of death in the United States is very much lower because of the widespread use of the Papanicolaou (Pap) test, which detects cervical cancer at an early and usually treatable stage.

But for those whose infection does not go away, the consequences are serious, especially if the infection comes from the high-risk strain of HPV. The high-risk strain is present in nearly all (99 percent) of cervical cancers. Still, if a young woman is infected with the lower-risk variation, the association with cervical cancer is relatively low.

Clearly, cervical cancer related to HPV infection in the developing world is a major public health problem. But what about the United States? The chances of becoming infected with HPV are quite high, but the chances of this infection leading to cervical cancer are relatively low.

This issue was moved from the theoretical to the real world in June 2006 when the Food and Drug Administration (FDA), which must approve the safety and effectiveness of a medication or vaccine before it is introduced to the general public, licensed a prophylactic (preventive) vaccine against four strains of HPV. The vaccine protects against 70 percent of cervical cancers linked to HPV, but not against all cancer-causing types of HPV. The vaccine was approved for females aged 9–26. Commonly known as Gardasil, its trade name, the vaccine is manufactured and marketed by Merck. In October 2009, the FDA approved a second HPV vaccine, Cervarix, which targets a different HPV strain and is manufactured by GlaxoSmithKline.

The Advisory Committee on Immunization Practices of the Centers for Disease Control and Prevention (CDC) then recommended routine vaccination of 11- and 12-year-old girls with three doses of the vaccine as well as vaccination of 13- to 26-year-olds who had no opportunity to receive the vaccine when they were younger. The three-dose vaccination costs $360, making it one of the most costly vaccines available.

The CDC's recommendations were just that—recommendations. The controversy began when Merck officials lobbied state legislatures to require the vaccine as a condition of school entry for girls entering the sixth grade. By executive order from the governor, in 2007 Texas became the first state to mandate this use of the vaccine, but the state legislature passed legislation to override the executive order and the governor did not veto it. As a result of the controversy, Merck withdrew its lobbying campaign.

As of October 2010 legislators in at least 41 states and the District of Columbia have introduced legislation to require, fund, or educate the public about HPV vaccines. At least 19 states have enacted such legislation.

The following selections explore this controversy from different perspectives. After analyzing the scientific and public health grounds for compulsory HPV vaccinations for teenage girls, health science professor Joseph E. Balog concludes that it can be defended on those grounds as well as moral principles. Gail Javitt and Lawrence O. Gostin, law professors, and Deena Berkowitz, a physician, based their objections on the lack of long-term data on safety and effectiveness and on the lack of imminent risk to others posed by HPV. They believe that mandates would undermine trust in the vaccine and contribute to the prevalent fear of vaccination in general.

YES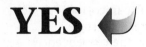

Joseph E. Balog

The Moral Justification for a Compulsory Human Papillomavirus Vaccination Program

Early in the 1950s, polio hysteria erupted across the United States in the wake of a rash of new cases. Thousands of people, mostly young children, were crippled. In 1952, more than 58,000 cases of polio were reported, including 21,000 cases of paralytic polio and more than 3000 deaths. Terrified parents, worried that polio would render their children unable to walk or force them into iron lungs,[1] kept their children away from beaches and movie theaters. Medical researchers conducted experimental studies in public schools. Polio became one of the most feared and studied diseases in the mid-20th century.[2,3]

In retrospect, the decision to implement a compulsory vaccination program for polio was an effective, legal, and ethical use of public health authority. The vaccine was effective: the incidence rate for polio was 3.6 times higher for unvaccinated than vaccinated children, the Salk vaccine was 80% to 90% successful in preventing paralytic poliomyelitis, and over the two- to three-year period after the Salk vaccine was introduced, an overall 60% to 70% prevention rate was achieved.[1,2,4] As a result, the elimination of poliomyelitis has been called one of the 10 great public health achievements of the twentieth century in the United States.[5] . . .

A compulsory HPV vaccination program also appears to be ethically permissible according to the harm principle proposed by John Stuart Mill in *On Liberty*.[6] Mill argued that "the only purpose for which power can be rightfully exercised over any member of a civilized community, against his will, is to prevent harm to others."[7] In the polio vaccination campaign, the diminution of individual autonomy and liberty was justified by the collective interest of the public in preventing harm from disease and promoting the common good. The ethical principles of beneficence and nonmaleficence and the desire to prevent harm overrode the ethical principles of autonomy and liberty. . . .

The desire of some health professionals to prevent illness and deaths from diseases that have low morbidity and mortality rates raises questions about whether the ends—lowered morbidity and mortality rates—justify the means—compulsory vaccinations. The key moral dilemma is whether a utilitarian perspective that weighs the social and health care consequences and costs should override a deontological perspective that it is always good to act

From *American Journal of Public Health*, April 2009. Copyright © 2009 by American Public Health Association. Reprinted by permission of American Public Health Association.

to prevent harm, disease, and death. In other words, is the utility and good of a compulsory vaccine in preventing harm greater than the utility and good of preserving individual liberty and choice? . . .

Ethics and Morality of Compulsory Vaccination

To begin the process of moral reasoning on this dilemma, it is reasonable to acknowledge that health professionals and members of society who support a compulsory vaccination program and their counterparts who oppose compulsory vaccination programs and prefer alternatives such as voluntary vaccinations, premarital abstinence programs, improved screening and treatment, and other options, appear virtuous. None of the proposed alternatives to compulsory vaccination are intended to do harm. Rather, all parties to the debate desire good, achieved through differing means. Furthermore, neither the act of making a compulsory HPV vaccination program available nor implementing alternative programs possesses any inherent or intrinsic feature that is wrong or harmful. Therefore, from a public health perspective, a judgment about the rightness or wrongness of a compulsory vaccination program should be determined by assessing whether key ethical principles justify such action, whether this action reduces harm to individuals and society, and whether this action produces consequences that are at least as good as, if not better than, alternative actions that are available for preventing disease and death.

Beneficence and Nonmaleficence

HPV infection can lead to suffering and harm. Scientific observations have documented that young people in the United States engage in sexual practices that place them at risk for STIs and subsequent illnesses such as cervical cancer. For example, it is estimated that 46% of high school students have sexual intercourse with another person by the time they graduate and 75% of young people have sexual relationships before they marry.[7–11] STIs are reportedly common among sexually active adolescent girls. For example, the Centers for Disease Control and Prevention estimates that 3.2 million adolescent girls have STIs, and of these, 18.3% are infected with HPV. . . .

Evidence about the rates of HPV infections and sexual activity among the young, the ineffectiveness of abstinence programs, and the quantity and quality of communications between parents and children on sexual issues demonstrates a need for public health interventions that prevent the harm that HPV causes among young people. A compulsory or voluntary vaccination program could greatly improve disease prevention over the status quo. It would be wrong to uphold a symbolic ideal of no sexual intercourse among youths by prohibiting an alternative that can alleviate a real harm. In an ideal world, all people would stop engaging in risky sexual behaviors and all parents would engage in meaningful and effective discussions with their children about sexual (and other important) matters. However, these worthy ideals are not realistic enough, nor likely to occur soon and often enough, to match the effectiveness of a vaccine that is available now to eliminate real and immediate harm. Reducing the transmission of HPV infection among youths is an act of beneficence, and the alternative—opposing vaccinations that can reduce real and probable harm or simply failing to provide them—is an act of malevolence.

Autonomy

An important question is, whose autonomy should have a higher priority, the child's or the parent's? It is reasonable to consider who is at greater risk and who stands to gain a greater benefit. In the case of HPV vaccination of youths who have not yet been exposed to HPV, the right of the child to receive the preventive measure should override respect for the parents' autonomy and the parents' desire to teach social beliefs that restrict health care action, because the health threat directly involves the life of the child. The rights, autonomy, and desires of parents are important, but the consequences of the decision affect them indirectly. If respect for parental autonomy leads to denying children access to effective health care, the probability of harm and the loss of benefits are much greater for the children than for their parents.

Disease, disability, and loss of life are burdens—for both individuals and society—that outweigh the benefits derived from upholding parental rights and authority. Furthermore, the availability of a voluntary or compulsory vaccination program does not deprive parents of the opportunity, or the right, to teach their own values to their children. It simply helps to ensure health care for all. As Colgrove pointed out in his essay on ethics and politics associated with an HPV vaccine,

> Minors have a right to be protected against vaccine-preventable illness, and society has an interest in safeguarding the welfare of children who may be harmed by the choices of their parents and guardians.[16]

Justice

The risks of polio, STIs, and cancer are present in society, and all people, regardless of age, are exposed to these health problems, albeit at different rates during different stages of life. It would be wrong, according to Rawls's principle of justice, to provide health care to one group and withhold health care from another group because of a bias about age, race, gender, socioeconomic status, religion, or other factors.[12] The opportunity for justice, according to Rawls, should be provided to all impartially. This principle implies that an HPV vaccine should be made available to everyone in need. Universal access is fair, and withholding the vaccine on grounds of age, potential sexual behavior, or competing values about sexual engagement among youths is unfair. . . .

A compulsory vaccination program will better serve populations that are at greatest risk and in most need of health care and social justice. A utilitarian cost–benefit approach may lead to the greatest good for the greatest number of people, but a compulsory approach may produce the greatest utility for populations who are at greatest risk of disease. A compulsory vaccination program, therefore, appears to be a better alternative for ensuring justice and a fair opportunity for all in reducing harm caused by HPV infections.

Scientific Concerns About Compulsory Vaccination

Concerns have been raised in the scientific literature about mandating an HPV vaccination. In general, these objections evolve from a traditional utilitarian public health perspective that assesses the costs, benefits, outcomes, and risks of a compulsory vaccination program aimed at preventing health problems associated with HPV infection, including cervical cancer, that have low morbidity and mortality rates.

Scientists who question the use of a compulsory program recognize that an HPV vaccination can provide a highly effective means of protection from cervical cancer but caution against mandatory measures before research provides evidence of the vaccine's relative value. For example, Gostin and DeAngelis argue that the benefits from reducing an already low incidence rate of cervical cancer may be minimal.[13] Others assert that no imminent harm exists,[13-15] an alternative method of screening has been effective in reducing this threat,[13,14] achieving universal uptake will be difficult,[14] the vaccine is expensive,[13-15] long-term efficacy is not known,[31,32] and the ethics of limiting autonomy remains an issue.[13-16] . . .

In the United States, it is common to use vaccinations to reduce disease, including mandatory vaccinations for diseases such as measles and polio that have relatively low incidence rates for serious harm. The difference with HPV infection is that vaccination is being recommended to prevent cancer and genital warts that are related to sexual behavior, which raises moral, social, and scientific concerns among some segments of society. But youths who face the threat of STIs and cancer are in as great a need of disease prevention as children who faced the threat of polio in the 1950s. To withhold available and effective measures that prevent disease and death is immoral, as is advocating for alternative programs such as abstinence education that are unrealistic and ineffective.

Opposition in the scientific literature to compulsory vaccination arises from important and valid objections to an unspecified definition of imminent harm, given low rates of morbidity and mortality from cervical cancer and lack of long-term evidence for the safety and efficacy of the vaccine. However, there is precedent for mandating vaccinations against diseases that have low incidence rates of serious harm. Although the vaccine is less effective for sexually active women, it is nonetheless an important preventive measure for young women who have not been exposed to HPV types 16 and 18.

The HPV vaccine is not a replacement for cervical cancer screening and treatment. Rather, as Saraiya suggested, it is an additional and valuable tool for fighting cancer.[17] Combining a 70% reduction of cervical cancer by vaccination with the 80% efficacy of screening and treatment of cervical cancer will achieve a greater good for society than can be produced by either of these health measures alone. In addition, although vaccination will not eliminate the continued need to improve screening methods for detecting cervical cancer, it could potentially reduce the need for the intrusive treatment required for cervical cancer.

As more becomes known about the long-term consequences of an HPV vaccine, it is reasonable to hope that the goals of science—development of a safe and effective vaccine—will ally with moral ideals to offer all citizens equal access to a vaccine that reduces harm, which will be especially valuable to the disadvantaged populations at greatest risk. Ideally, this would occur on a voluntary basis, but history teaches us that it will be best accomplished by implementation of a compulsory vaccination program.

Some have proposed as an ethical test for mandatory public health polices that such policies can only be justified if voluntary measures have failed, no less coercive alternatives exist, the scientific rationale is compelling, and members of the general public are unknowingly at risk. I propose that the rightness or wrongness of a compulsory vaccination program should be determined from a public health perspective by assessing whether key ethical principles justify such action, whether the action reduces harm to individuals and society, and whether the action produces consequences that are at least as good as, if not better than, alternative actions that are present in society for preventing disease and death. Compulsory HPV vaccination meets this test.

Human Participant Protection

No protocol approval was required because no human participants were involved.

References

1. Smith JS. *Patenting the Sun: Polio and the Salk Vaccine.* New York, NY: William Morrow; 1990.
2. Centers for Disease Control and Prevention. *Epidemiology and Prevention of Vaccine-Preventable Diseases: The Pink Book.* 9th ed. Washington, DC: Public Health Foundation; 2006. Available at: http://www.cdc.gov/vaccine/pubs/pinkbook/pink-test.htm. Accessed June 15, 2007.
3. Cono J, Alexander LN. Poliomyelitis. In: Roush SW, McIntyre L, Baldy LM, eds. *VPD Surveillance Manual.* 3rd ed. Atlanta, GA: Centers for Disease Control and Prevention; 2002. http://www.cdc.gov/vaccines/pubs/sur-manual/downloads/chpt10_polio.pdf. Accessed November 20, 2007.
4. Meldrum M. "A calculated risk": The Salk polio vaccine field trials of 1954. *BMJ.* 1998;317(31):1233–1236.
5. Centers for Disease Control and Prevention. Ten great public health achievements—United States, 1900–1999. *MMWR Morb Mortal Wkly Rep.* 1999;48:241–243. http://www.cdc.gov/mmwr/preview/mmwrhtlm/00056796.htm. Accessed April 10, 1999.
6. Mill JS. *On Liberty.* New York, NY: Bobbs-Merrill; 1956.
7. Blake SM, Ledsky R, Goodenow C, Sawyer R, Lohrmann D, Windsor R. Condom availability programs in Massachusetts high schools: relationships with condom use and sexual behavior. *Am J Public Health.* 2003;93:955–962.
8. Centers for Disease Control and Prevention. National and state-specific pregnancy rates among adolescents—United States, 1995–1997. *MMWR Morb Mortal Wkly Rep.* 2000;49:605–611.

9. Eaton DK, Kann L, Kinchen S, et al. Youth risk behavior surveillance—United States, 2005. *J Sch Health*. 2006;76:353–372.

10. Finer LB. Trends in premarital sex in the United States, 1954–2003. *Public Health Rep*. 2007;122(1):73–78.

11. Kann L, Kinchen SA, Williams BI, Ross JG, Lowry R, Grunbaum JA, Kolbe LJ. Youth risk behavior surveillance United States, 1999. *MMWR Morb Mortal Surveill Summ*. 2000;49(SS-5):1–96. http://www.cdc.gov/mmwr/preview/mmwrhtml/ss4905a1.htm. Accessed December 31, 2008.

12. Rawls J. *Theory of Justice*. Cambridge, MA: Harvard University Press; 1971.

13. Gostin LO, DeAngelis CD. Mandatory HPV vaccination: public health vs private wealth. *JAMA*. 2007;297(17):1921–1923.

14. Raffle AE. Challenges of implementing human papillomavirus (HPV) vaccination policy. *BMJ*. 2007;335(7616):375–377.

15. Udesky L. Push to mandate HPV vaccine triggers backlash in USA. *Lancet*. 2007;369:979–980.

16. Colgrove J. The ethics and politics of compulsory HPV vaccination. *N Engl J Med*. 2006;355(23):2389–2391.

17. Saraiya M, Ahmed F, Krishnan S, Richards TB, Unger ER, Lawson HW. Cervical cancer incidence in a prevaccine era in the United States, 1998–2002. *Obstet Gynecol*. 2007;109(2 pt 1):60–70.

Gail Javitt, Deena Berkowitz,
and Lawrence O. Gostin

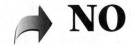

Assessing Mandatory HPV Vaccination: Who Should Call the Shots?

Why Mandating HPV Is Premature

The approval of a vaccine against cancer-causing HPV strains is a significant public health advance. Particularly in developing countries, which lack the health care resources for routine cervical cancer screening, preventing HPV infection has the potential to save millions of lives. In the face of such a dramatic advance, opposing government-mandated HPV vaccination may seem foolhardy, if not heretical. Yet strong legal, ethical, and policy arguments underlie our position that state-mandated HPV vaccination of minor females is premature.

A. Long-Term Safety and Effectiveness of the Vaccine Is Unknown

Although the aim of clinical trials is to generate safety and effectiveness data that can be extrapolated to the general population, it is widely understood that such trials cannot reveal all possible adverse events related to a product. For this reason, post-market adverse event reporting is required for all manufacturers of FDA-approved products, and post-market surveillance (also called "phase IV studies") may be required in certain circumstances. There have been numerous examples in recent years in which unforeseen adverse reactions following product approval led manufacturers to withdraw their product from the market. . . .

In the case of HPV vaccine, short-term clinical trials in thousands of young women did not reveal serious adverse effects. However, the adverse events reported since the vaccine's approval are, at the very least, a sobering reminder that rare adverse events may surface as the vaccine is administered to millions of girls and young women. Concerns have also been raised that other carcinogenic HPV types not contained in the vaccines will replace HPV types 16 and 18 in the pathological niche.

The duration of HPV vaccine-induced immunity is unclear. The average follow-up period for Gardasil during clinical trials was 15 months after the third dose of the vaccine. Determining long-term efficacy is complicated by

From *Journal of Law, Medicine and Ethics,* Summer 2008, pp. 384–395 (excerpts). Copyright © 2008 by American Society of Law, Medicine & Ethics. Reprinted by permission of Wiley-Blackwell via Rightslink.

the fact that even during naturally occurring HPV infection, HPV antibodies are not detected in many women. Thus, long-term, follow-up post-licensure studies cannot rely solely upon serologic measurement of HPV-induced antibody titers. . . .

The current ACIP recommendation is based on assumptions about duration of immunity and age of sexual debut, among other factors. As the vaccine is used for a longer time period, it may turn out that a different vaccine schedule is more effective. In addition, the effect on co-administration of other vaccines with regard to safety is unknown, as is the vaccines' efficacy with varying dose intervals. Some have also raised concerns about a negative impact of vaccination on cervical cancer screening programs, which are highly effective at reducing cervical cancer mortality. These unknowns must be studied as the vaccine is introduced in the broader population.

At present, therefore, questions remain about the vaccine's safety and the duration of its immunity, which call into question the wisdom of mandated vaccination. Girls receiving the vaccine face some risk of potential adverse events as well as risk that the vaccine will not be completely protective. These risks must be weighed against the state's interest in protecting the public from the harms associated with HPV. As discussed in the next section, the state's interest in protecting the public health does not support mandating HPV vaccination.

B. Historical Justifications for Mandated Vaccination Are Not Met

HPV is different in several respects from the vaccines that first led to state-mandated vaccination. Compulsory vaccination laws originated in the early 1800s and were driven by fears of the centuries-old scourge of smallpox and the advent of the vaccine developed by Edward Jenner in 1796. By the 1900s, the vast majority of states had enacted compulsory smallpox vaccination laws.[1] While such laws were not initially tied to school attendance, the coincidental rise of smallpox outbreaks, growth in the number of public schools, and compulsory school attendance laws provided a rationale for compulsory vaccination to prevent the spread of smallpox among school children as well as a means to enforce the requirement by barring unvaccinated children from school.[2] In 1827, Boston became the first city to require all children entering public school to provide evidence of vaccination.[3] Similar laws were enacted by several states during the latter half of the 19th century.[4]

The theory of herd immunity, in which the protective effect of vaccines extends beyond the vaccinated individual to others in the population, is the driving force behind mass immunization programs. Herd immunity theory proposes that, in diseases passed from person to person, it is difficult to maintain a chain of infection when large numbers of a population are immune. With the increase in number of immune individuals present in a population, the lower the likelihood that a susceptible person will come into contact with an infected individual. There is no threshold value above which herd immunity exists, but as vaccination rates increase, indirect protection also increases until the infection is eliminated. . . .

The smallpox laws of the 19th century, which were almost without exception upheld by the courts, helped lay the foundation for modern immunization statutes. Many modern-era laws were enacted in response to the transmission of measles in schools in the 1960s and 1970s. In 1977, the federal government launched the Childhood Immunization Initiative, which stressed the importance of strict enforcement of school immunization laws.[5] Currently, all states mandate vaccination as a condition for school entry, and in deciding whether to mandate vaccines, are guided by ACIP recommendations. At present, ACIP recommends vaccination for diphtheria, tetanus, and acellular pertussis (DTaP), Hepatitis B, polio, measles, mumps, and rubella (MMR), varicella (chicken pox), influenza, rotavirus, haemophilus Influenza B (HiB), pneumococcus, Hepatitis A, meningococcus, and, most recently HPV. State mandates differ; for example, whereas all states require DTaP, polio, and measles in order to enter kindergarten, most do not require Hepatitis A.[6]

HPV is different from the vaccines that have previously been mandated by the states. With the exception of tetanus, all of these vaccines fit comfortably within the "public health necessity" principle articulated in *Jacobson* [v. *Massachusetts* (1905)], in that the diseases they prevent are highly contagious and are associated with significant morbidity and mortality occurring shortly after exposure. And, while tetanus is not contagious, exposure to *Clostridium tetani* is both virtually unavoidable (particularly by children, given their propensity to both play in the dirt and get scratches), life threatening, and fully preventable only through vaccination. Thus, the public health necessity argument plausibly extends to tetanus, albeit for different reasons.

Jacobson's "reasonable relationship" principle is also clearly met by vaccine mandates for the other ACIP recommended vaccines. School-aged children are most at risk while in school because they are more likely to be in close proximity to each other in that setting. All children who attend school are equally at risk of both transmitting and contracting the diseases. Thus, a clear relationship exists between conditioning school attendance on vaccination and the avoidance of the spread of infectious disease within the school environment. Tetanus, a non-contagious disease, is somewhat different, but school-based vaccination can nevertheless be justified in that children will foreseeably be exposed within the school environment (e.g., on the playground) and, if exposed, face a high risk of mortality.

HPV vaccination, in contrast, does not satisfy these two principles. HPV infection presents no public health necessity, as that term was used in the context of *Jacobson*. While non-sexual transmission routes are theoretically possible, they have not been demonstrated. Like other sexually transmitted diseases which primarily affect adults, it is not immediately life threatening; as such, cervical cancer, if developed, will not manifest for years if not decades. Many women will never be exposed to the cancer-causing strains of HPV; indeed the prevalence of these strains in the U.S. is quite low. Furthermore, many who are exposed will not go on to develop cervical cancer. Thus, conditioning school attendance on HPV vaccination serves only to coerce compliance in the absence of a public health emergency.[7]

The relationship between the government's objective of preventing cervical cancer in women and the means used to achieve it—that is, vaccination of all girls as a condition of school attendance—lacks sufficient rationality. First, given that HPV is transmitted through sexual activity, exposure to HPV is not directly related to school attendance.[8] Second, not all children who attend school are at equal risk of exposure to or transmission of the virus. Those who abstain from sexual conduct are not at risk for transmitting or contracting HPV. Moreover, because HPV screening tests are available, the risk to those who choose to engage in sexual activity is significantly minimized. Because it is questionable how many school-aged children are actually at risk— and for those who are at risk, the risk is not linked to school attendance— there is not a sufficiently rational reason to tie mandatory vaccination to school attendance.

To be sure, the public health objective that proponents of mandatory HPV vaccination seek to achieve is compelling. Vaccinating girls before sexual debut provides an opportunity to provide protection against an adult onset disease. This opportunity is lost once sexual activity begins and exposure to HPV occurs. However, that HPV vaccination may be both medically justified and a prudent public health measure is an insufficient basis for the state to compel children to receive the vaccine as a condition of school attendance.

C. In the Absence of Historical Justification, the Government Risks Public Backlash by Mandating HPV Vaccination

Childhood vaccination rates in the United States are very high; more than half of the states report meeting the Department of Health and Human Services (HHS) Healthy People 2010 initiative's goal of ≥95 percent vaccination coverage for childhood vaccination.[9] However, from its inception, state mandated vaccination has been accompanied by a small but vocal anti-vaccination movement. Opposition has historically been "fueled by general distrust of government, a rugged sense of individualism, and concerns about the efficacy and safety of vaccines."[10] In recent years, vaccination programs also have been a "victim of their tremendous success,"[11] as dreaded diseases such as measles and polio have largely disappeared in the United States, taking with them the fear that motivated past generations. Some have noted with alarm the rise in the number of parents opting out of vaccination and of resurgence in anti-vaccination rhetoric making scientifically unsupported allegations that vaccination causes adverse events such as autism.[12]

The rash of state legislation to mandate HPV has led to significant public concern that the government is overreaching its police powers authority. As one conservative columnist has written, "[F]or the government to mandate the expensive vaccine for children would be for Big Brother to reach past the parents and into the home."[13] While some dismiss sentiments such as this one as simply motivated by right wing moral politics, trivializing these concerns is both inappropriate and unwise as a policy matter. Because sexual behavior is involved in transmission, not all children are equally at risk. Thus, it is a reasonable exercise of a parent's judgment to consider his or her child's specific risk and weigh that against the risk of vaccination.

To remove parental autonomy in this case is not warranted and also risks parental rejection of the vaccine because it is perceived as coercive. In contrast, educating the public about the value of the vaccine may be highly effective without risking public backlash. According to one poll, 61 percent of parents with daughters under 18 prefer vaccination, 72 percent would support the inclusion of information about the vaccine in school health classes, and just 45 percent agreed that the vaccine should be included as part of the vaccination routine for all children and adolescents.[14]

Additionally, Merck's aggressive role in lobbying for the passage of state laws mandating HPV has led to some skepticism about whether profit rather than public health has driven the push for state mandates.[15] Even one proponent of state-mandated HPV vaccination acknowledges that Merck "overplayed its hand" by pushing hard for legislation mandating the vaccine.[16] In the face of such criticisms, the company thus ceased its lobbying efforts but indicated it would continue to educate health officials and legislators about the vaccine.[17]

Some argue that liberal opt-out provisions will take care of the coercion and distrust issues. Whether this is true will depend in part on the reasons for which a parent may opt out and the ease of opting out. For example, a parent may not have a religious objection to vaccination in general, but nevertheless may not feel her 11-year-old daughter is at sufficient risk for HPV to warrant vaccination. This sentiment may or may not be captured in a "religious or philosophical" opt-out provision.

Even if opt-out provisions do reduce public distrust issues for HPV, however, liberal opt outs for one vaccine may have a negative impact on other vaccine programs. Currently, with the exception of those who opt out of all vaccines on religious or philosophical grounds, parents must accept all mandated vaccines because no vaccine-by-vaccine selection process exists, which leads to a high rate of vaccine coverage. Switching to an "a la carte" approach, in which parents can consider the risks and benefits of vaccines on a vaccine-by-vaccine basis, would set a dangerous precedent and may lead them to opt out of other vaccines, causing a rise in the transmission of these diseases. In contrast, an "opt in" approach to HPV vaccine would not require a change in the existing paradigm and would still likely lead to a high coverage rate.

Conclusion

Based on the current scientific evidence, vaccinating girls against HPV before they are sexually active appears to provide significant protection against cervical cancer. The vaccine thus represents a significant public health advance. Nevertheless, mandating HPV vaccination at the present time would be premature and ill-advised. The vaccine is relatively new, and long-term safety and effectiveness in the general population is unknown. Vaccination outcomes of those voluntarily vaccinated should be followed for several years before mandates are imposed. Additionally, the HPV vaccine does not represent a public health necessity of the type that has justified previous vaccine mandates. State mandates could therefore lead to a public backlash that will undermine both HPV vaccination efforts and existing vaccination programs. Finally, the economic consequences of mandating HPV are significant and could have a negative impact on financial support for other vaccines as well as other public health programs. These consequences should be considered before HPV is mandated.

The success of childhood vaccination programs makes them a tempting target for the addition of new vaccines that, while beneficial to public health, exceed the original justifications for the development of such programs and impose new financial burdens on both the government, private physicians, and, ultimately, the public. HPV will not be the last disease that state legislatures will attempt to prevent through mandatory vaccination. Thus, legislatures and public health advocates should consider carefully the consequences of altering the current paradigm for mandatory childhood vaccination and should not mandate HPV vaccination in the absence of a new paradigm to justify such an expansion.

Note

The views expressed in this article are those of the author and do not reflect those of the Genetics and Public Policy Center or its staff.

References

1. J. G. Hodge and L. O. Gostin, "School Vaccination Requirements: Historical, Social, and Legal Perspectives," *Kentucky Law Journal* 90, no. 4 (2001–2002): 831–890.

2. J. Duffy, "School Vaccination: The Precursor to School Medical Inspection," *Journal of the History of Medicine and Allied Sciences* 33, no. 3 (1978): 344–355.

3. See Hodge and Gostin, *supra* note 1.

4. *Id.*

5. A. R. Hinman et al., "Childhood Immunization: Laws that Work," *Journal of Law, Medicine & Ethics* 30, no. 3 (2002): 122–127; K. M. Malone and A. R. Hinman, "Vaccination Mandates: The Public Health Imperative and Individual Rights," in R. A. Goodman et al., *Law in Public Health Practice* (New York: Oxford University Press, 2006).

6. Centers for Disease Control and Prevention, *Childcare and School Immunization Requirements, 2005–2006*, August 2006, *available at* <http://www.immunize.org/laws/2005-06_izrequirements.pdf> (last visited March 5, 2008).

7. B. Lo, "HPV Vaccine and Adolescents' Sexual Activity: It Would Be a Shame If Unresolved Ethical Dilemmas Hampered This Breakthrough," *BMJ* 332, no. 7550 (2006): 1106–1107.

8. R. K. Zimmerman, "Ethical Analysis of HPV Vaccine Policy Options," *Vaccine* 24, no. 22 (2006): 4812–4820.

9. C. Stanwyck et al., "Vaccination Coverage Among Children Entering School—United States, 2005–06 School Year," *JAMA* 296, no. 21 (2006): 2544–2547.

10. See Hodge and Gostin, *supra* note 1.

11. S. P. Calandrillo, "Vanishing Vaccinations: Why Are So Many Americans Opting Out of Vaccinating Their Children?" *University of Michigan Journal of Legal Reform* 37 (2004): 353–440.

12. *Id.*

13. B. Hart, "My Daughter Won't Get HPV Vaccine," *Chicago Sun Times,* February 25, 2007, at B6.

14. J. Cummings, "Seventy Percent of U.S. Adults Support Use of the Human Papillomavirus (HPV) Vaccine: Majority of Parents of Girls under 18 Would Want Daughters to Receive It," *Wall Street Journal Online* 5, no. 13 (2006). . . .

15. J. Marbella, "Sense of Rush Infects Plan to Require HPV Shots," *Baltimore Sun*, January 30, 2007. . . .

16. S. Reimer, "Readers Worry About HPV Vaccine: Doctors Say It's Safe," *Baltimore Sun*, April 3, 2007.

17. A. Pollack and S. Saul, "Lobbying for Vaccine to Be Halted," *New York Times*, February 21, 2007. . . .

POSTSCRIPT

Should Vaccination for HPV Be Mandated for Teenage Girls?

In October 2008, the CDC announced that one in four girls aged 13–17 have been vaccinated with Gardasil since its introduction. This is a lower percentage that vaccine advocates had anticipated.

According to the National Conference of State Legislatures, in 2007 at least 24 states and the District of Columbia introduced legislation specifically mandating a school HPV vaccine requirement. Of these, only the District of Columbia's bill was enacted, with enforcement to start 30 days after the Congressional Review Period expired. Other state legislatures are moving more slowly; although most legislatures have considered the issue, when they have acted, they have mostly provided funds for voluntary vaccination or for educational programs for the public. For a complete list of state legislation, go to http://www.ncsl.org/programs/health/HPVVaccine.htm.

On August 1, 2008, the HPV vaccine became one of the required vaccinations for young immigrant females. A 1996 immigration law requires applicants for a green card (legal entry into the United States) have all the vaccinations recommended (not required) by the CDC. This action has been criticized by many immigration advocates and even members of the original CDC panel that recommended the use of the vaccine, as well as Merck representatives. Even though only one dose is required, this adds about $120 to an already expensive list of requirements (*Wall Street Journal,* October 1, 2008).

Although the European Union has approved the use of another HPV vaccine, GlaxoSmithKline's Cervarix, the FDA has not done so yet.

J. L. Schwartz, A. L. Caplan, R. R. Faden, and J. Sugarman review the "unexpectedly early" activity in state legislatures from an ethical perspective ("Lessons from the Failure of Human Papillomavirus Vaccine State Requirments," *Clinical Pharmacological Therapy,* December 2007). R. I. Field and A. L. Caplan see the controversy as one between autonomy (in this case freedom from government intrusion) and beneficence, utilitarianism, and justice, all of which lend support to intervention. They would support a mandate based on utilitarianism if certain conditions are met and if "herd immunity" (protecting the community by vaccinating the few) is a realistic objective ("A Proposed Ethical Framework for Vaccine Mandates: Competing Values and the Case of HPV," *Kennedy Institute of Ethical Journal,* June 2008).

For additional commentary on the HPV vaccine, see these articles in the May 10, 2007, issue of *The New England Journal of Medicine*: George F. Sawaya and Karen Smith-McCune, "HPV Vaccination—More Answers, More Questions"; Lindsey R. Baden, Gregory D. Curfman, Stephen Morrissey, and

Jeffry M. Drazen, "Human Papillomavirus Vaccine—Opportunity and Challenge"; Jan M. Agosti and Sue J. Goldie, "Introducing HPV Vaccine in Developing Countries—Key Challenges and Issues." The scientific report that inspired these commentaries, also in this issue, is "Quadrivalent Vaccine against Human Papillomavirus to Prevent High-Grade Cervical Lesions," by The FUTURE II Study Group.

Internet References . . .

Human Genome Project Information

This site contains information on the ethics, legal, and social issues related to advances in genetics.

http://www.ornl.gov/sci/techresources/Human_Genome/elsi.shtml

President's Council on Bioethics

This site has all the reports on cloning and stem cell research of this council, as well as those of prior commissions.

http://www.bioethics.gov

Council for Responsible Genetics

This organization has a newsletter and articles on the political, medical, consumer, and scientific aspects of genetics.

http://www.gene-watch.org

Genetics

*T*he explosion of technology for unraveling the mysteries of human genetics has created enormous possibilities for the future in terms of understanding heredity and its influence on disease, of identifying people who are at risk for genetic diseases, and eventually of treating at-risk people. All scientific and technical breakthroughs bring unresolved problems. The ability to replicate basic genetic material raises fundamental questions about the ethics of creating and using human embryos and what limits should be set on use of genetic material, even in the advance of scientific knowledge that might be used to treat devastating diseases or to enhance existing characteristics. Earlier abuses of genetic information (much of it misinformation) haunt efforts today to use this information wisely and compassionately. What impact will this knowledge have on individuals' lives and futures, and on the lives and futures of their children? These are some of the challenging issues raised in this section.

- Is Genetic Enhancement an Unacceptable Use of Technology?

- Do the Potential Benefits of Synthetic Biology Outweigh the Possible Risks?

ISSUE 12

Is Genetic Enhancement an Unacceptable Use of Technology?

YES: Michael J. Sandel, from "The Case Against Perfection," *The Atlantic Monthly* (April 2004)

NO: Howard Trachtman, from "A Man Is a Man Is a Man," *The American Journal of Bioethics* (May/June 2005)

ISSUE SUMMARY

YES: Political philosopher Michael J. Sandel believes that using genetic technology to enhance performance, design children, and perfect human nature is a flawed attempt at human mastery, and banishes appreciation of life as a gift.

NO: Physician Howard Trachtman says that the medical community should embrace enhancement as a never-ending quest for health that recognizes that perfection can never be achieved.

Perhaps more than any other people, Americans seem to be obsessed with self-improvement. Each year there is a flood of new books and television commercials promoting ways to be richer, thinner, smarter, happier, healthier, more successful, attractive, or all of the above. Whatever one's presumed character or bodily flaw, there is a remedy. And for parents, there is an additional opportunity (sometimes presented as an obligation) to make one's children richer, thinner, smarter, happier, or all of the above.

Most of these "solutions" are things that individuals do to themselves or with others. Some, such as taking performance-enhancing drugs in sports, involve chemical interventions (see Issue 20). But all at some point encounter the natural limits of an individual's intelligence, physical structure, and inherited or acquired traits, as well as the economic and social context that determines availability and acceptability. A short, slow-moving man is unlikely to become a professional basketball player, no matter how many steroids he takes or how much he trains. Cosmetic surgery can only do so much to alter an aging face or body. Without a natural vocal talent, a woman is unlikely to become an international opera star.

But what if we could change all that? And, if not for ourselves, for our children? The basic idea is not new, and has been practiced for centuries in animal husbandry and agriculture. By breeding for certain characteristics, animals and plants have been created to better meet human purposes. The largest Great Dane and the smallest Pekinese, and all the dog breeds in between, are descended from a handful of wolves tamed by humans in Asia nearly 15,000 years ago. Over the last 500 years humans have practiced breeding techniques that account for the vastly different appearances and characteristics of modern dogs.

Applying these techniques to humans—the theory of eugenics or "better genes"—also has a long but disastrous history. Its advocates, many of them in the United States in the twentieth century, advocated the elimination of "undesirable" people by preventing them from reproducing through involuntary sterilization. In the most malevolent form of eugenics, of course, the Nazi regime in Germany in the 1930s wanted to create a "master race" by encouraging reproduction among blonde, blue-eyed, tall Aryan types and eliminating from the gene pool by murder those from other population groups, such as Jews and gypsies.

While these eugenics methods are not only barbarous and morally corrupt, the idea of enhancing one's capacities and those of future generations has been given new life by scientific advances in genetics. Being able to manipulate genes—the very core of human inheritance—opens up a new world of possibilities. Already animals like sheep and cows have been cloned, that is, reproduced in exact copies. Is it possible to enhance an individual's intelligence or height or beauty—through genetic manipulation? Can a smart person be made smarter? A strong person stronger? Can people be programmed to live two hundred years in good health? Can children be "designed" with particular talents, appearances, and futures? Can "bad" genes—those linked to disease or, more speculatively, criminal tendencies—be eliminated? And if these things are indeed possible, are they a valid use of technology? If these techniques proved to be safe and effective, would they be distributed fairly throughout society?

These questions are at the core of the selections that follow. Political philosopher Michael J. Sandel argues that there is a moral problem with enhancement, whether it is undertaken for one's own benefit or for one's children. These goals express a desire for human mastery over life, which is essentially a gift, and destroys the natural relationship between parents and children. Physician Howard Trachtman, on the other hand, accepts enhancement as a new way of expressing a natural desire to improve health and well-being. He believes that we should not fear progress or try to limit medical manipulations.

YES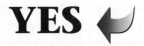

Michael J. Sandel

The Case Against Perfection

Breakthroughs in genetics present us with a promise and a predicament. The promise is that we may soon be able to treat and prevent a host of debilitating diseases. The predicament is that our newfound genetic knowledge may also enable us to manipulate our own nature—to enhance our muscles, memories, and moods; to choose the sex, height, and other genetic traits of our children; to make ourselves "better than well." When science moves faster than moral understanding, as it does today, men and women struggle to articulate their unease. In liberal societies they reach first for the language of autonomy, fairness, and individual rights. But this part of our moral vocabulary is ill equipped to address the hardest questions posed by genetic engineering. The genomic revolution has induced a kind of moral vertigo. . . .

In order to grapple with the ethics of enhancement, we need to confront questions largely lost from view—questions about the moral status of nature, and about the proper stance of human beings toward the given world. Since these questions verge on theology, modern philosophers and political theorists tend to shrink from them. But our new powers of biotechnology make them unavoidable. To see why this is so, consider four examples already on the horizon: muscle enhancement, memory enhancement, growth-hormone treatment, and reproductive technologies that enable parents to choose the sex and some genetic traits of their children. In each case what began as an attempt to treat a disease or prevent a genetic disorder now beckons as an instrument of improvement and consumer choice.

Muscles   Everyone would welcome a gene therapy to alleviate muscular dystrophy and to reverse the debilitating muscle loss that comes with old age. But what if the same therapy were used to improve athletic performance? Researchers have developed a synthetic gene that, when injected into the muscle cells of mice, prevents and even reverses natural muscle deterioration. The gene not only repairs wasted or injured muscles but also strengthens healthy ones. This success bodes well for human applications. H. Lee Sweeney, of the University of Pennsylvania, who leads the research, hopes his discovery will cure the immobility that afflicts the elderly. But Sweeney's bulked-up mice have already attracted the attention of athletes seeking a competitive edge. Although the therapy is not yet approved for human use, the prospect of genetically enhanced weight lifters, home-run sluggers, linebackers, and sprinters is easy to imagine. The widespread use of steroids and other performance-improving drugs in professional sports suggests that many athletes will be eager to avail themselves of genetic enhancement. . . .

Memory   Genetic enhancement is possible for brains as well as brawn. In the mid-1990s scientists managed to manipulate a memory-linked gene in fruit flies, creating flies with photographic memories. More recently researchers have produced smart mice by inserting extra copies of a memory-related gene into mouse embryos. The altered mice learn more quickly and remember things longer than normal mice. The extra copies were programmed to remain active even in old age, and the improvement was passed on to offspring.

Human memory is more complicated, but biotech companies, including Memory Pharmaceuticals, are in hot pursuit of memory-enhancing drugs, or "cognition enhancers," for human beings. The obvious market for such drugs consists of those who suffer from Alzheimer's and other serious memory disorders. The companies also have their sights on a bigger market: the 81 million Americans over fifty, who are beginning to encounter the memory loss that comes naturally with age. A drug that reversed age-related memory loss would be a bonanza for the pharmaceutical industry: a Viagra for the brain. Such use would straddle the line between remedy and enhancement. Unlike a treatment for Alzheimer's, it would cure no disease; but insofar as it restored capacities a person once possessed, it would have a remedial aspect. It could also have purely nonmedical uses: for example, by a lawyer cramming to memorize facts for an upcoming trial, or by a business executive eager to learn Mandarin on the eve of his departure for Shanghai.

Some who worry about the ethics of cognitive enhancement point to the danger of creating two classes of human beings: those with access to enhancement technologies, and those who must make do with their natural capacities. And if the enhancements could be passed down the generations, the two classes might eventually become subspecies—the enhanced and the merely natural. But worry about access ignores the moral status of enhancement itself. Is the scenario troubling because the unenhanced poor would be denied the benefits of bioengineering, or because the enhanced affluent would somehow be dehumanized? As with muscles, so with memory: the fundamental question is not how to ensure equal access to enhancement but whether we should aspire to it in the first place.

Height   Pediatricians already struggle with the ethics of enhancement when confronted by parents who want to make their children taller. Since the 1980s human growth hormone has been approved for children with a hormone deficiency that makes them much shorter than average. But the treatment also increases the height of healthy children. Some parents of healthy children who are unhappy with their stature (typically boys) ask why it should make a difference whether a child is short because of a hormone deficiency or because his parents happen to be short. Whatever the cause, the social consequences are the same.

In the face of this argument some doctors began prescribing hormone treatments for children whose short stature was unrelated to any medical problem. By 1996 such "off-label" use accounted for 40 percent of human-growth-hormone prescriptions. Although it is legal to prescribe drugs for purposes not approved by the Food and Drug Administration, pharmaceutical companies cannot promote such use. Seeking to expand its market, Eli Lilly & Co. recently persuaded the FDA to approve its human growth hormone for healthy children whose projected adult height is in the bottom one percentile—under five feet three inches for boys and four feet eleven inches for girls. This concession raises a large question about the ethics of enhancement: If hormone treatments need not be limited to those with hormone deficiencies, why should they be available only to very short children? Why shouldn't all shorter-than-average children be able to seek treatment? And what about a child of average height who wants to be taller so that he can make the basketball team?

Some oppose height enhancement on the grounds that it is collectively self-defeating; as some become taller, others become shorter relative to the norm. Except in Lake Wobegon, not every child can be above average. As the unenhanced began to feel shorter, they, too, might seek treatment, leading to a hormonal arms race that left everyone worse off, especially those who couldn't afford to buy their way up from shortness.

But the arms-race objection is not decisive on its own. Like the fairness objection to bioengineered muscles and memory, it leaves unexamined the attitudes and dispositions that prompt the drive for enhancement. If we were bothered only by the injustice of adding shortness to the problems of the poor, we could remedy that unfairness by publicly subsidizing height enhancements. As for the relative height deprivation suffered by innocent bystanders, we could compensate them by taxing those who buy their way to greater height. The real question is whether we want to live in a society where parents feel compelled to spend a fortune to make perfectly healthy kids a few inches taller.

Sex selection   Perhaps the most inevitable nonmedical use of bioengineering is sex selection. For centuries parents have been trying to choose the sex of their children. Today biotech succeeds where folk remedies failed.

One technique for sex selection arose with prenatal tests using amniocentesis and ultrasound. These medical technologies were developed to detect genetic abnormalities such as spina bifida and Down syndrome. But they can also reveal the sex of the fetus—allowing for the abortion of a fetus of an undesired sex. Even among those who favor abortion rights, few advocate abortion simply because the parents do not want a girl. Nevertheless, in traditional societies with a powerful cultural preference for boys, this practice has become widespread. . . .

It is commonly said that genetic enhancements undermine our humanity by threatening our capacity to act freely, to succeed by our own efforts, and to consider ourselves responsible—worthy of praise or blame—for the things we do and for the way we are. . . .

Though there is much to be said for this argument, I do not think the main problem with enhancement and genetic engineering is that they undermine effort and erode human agency. The deeper danger is that they represent a kind of hyperagency—a Promethean aspiration to remake nature, including human nature, to serve our purposes and satisfy our desires. The problem is not the drift to mechanism but the drive to mastery. And what the drive to mastery misses and may even destroy is an appreciation of the gifted character of human powers and achievements.

To acknowledge the giftedness of life is to recognize that our talents and powers are not wholly our own doing, despite the effort we expend to develop and to exercise them. It is also to recognize that not everything in the world is open to whatever use we may desire or devise. Appreciating the gifted quality of life constrains the Promethean project and conduces to a certain humility. It is in part a religious sensibility. But its resonance reaches beyond religion. . . .

The ethic of giftedness, under siege in sports, persists in the practice of parenting. But here, too, bioengineering and genetic enhancement threaten to dislodge it. To appreciate children as gifts is to accept them as they come, not as objects of our design or products of our will or instruments of our ambition. Parental love is not contingent on the talents and attributes a child happens to have. We choose our friends and spouses at least partly on the basis of qualities we find attractive. But we do not choose our children. Their qualities are unpredictable, and even the most conscientious parents cannot be held wholly responsible for the kind of children they have. That is why parenthood, more than other human relationships, teaches what the theologian William F. May calls an "openness to the unbidden."

May's resonant phrase helps us see that the deepest moral objection to enhancement lies less in the perfection it seeks than in the human disposition it expresses and promotes. The problem is not that parents usurp the autonomy of a child they design. The problem lies in the hubris of the designing parents, in their drive to master the mystery of birth. Even if this disposition did not make parents tyrants to their children, it would disfigure the relation between parent and child, and deprive the parent of the humility and enlarged human sympathies that an openness to the unbidden can cultivate.

To appreciate children as gifts or blessings is not, of course, to be passive in the face of illness or disease. Medical intervention to cure or prevent illness or restore the injured to health does not desecrate nature but honors it. Healing sickness or injury does not override a child's natural capacities but permits them to flourish.

Nor does the sense of life as a gift mean that parents must shrink from shaping and directing the development of their child. Just as athletes and artists have an obligation to cultivate their talents, so parents have an obligation to cultivate their children, to help them discover and develop their talents and gifts. As May points out, parents give their children two kinds of love: accepting love and transforming love. Accepting love affirms the being of the child, whereas transforming love seeks the well-being of the child. Each aspect corrects the excesses of the other, he writes: "Attachment becomes too quietistic if it slackens into mere acceptance of the child as he is." Parents have a duty to promote their children's excellence.

These days, however, overly ambitious parents are prone to get carried away with transforming love—promoting and demanding all manner of accomplishments from their children, seeking perfection. "Parents find it difficult to maintain an equilibrium between the two sides of love," May observes. "Accepting love, without transforming love, slides into indulgence and finally neglect. Transforming love, without accepting love, badgers and finally rejects." May finds in these competing impulses a parallel with modern science: it, too, engages us in beholding the given world, studying and savoring it, and also in molding the world, transforming and perfecting it.

The mandate to mold our children, to cultivate and improve them, complicates the case against enhancement. We usually admire parents who seek the best for their children, who spare no effort to help them achieve happiness and success. Some parents confer advantages on their children by enrolling them in expensive schools, hiring private tutors, sending them to tennis camp, providing them with piano lessons, ballet lessons, swimming lessons, SAT-prep courses, and so on. If it is permissible and even admirable for parents to help their children in these ways, why isn't it equally admirable for parents to use whatever genetic technologies may emerge (provided they are safe) to enhance their children's intelligence, musical ability, or athletic prowess?

The defenders of enhancement are right to this extent: improving children through genetic engineering is similar in spirit to the heavily managed, high-pressure child-rearing that is now common. But this similarity does not vindicate genetic enhancement. On the contrary, it highlights a problem with the trend toward hyperparenting. One conspicuous example of this trend is sports-crazed parents bent on making champions of their children. Another is the frenzied drive of overbearing parents to mold and manage their children's academic careers. . . .

Some see a clear line between genetic enhancement and other ways that people seek improvement in their children and themselves. Genetic manipulation seems somehow worse—more intrusive, more sinister—than other ways of enhancing performance and seeking success. But morally speaking, the difference is less significant than it seems. Bioengineering gives us reason to question the low-tech, high-pressure child-rearing practices we commonly accept. The hyperparenting familiar in our time represents an anxious excess of mastery and dominion that misses the sense of life as a gift. . . .

In a social world that prizes mastery and control, parenthood is a school for humility. That we care deeply about our children and yet cannot choose the kind we want teaches parents to be open to the unbidden. Such openness is a disposition worth affirming, not only within families but in the wider world as well. It invites us to abide the unexpected, to live with dissonance, to rein in the impulse to control. A *Gattaca*-like world in which parents became accustomed to specifying the sex and genetic traits of their children would be a world inhospitable to the unbidden, a gated community writ large. The awareness that our talents and abilities are not wholly our own doing restrains our tendency toward hubris. . . .

There is something appealing, even intoxicating, about a vision of human freedom unfettered by the given. It may even be the case that the allure of that vision played a part in summoning the genomic age into being. It is often assumed that the powers of enhancement we now possess arose as an inadvertent by-product of biomedical progress—the genetic revolution came, so to speak, to cure disease, and stayed to tempt us with the prospect of enhancing our performance, designing our children, and perfecting our nature. That may have the story backwards. It is more plausible to view genetic engineering as the ultimate expression of our resolve to see ourselves astride the world, the masters of our nature. But that promise of mastery is flawed. It threatens to banish our appreciation of life as a gift, and to leave us with nothing to affirm or behold outside our own will.

Howard Trachtman 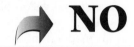 **NO**

A Man Is a Man Is a Man

Every field of human endeavor goes through a period of great anticipation in which the leading lights predict that the end of the discipline is near and that acquisition of new knowledge in the area is almost complete. Thus, at the end of the nineteenth century, physicists were confident that they had natural order of things under control and that mastery of the physical world was just a matter of time. A few decades later, David Hilbert and colleagues asserted that they were closing in on verification of the internal consistency and validity of mathematics and by inference all of philosophy (Goldstein 2005). In the early 1970s, as immunization practice and administration of antibiotics became standard and scourges of earlier eras like smallpox and polio were vanishing, specialists in infectious disease were sure that their field had things well in hand. Finally, after the fall of the Berlin Wall, Francis Fukuyama (1992) wrote confidently that history was at an end and that the global community was entering a phase of prosperity and harmony.

From the privileged vantage point of the early 21st century, we know how grandiose these predictions were. Einstein and his relativistic quanta, Godel and his incompleteness theorem, AIDS and Ebola, and the attack on the World Trade Center demonstrate that nothing ever goes quite exactly according to plan and that human beings still have plenty of work cut out for them.

In light of all of this sobering experience, it is surprising that physicians and bioethicists should have such unrealistic views and apprehensions about prospective therapeutic interventions that may arise from the remarkable advances in genetics or neurobiology. Michael Sandel's (2004) article is representative of this literature and Kamm's (2005) review is an insightful analysis of this position. However, I think it falls short on several practical points that should disarm anxious critics of enhancement.

Enhancement is a new term that is in vogue to describe what doctors have been doing since time immemorial, namely working to improve the lot of the patients they care for. Each medical advance from X-rays to imatinib has always been heralded as the advent of the new millennium only to be replaced by new problems or unexpected complications of old problems (Kantarjian et al. 2002). But, despite rapid approval and grand hopes, no enhancement or treatment has ever turned out to be all it was cracked up to be. Outcomes in real patients hardly ever live up to the exaggerated claims of the advanced sales

From *The American Journal of Bioethics*, vol. 5, no. 3, May/June 2005, pp. 31–33. Copyright © 2005 by Routledge/Taylor & Francis Group. Reprinted by permission via Rightslink. www.informaworld.com

pitch. With each answer that emerges from a clinical trial, there are even more questions that are raised about optimal efficacy, the best target population, and the appropriate balance of benefits and risks. Longer life spans means more cancer and dementia, more antibiotics mean more virulent organisms, improvements in neonatal care mean more damaged low birth weight survivors. Programs for medical enhancement will never deliver on all great expectations, either good or bad. As such there appears to be no inherent reason to fear enhancement or limit its application.

If enhancement represents the intrinsic nature of man to reach out and control his own fate by manipulating his environment and to reverse any adverse effects of his surroundings, then it is inappropriate to use the term mastery in describing this defining human capacity. Instead of considering enhancement an activity with automatic winners and losers, I suggest that it would clarify the discussion if it was viewed as a hard wired human trait that we all engage in. Some do it better than others but all of us try to enhance our lot in life as best as we can. It is undoubtedly true that knowledge can and will be misdirected and even abused by those interested in self-aggrandizement. However, again this is not a unique feature of the remarkable advances in genomics or imaging technology. The fact that there are Harry Limes in the world does not take away from the benefits of antibiotics. The abuse of erythropoietin by athletes does not detract from the qualitative improvement in the lives of patients with end stage renal disease who are treated with this drug (Schumacher et al. 2001).

Moreover, intent has always been a difficult barometer to gauge the behavior of any professional. Most patients are only interested in getting better or improving their health. They rarely concern themselves with the motivation of the care provider, be it money, fame, fortune, or an altruistic desire to help others. Similarly, physicians rarely question why people want to get better as long as they follow instructions and balance the risks and benefits reasonably in their health care judgments. Even in judging religious behavior, which must comply with extralegal concerns and varying standards of dogma, intent is usually implicitly assumed to be appropriate or ignored provided the outcome is not destructive to the individual or community. One would be hard pressed to see any advantage for the patients if individual doctors or the health profession as a whole got into the business of judging patients' intention when they seek a medical treatment to cure disease or enhance health. If there are any lessons to be drawn from the endless discussions about active and passive euthanasia, it may be that no one is served by making this fine distinction in clinical practice (Kamisar 1969).

Finally, the distinction that is being made between treatment which is justified and permissible *versus* enhancement which smacks of hubris and should be constrained may prove to be irrelevant in real life situations where the boundaries are blurred by rapid advances in medical therapeutics and the definition of disease itself. When is failure to concentrate a sign of disease worthy of treatment and when does it indicate a lazy student who is not willing to work hard enough in school? Is erectile dysfunction an ailment like salmonella enteritis or a failure to perform? If I can confidently help the patient with their problem safely and effectively, I for one would just as soon avoid categorizing their complaint into an acceptable *versus* unacceptable category.

Finally, what is intriguing is that those who frown upon physicians who would dispense treatments that enhance patients rather than treat a disease is the assumption that there will be near unanimous acceptance of the treatment and a groundswell of people requesting the therapy. However, a survey of the history of public health interventions indicates that people, at least in this country, are reluctant to take the words of doctors on faith. Although each advance reported in the press is greeted by the public with great fanfare and anticipation, in reality many treatments are rejected by large segments of the population. Think of the people who refuse immunizations for their child, who place greater credence in alternative medications instead of chemotherapy (Frederickson 2004). There will always be people in search for the quick fix to treat obesity, prevent dementia, or win an Olympic medal. But, I think it is contrary to experience to think that everyone will line up for each new genetic treatment or enhancement. Doctors would do well to remind themselves of how varied their patients really are and that application of any therapeutic advance will still begin with a sensitive dialogue between doctor and patient.

In conclusion, I would encourage the medical community to embrace enhancement as a never ending quest for health that will make us healthier but never perfect. We should not fear progress in diagnostics or try to limit medical manipulations. This is because experience teaches us that they will never meet their goals and always leave us striving for more. I endorse Kamm's proposal to promote education about appropriate utilization of advances in genetics and medical science, insure equitable use of these resources, and maintain surveillance for unanticipated and undesirable consequences. However, as it says in Ethics of the Fathers, "The day is short, the work is hard, the employees are tired, the reward is great, and the boss is pressing" (Babylonian Talmud, Ch. 2, Mishna, 20). But, at the end of the day, we will still be human and knowing that should give us the confidence to proceed.

Acknowledgement

The author wishes to thank Rachel Frank, R.N. for her thoughtful comments about this essay.

References

Frederickson, D. D., T. C. Davis, C. L. Arnould, et al. 2004. Childhood immunization refusal: Provider and parent perceptions. *Family Medicine* 36:431–439.

Fukuyama, F. 1992. *The end of history and the last man.* New York: Free Press.

Goldstein, R. 2005. Incompleteness: The proof and paradox of Kort Godel. New York: W.W. Norton & Co.

Kamisar, Y. 1969. Euthanasia legislation: Some non-religious objections. In *Euthanasia and the right to death,* ed. A. B. Downing, Los Angeles, CA: Nash Publishing Company.

Kamm, F. M. 2005. Is there a problem with enhancement? *Am. J. Bioethics* 5–14.

Kantarjian H., C. Sawyers, A. Hochhaus, et al. 2002. Hematologic and cytogenetic responses to imatinib mesylate in chronic myelogenous leukemia. *New England Journal of Medicine* 346:645–652.

Sandel, M. 2004. The case against perfection. *The Atlantic Monthly* 293(3): 51–62.

Schumacher, Y. O., A. Schmid, and T. Lenz. 2001. Blood testing in sports: Hematological profile of a convicted athlete. *Clinical Journal of Sport Medicine* 11:115–117.

POSTSCRIPT

Is Genetic Enhancement an Unacceptable Use of Technology?

None of the genetic enhancements that arouse either fear or anticipation are possible with current technologies. Some say that they will never be possible since most of the desired or unwelcome characteristics are not controlled by a single gene and are also affected by many other background factors. Still, the future may bring still-undreamed-of possibilities.

The issue of *The American Journal of Bioethics* (vol. 5, no. 3, 2005), from which Howard Trachtman's essay is drawn, also contains several other articles on enhancement. The lead article by Frances M. Kamm, "Is There a Problem with Enhancement?" analyzes Sandel's article from a philosophical perspective.

For a fuller explanation of Sandel's views, see his book *The Case Against Perfection: Ethics in the Age of Genetic Engineering* (Belknap Press, 2007). Also see Jonathan Glover, *Choosing Children: Genes, Disability, and Design* (Oxford University Press, 2008) for a perspective incorporating the viewpoints of people with disabilities.

Julian Savulescu argues that we have a moral obligation to enhance human beings and that "to be human is to strive to be better" ("New Breeds of Humans: The Moral Obligation to Enhance," *Reproductive Medicine Online*, March 2005). In "Enhancements and Justice: Problems in Determining the Requirements of Justice in a Genetically Transformed Society," Ronald A. Lindsay asserts that concern about the "threat of a genetic aristocracy" appears misplaced, given the already existing disparities in society (*Kennedy Institute of Ethics Journal*, vol. 15, no. 1, 2005).

Wondergenes: Genetic Enhancement and the Future of Society by Maxwell J. Mehlman (Indiana University Press, 2003) is an accessible introduction to the social and personal implications of genetic engineering. See also Erik Parens, "Authenticity and Ambivalence: Toward Understanding the Enhancement Debate," *Hastings Center Report* (May–June 2005).

Genetic enhancement to improve performance in sports is often rumored but not yet a reality, according to Thomas H. Murray in "Gene Doping and Olympic Sport" (*Play True*, issue 1, 2005). He points to the dangers of untested technologies to alter genetic makeup. See Issue 20, "Should Performance-Enhancing Drugs Be Banned from Sports?"

On the Web: "Genetic Enhancement" from the National Human Genome Research Institute, http://www.genome.gov/10004767.

ISSUE 13

Do the Potential Benefits of Synthetic Biology Outweigh the Possible Risks?

YES: **Gregory E. Kaebnick,** from Prepared Statement before the U.S. House of Representatives Committee on Energy and Commerce (May 27, 2010)

NO: **Christopher J. Preston,** from "Synthetic Biology: Drawing a Line in Darwin's Sand," *Environmental Values* (February 2008)

ISSUE SUMMARY

YES: Philosopher Gregory E. Kaebnick believes that the potential societal benefits of the new technology of synthetic biology are too great to delay its use.

NO: Christopher J. Preston, an environmental ethicist, warns that synthetic biology is a threat to the concept of "natural" that has guided moral thinking about the environment in North America.

On May 20, 2010, the Craig J. Venter Institute announced that it had engineered the "first self-replicating synthetic bacterial cell." This achievement was described in some media reports as "creating life" or "playing God." Although the achievement was indeed significant, it did not create human or animal life. It built new cellular life-form in the laboratory by assembling and programming blocks of genes, chromosomes, and proteins ("biobricks") so that the microorganism could give instructions that control the cell's function. The Venter Institute's self-replicating cell involved the complete replacement of genetic material, including more than one million base pairs of DNA and almost 1,000 genes.

Unlike genetic engineering, which modifies biological systems by combining existing genes, synthetic biology (sometimes called "synbio") engineers new systems, which may have never existed before. Synthetic biology begins in the computer, not in nature. As Joachim Boldt and Oliver Müller from Freiburg University explain, "If we look at nature through the glasses of genetic engineering, we see a world filled with entities that are already useful to us in many respects and that just need some reshaping here and there to perfectly match our interests. In contrast, synthetic biology does not soften edges, but creates life-forms that are meant not to have any edges from the start. . . . Nature is a blank space to be filled with whatever we wish." (*Nature Biotechnology,* April 2008, p. 388). These new microorganisms will be designed to serve a specific purpose such as creating new biofuels or clean water. There are potential medical uses as well, such as developing new medications or destroying cancer cells.

The field of synthetic biology has accelerated in recent years because of the increased sophistication and power of genetic sequencing technologies. At the same time, these technologies have become much cheaper. The basic components are readily available.

The introduction of a new technology raises both hopes and fears. While many scientists see enormous possibilities in synthetic biology, others worry about the risk that the engineered cell will escape the laboratory, cause environmental havoc, or be used by terrorists. Other worries are more philosophical—that the very enterprise will somehow imperil other important societal values, such as environmentalism and protection of nature.

This discussion has historical roots. In the early 1970s, when genetic engineering was introduced, the scientists who had developed the ability to splice and combine genes were themselves concerned about the implications, primarily risk to laboratory workers. They agreed on a voluntary moratorium (delay) on conducting the most dangerous experiments and convened a conference at Asilomar in Pacific Grove, California, in 1975 to discuss the potential hazards. They agreed to lift the moratorium but established safety guidelines, including containment standards, and a review system. Over the years, with the benefit of extensive experience, scientists and government agencies have modified the restrictions. One of the current questions is whether existing government oversight for genetic engineering is adequate for synbio.

The selections that follow provide two opposing views of this new technology. Gregory E. Kaebnick, a philosopher and editor, acknowledges the unknowns but concludes on balance that the potential benefits of synthetic biology outweigh the possible risks. Christopher J. Preston, a philosopher and environmentalist, addresses the question of "natural" as it relates to the environment. He fears that the newly created forms depart so radically from the core principle of Darwinian natural selection—descent through modification—that there will be a direct negative impact on environmental ethics.

YES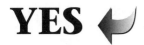

Gregory E. Kaebnick

Prepared Statement before the U.S. House of Representatives Committee on Energy and Commerce

The ethical issues raised by synthetic biology are familiar themes in an ongoing conversation this nation has been having about biotechnologies for several decades. . . .

The concerns fall into two general categories. One has to do with whether the creation of synthetic organisms is a good or a bad thing in and of itself, aside from the consequences. These are thought of as intrinsic concerns. Many people had similar intrinsic concerns about reproductive cloning, for example, they just felt it was wrong to do, regardless of benefits. Another has to do with potential consequences—that is, with risks and benefits. The distinction between these categories can be difficult to maintain in practice, but it provides a useful organizational structure.

Intrinsic Concerns

I will start with the more philosophical, maybe more baffling, kind of concern— the intrinsic concerns. They are an appropriate place to start because the work just published by researchers at Synthetic Genomics, Inc., has been billed as advancing our understanding of these issues in addition to making a scientific advance.

This announcement is not the first time we have had a debate about whether biotechnology challenges deeply held views about the status of life and the power that biotechnology and medicine give us over it. There was a similar debate about gene transfer research in the 1970s and 1980s, about cloning and stem cell research in the 1990s, and—particularly in the last decade but also earlier—about various tools for enhancing human beings. They have been addressed by the President's Commission for the Study of Ethical Problems in Medicine and Biomedical and Behavioral Research in 1983, by President Clinton's National Bioethics Advisory Council, and by President Bush's President's Council on Bioethics. These concerns are related to even older concerns in medicine about decisions to withhold or withdraw medical treatment at the end of life.

The fact that we have had this debate before speaks to its importance. I believe the intrinsic concerns deserve respect, and with some kinds of

U.S. House of Representatives Committee on Energy and Commerce, May 27, 2010 biotechnology I think they are very important, but for synthetic biology, I do not think they provide a basis for decisions about governance.

Religious or Metaphysical Concerns

The classic concern about synthetic biology is that it puts human beings in a role properly held by God—that scientists who do it are "playing God," as people say. Some may also believe that life is sacred, and that scientists are violating its sacredness. Prince Charles had this in mind in a famous polemic some years ago when he lamented that biotechnology was leading to "the industrialisation of Life."

To object to synthetic biology along these lines is to see a serious moral mistake in it. This kind of objection may be grounded in deeply held beliefs about God's goals in creating the world and the proper role of human beings within God's plan. But these views would belong to particular faiths—not everybody would share them. Moreover, there is a range of opinions even within religious traditions about what human beings may and may not do. Some people celebrate human creativity and science. They may see science as a gift from God that God intends human beings to develop and use.

The announcement that Synthetic Genomics, Inc., has created a synthetic cell appears to some to disprove the view that life is sacred, but I do not agree. Arguably, what has been created is a synthetic genome, not a completely synthetic cell. Even if scientists manage to create a fully synthetic cell, however, people who believe that life is sacred, that it is something more than interacting chemicals, could continue to defend that belief. A similar question arises about the existence of souls in cloned people: If people have souls, then surely they would have souls even if they were created in the laboratory by means of cloning techniques. By the same reasoning, if microbial life is more than a combination of chemicals, then even microbial life created in the laboratory would be more than just chemicals. In general, beliefs about the sacredness of life are not undermined by science. Moreover, even the creation of a truly synthetic cell would still start with existing materials. It would not be the kind of creating with which God is credited, which is creating something from nothing—creation ex nihilo.

Concerns that Synthetic Biology Will Undermine Morally Significant Concepts

A related but different kind of concern is that synthetic biology will simply undermine our shared understanding of important moral concepts. For example, perhaps it will lead us to think that life does not have the specialness we have often found in it, or that we humans are more powerful than we have thought in the past. This kind of concern can be expressed without talking about God's plan.

Synthetic biology need not change our understanding of the value of life, however. The fact that living things are created naturally, rather than by people, would be only one reason for seeing them as valuable, and we could continue to see them as valuable when they are created by people. Further, in its current form, synthetic biology is almost exclusively about engineering single-celled organisms, which may be less troubling to people than engineering more complex organisms. If the work is contained within the laboratory and the factory, then it might not end up broadly changing humans' views of the value of life.

Also, of course, the fact that the work challenges our ideas may not really be a moral problem. It would not be the first time that science has challenged our views of life or our place in the cosmos, and we have weathered these challenges in the past.

Concerns about the Human Relationship to Nature

Another way of saying that there's something intrinsically troubling about synthetic biology, again without necessarily talking about the possibility that people are treading on God's turf, is to see it as a kind of environmentalist concern. Many environmentalists want to do more than make the environment good for humans; they also want to save nature from humans—they want to save endangered species, wildernesses, "wild rivers," old-growth forests, and mountains, canyons, and caves, for example. We should approach the natural world, many feel, with a kind of reverence or gratitude, and some worry that synthetic biology—perhaps along with many other kinds of biotechnology—does not square with this value.

Of course, human beings have been altering nature throughout human history. They have been altering ecosystems, affecting the survival of species, affecting the evolution of species, and even creating new species. Most agricultural crop species, for example, are dramatically different from their ancestral forebears. The issue, then, is where to draw the line. Even people who want to preserve nature accept that there is a balance to be struck between saving trees and harvesting them for wood. There might also be a balance when it comes to biotechnology. The misgiving is that synthetic biology goes too far—it takes human control over nature to the ultimate level, where we are not merely altering existing life-forms but creating new forms.

Another environmentalist perspective, however, is that synthetic biology could be developed so that it is beneficial to the environment. Synthetic Genomics, Inc. recently contracted with Exxon Mobil to engineer algae that produce gasoline in ways that not only eliminate some of the usual environmental costs of producing and transporting fuel but simultaneously absorb large amounts of carbon dioxide, thereby offsetting some of the environmental costs of burning fuel (no matter how it is produced). If that could be achieved, many who feel deeply that we should tread more lightly on the natural world might well find synthetic biology attractive. In order to achieve this benefit, however, we must be confident that synthetic organisms will not escape into the environment and cause harms there.

Concerns Involving Consequences

The second category of moral concerns is about consequences—that is, risks and benefits. The promise of synthetic biology includes, for example, better ways of producing medicine, environmentally friendlier ways of producing fuel and other substances, and remediation of past environmental damage. These are not morally trivial considerations. There are also, however, morally serious risks. These, too, fall into three categories.

Concerns about Social Justice

Synthetic biology is sometimes heralded as the start of a new industrial age. Not only will it lead to new products, but it will lead to new modes of production and distribution; instead of pumping oil out of the ground and shipping it around the world, we might be able to produce it from algae in places closer to where it will be used. Inevitably, then, it would have all sorts of large-scale economic and social consequences, some of which could be harmful and unjust. Some commentators hold, for example, that if synthetic biology generates effective ways of producing biofuels from feedstocks such as sugar cane, then farmland in poor countries would be converted from food production to sugar cane production. Another set of concerns arises over the intellectual property rights in synthetic biology. If synthetic biology is the beginning of a new industrial age, and a handful of companies received patents giving them broad control over it, the results could be unjust.

Surely we ought to avoid these consequences. It is my belief that we can do so without avoiding the technology. Also, traditional industrial methods themselves seem to be leading to disastrous long-term social consequences; if so, synthetic biology might provide a way toward better social outcomes.

Concerns about Biosafety

Another concern is about biosafety—about mechanisms for containing and controlling synthetic organisms, both during research and development and in industrial applications. The concern is that organisms will escape, turn out to have properties, at least in their new environment, different from what was intended and predicted, or maybe mutate to acquire them, and then pose a threat to public health, agriculture, or the environment. Alternatively, some of their genes might be transferred to other, wild microbes, producing wild microbes with new properties.

Controlling this risk means controlling the organisms—trying to prevent industrial or laboratory accidents, and then trying to make sure that, when organisms do escape, they are not dangerous. Many synthetic biologists argue that an organism that devotes most of its energy to producing jet fuel or medicine, that is greatly simplified (so that it lacks the genetic complexity and therefore the adaptability of a wild form), and that is designed to work in a controlled, contained environment, will simply be too weak to survive in the wild. For added assurance, perhaps engineering them with failsafe mechanisms will *ensure* that they are incapable of surviving in the wild.

Concerns about Deliberate Misuse

I once heard a well-respected microbiologist say that he was very enthusiastic about synthetic biology, and that the only thing that worries him is the possibility of catastrophe. The kind of thing that worries him is certainly possible.

The 1918 flu virus has been recreated in the laboratory. In 2002, a scientist in New York stitched together stretches of nucleotides to produce a string of DNA that was equivalent to RNA polio virus and eventually produced the RNA virus using the DNA string. More recently, the SARS virus was also created in the laboratory. Eventually, it will almost certainly be possible to recreate bacterial pathogens like smallpox. We might also be able to enhance these pathogens. Some work in Australia on mousepox suggests ways of making smallpox more potent, for example. In theory, entirely new pathogens could be created. Pathogens that target crops or livestock are also possible.

Controlling this risk means controlling the people and companies who have access to DNA synthesis or the tools they could use to synthesize DNA themselves. There are some reasons to think that the worst will never actually happen. To be wielded effectively, destructive synthetic organisms would also have to be weaponized; for example, methods must be found to disperse pathogens in forms that will lead to epidemic infection in the target population while sparing one's own population. Arguably, terrorists have better forms of attacking their enemies than with bioweapons, which are still comparatively hard to make and are very hard to control. However, our policy should amount to more than hoping for the best. . . .

Concluding Comments

I take seriously concerns that synthetic biology is bad in and of itself, and I believe that they warrant a thorough public airing, but I do not believe that they provide a good basis for restraining the technology, at least if we can be confident that the organisms will not lead to environmental damage. Better yet would be to get out in front of the technology and ensure that it benefits the environment. Possibly, some potential applications of synthetic biology are more troubling than others and should be treated differently.

Ultimately, I think the field should be assessed on its possible outcomes. At the moment, we do not understand the possible outcomes well enough. We need, I believe:

- more study of the emergence, plausibility, and impact of potential risks;
- a strategy for studying the risks that is multidisciplinary, rather than one conducted entirely within the field;
- a strategy that is grounded in good science rather than sheer speculation, yet flexible enough to look for the unexpected; and
- an analysis of whether our current regulatory framework is adequate to deal with these risks and how the framework should be augmented.

Different kinds of applications pose different risks and may call for different responses. Microbes intended for release into the environment, for example, would pose a different set of concerns than microbes designed to be kept in specialized, contained settings. Overall, however, while the risks of synthetic biology are too significant to leave the field alone, its potential benefits are too great to call for a general moratorium.

Christopher J. Preston 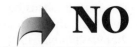 **NO**

Synthetic Biology: Drawing a Line in Darwin's Sand

Introduction

Two years shy of celebrating the 150 year anniversary of the publication *Origin of Species*—a book without which it is hard to imagine either modern biology or modern environmentalism existing in any recognisable form—synthetic biology and nanotechnology threaten to usurp the most important principle of Darwinian natural selection. These emerging technologies strike at the very heart of the distinction between biotic nature and artefact. They create organisms that lack significant connections to the historical evolutionary process. With the threat provided by these technologies looming, those for whom the ideas of 'nature' and the 'historical evolutionary process'comes with any kind of normative punch have some serious self-reflection to do. Many environmental ethicists are about to lose the ground from underneath one of their favourite philosophical ideas. . . .

At Stake for Environmental Ethics

A large number of positions in environmental ethics rest on a substantial normative commitment to the value of what is biologically natural over what is artefactual. In environmental philosophy the term the 'natural' generally prompts some form of moral approbation while objects classed as 'unnatural' or 'artefactual' are viewed more suspiciously. Aldo Leopold introduced his landmark Sand County Almanac with a request for a re-appraisal of things 'unnatural, tame, and confined' in terms of things 'wild, natural, and free' (Leopold, 1949: ix). Contemporary environmental ethicist Holmes Rolston, III, captured a similar sentiment in his statement that '[m]y concept of the good is not coextensive with the natural, but it does greatly overlap it', adding '[N]o one has learned the full scope of what it means to be moral until he has learned to respect the integrity and worth of those things we call wild' (Rolston, 1986: 49,46). Both theorists point to the fact that the *naturalness* of wild nature carries moral weight.

To sustain this line of thinking, the small matter of how to delimit the natural and mark it off from the non-natural (or artefactual) has always been central to environmental philosophy. Typically, environmental ethicists have

From *Environmental Values*, vol. 17, no. 1, February 2008. Copyright © 2008 by The White Horse Press. Reprinted by permission.

put great stock in the distinction tidily made by Aristotle more than two thousand years ago. Aristotle characterised a natural object in *The Physics* as one which 'has within itself a principle of movement and of stationariness (in respect of place, or of growth and decrease, or by way of alteration)' (192b8-11) (Aristotle, 1941). Any change the object undergoes over time is determined from wholly within that object's nature. Acorns grow into oaks, silverback gorillas grow grey and arthritic, and mountains slowly erode. An artefact, by contrast, lacks 'the source of its own production . . . that principle is in something else external to the thing' (192b28). The external source to which Aristotle refers is the intentional action of a human. Artefacts thus display the presence of human intention. Natural objects do not. Keekok Lee, anchoring a good deal of her work entirely on Aristotle's distinction, usefully summarised the point this way:

> '[T]he natural' . . . refers to whatever exists which is not the result of deliberate human intervention, design, and creation in terms of its material efficient, formal, and final causes . . . The natural comes into existence, continues to exist, and goes out of existence entirely independent of human volition and manipulation . . . [B]y contrast, 'the artefactual' embodies a human intentional structure. (Lee, 1999: 82) . . .

The apparent simplicity of Aristotle's distinction turns out, of course, to be an illusion. The problems inherent in distinguishing the natural from the artefactual have long been known to environmental philosophers. In his 1874 essay 'Nature', John Stuart Mill noticed immediately what appears to be the most central paradox. On the one hand, all human actions are natural because humans have a natural origin and none of their actions transcend natural laws. Yet at the same time, Mill saw how everything a human does, by Aristotle's definition, leaves nature in a non-natural state. . . .

Despite its problems, the idea of nature unmodified by human activity is so central to environmentalism that it is almost impossible to imagine letting it go. Certainly the history of the North American environmental movement could hardly be so abruptly rewritten. The emotional connections run deep. As a matter of political reality, the idea that wild nature is morally significant is one that motivates millions. Images of polar bears prowling arctic ice-flows, humpback whales breaching in front of snow-capped mountains, and lionesses lounging with their young on the African savannah adorn the walls of bedrooms and boardrooms across the world. Denying the moral significance of the biologically natural is almost inconceivable for environmentalists.

In addition to the politics of the matter, there are also important non-pragmatic reasons to retain the Aristotelian idea of 'nature'. Nature unmodified by human intention may be increasingly hard to find today but, as a matter of historical fact, there were close to 4.6 billion years of geological history on Earth that preceded the arrival of our first, artefact-creating ancestor, *Homo habilis*, approximately 2 million years ago. During these 4.598 billion years of earth's history there were independent processes at work ultimately responsible for creating everything environmentalists find of value today. For 4.598 billion years, there really did exist—as a matter of historical fact—something one could call 'nature' in an unproblematically Aristotelian sense.

For almost 80 per cent of that long reach of time, there was also something one could call the 'natural historical evolutionary process' slowly working its effects on living beings. As Charles Darwin explained in 1859, natural variations appearing in successive generations of biological organisms would tend to be preserved if those variations provided survival and breeding advantage. Over the millions of years of evolutionary history before the arrival of early hominids, Darwinian processes were responsible for creating great biological diversity and complexity, progenitors of the same diversity and complexity environmentalists seek to preserve today. It is for good reason that many environmental philosophers think this historical process morally important. Part of the reason we protect wildlands, claims Holmes Rolston, III, is that they provide 'the profoundest historical museum of all, a relic of the way the world was during 99.9% of past time' (Rolston, 1988: 14). Eugene Hargrove, pushing a quite different aesthetics-based approach to environmental protection, also suggests 'nature aesthetically is not simply what exists at this point in time; it is also the entire series of events and undertakings that have brought it to that point. When we admire nature, we also admire that history' (Hargrove, 1989: 195). This blending of historical fact and normative overlay is why the idea of non-humanised nature, despite the objections of Steven Vogel and the gloomy outlook of Bill McKibben, still serves a valuable purpose. The pertinent question to ask is how today's environmentalist might effectively use Aristotle's distinction between nature and artefact in the light of its numerous acknowledged problems. . . .

The Last Stand for Aristotle's Distinction

Synthetic biologists assemble short DNA sequences with known properties to create synthetic organisms that perform desirable functions. The self-appointed task of a synthetic biologist is to 'create living systems from the scratch and then endow these systems with new and novel functions' (Chopra and Kamma, 2006). The products of the technology potentially include drugs for medical applications, vehicles for targeted drug delivery, biosensors to detect and neutralise contamination in the environment, biotic components for information technology applications, new biodegradable materials, and the environmentally sensitive generation of methane or ethanol for energy projects. Due to the scale at which this work is carried out, some synthetic biologists call the technique 'natural nanotechnology'.

These are still relatively early days for the research. Nevertheless, Israeli scientists have engineered DNA to carry out basic mathematical functions that could theoretically be integrated into functioning computers. A Princeton University team has made an artificial organism within an *E. coli* bacterium that blinked predictably. Both teams in effect designed a biological machine to perform a chosen function, with the product of their efforts located entirely within a living cell. This form of engineering seems to successfully blur the line between a living biological organism and a purpose-built machine.

One of the major preliminary tasks for synthetic biologists is to isolate the properties of particular DNA sequences so that those sequences might be used as 'bio-bricks' to build future synthetic organisms. MIT has set up a Registry of Standard Biological Parts in order to catalogue these bio-bricks. This element of synthetic biology is sometimes characterised in terms of the bioscientific project of 'understanding life'. But the project of gaining more knowledge about living systems takes on a different hue when bio-bricks are used to engineer functional synthetic bio-systems. In these endeavours, synthetic biology is more appropriately characterised as the engineering of life (Endy, 2005). The goal of redesigning life using engineering principles is the true framework under which synthetic biology operates.

Environmental ethicists have long recognised that not all biological organisms are created equal. Most agree that there is a significant moral difference between wild genomes and genomes influenced by conscious human intention. Nineteenth century environmental advocate John Muir was one of the first to take up this point when he decried the artificially created stupidity of domestic sheep, famously calling them the 'hooved locusts' of the High Sierra. Contemporary environmental philosopher J. Baird Callicott, thinking along similar lines, categorises domestic animals as 'living artefacts' constituting 'yet another mode of extension of the works of man into the ecosystem' (Callicott, 1980: 330). Callicott's attack against biological organisms that are not 'wild, natural, and free' is even more vitriolic than Muir's. 'From the perspective of the land ethic', Callicott has insisted, 'a herd of cattle, sheep, or pigs is as much or more a ruinous blight on the landscape as a fleet of four-wheel drive off-road vehicles' (Callicott, 1980: 330). But however much both these theorists condemn domestic animals as 'biotic artefacts', the products of future synthetic biology will reach a whole new level of artificity.

One of Keekok Lee's main objections to molecular nanotechnology was its ability to 'construct *de novo* synthetic, abiotic kinds, from the design board' (Lee, 1999: 118). Synthetic biologists do exactly this but with biotic, rather than abiotic, kinds. The rhetoric used by synthetic biologists reveals just how ambitious are their construction projects. 'Think of it as Life, version 2.0' suggested the author of an article in *Scientific American* in 2004. The side-stepping manoeuvre synthetic biology makes around the historical evolutionary process is unique. Craig Venter, a synthetic biologist who earlier headed the consortium that mapped the human genome, is described as desiring to 'short-circuit millions of years of evolution and create his own version of a second genesis'. Other researchers share the goal of replacing evolution with something better. 'It will be a marvelous challenge to see if we can outdesign evolution' offered George Whitesides (2001).

Statements such as these bring out the difference between synthetic biology and traditional biotechnology. The relevant difference is that traditional biotechnology has always started with the genome of an existing organism and modified it by deleting or adding genes. The biologist has always taken a viable organism and made a selective change, hoping in the process not to modify the existing organism to such a degree that it is no longer able to survive. In every case of traditional biotechnology—even in the case of transgenic organisms—the genome on which the modification takes place is either the product of natural evolutionary processes or is the descendent of such a product. In every case in traditional biotechnology, there exists prior to the modification a viable organism on which the manipulation takes place.

This is not the case in synthetic biology. Synthetic biology does not start with a viable genome and modify it. It starts afresh with bio-bricks possessing known properties. There is no existing genome that undergoes modification. In the current state of the technology, the synthetically engineered DNA sequences have all been inserted into existing single-celled organisms. The idea, however, is not to preserve properties of the existing bacteria with modified behaviour. It is to create an entirely new organism with DNA constructed in its entirety according to human plan. The products of synthetic biology do not borrow any genetic function from genomes produced by the historical evolutionary process. To the contrary, synthetic biology is guided by the idea of leaving evolution and existing genomes behind in order to do a better job of creation with human goals in mind.

There are a number of familiar prudential worries that immediately arise with synthetic biology. Environmentalists might be concerned about risks that range from bioterrorism to the havoc such synthetic organisms might potentially wreak on the natural world. Synthetic biologists themselves already recognise this latter worry. The Venter Institute in California states on its website that '[T]he group has long been committed to fully exploring and educating the public about the ethical issues surrounding synthetic life. As such the team is dedicated to developing only synthetic organisms that completely lack the ability to survive outside the lab.' Steve Benner, a synthetic biology pioneer at the University of Florida, tries to create similar reassurance with his claim that the more different an artificial system is from a natural biological system, the less likely it is to survive in the wild. But in addition to the important prudential arguments, it seems there is also a clear basis for a deontological argument against synthetic biology.

In a famous article against the coupling of nanotechnology with biotechnology in *Wired Magazine* in 2000, Bill Joy, founder of Sun Microsystems, came close to articulating the problem. Joy claimed that future bio-nano technologies will cross a fundamental line when they allow the 'replicating and evolving processes that have been confined to the natural world . . . to become realms of human endeavor' (Joy, 2000). Joy's worry can be refined to apply to synthetic biology. Arteficity is again the problem. But the reason that the arteficity in synthetic biology is particularly worrisome is that it is a kind of arteficity that departs from the fundamental principle of Darwinian evolution, namely, descent through modification.

Charles Darwin himself, when searching for clues as to how the transmutation of species occurred in nature, spent many hours amongst dog and pigeon breeders admiring what these breeders had created using selective breeding techniques. His comfort level in this company is revealing. Darwin appreciated that when an experimenter modifies an existing genome through selective breeding he or she is doing much the same thing as natural selection has been doing continuously for over 3 billion years. In fact, it was because these breeders were doing something so similar to natural selection that Darwin was able to gain important insights he incorporated into his emerging theory.

Since natural selection works by taking an existing viable genome and modifying it incrementally, it seems plausible to characterise many previous types of biotechnology the same way. We might accept selective breeding, hybridisation and genetic technologies on the basis that they, like natural selection, work with the fundamental principle of descent through modification. They take existing genomes and modify them, even though they do it intentionally rather than randomly. All late twentieth century molecular biotechnology, including (perhaps rather surprisingly) the creation of transgenic organisms, follows this basic pattern. Viable genomes are modified with humans in laboratories now playing an integral role in making it happen. Clearly the modifications are not as incremental as they were in the case of pigeon breeding. Many of today's modifications would likely never have happened through natural selection or selective breeding. Nevertheless the biotechnology of the late twentieth century might charitably be recognised to retain the essence of Darwinian descent through modification.

As a result of retaining this Darwinian essence, genetically modified organisms possess a continuous causal chain between the genome currently being manipulated and the historical evolutionary process. At every point in this chain, there has existed a viable organism. This is true even if the organism being modified is itself the product or selective breeding or is transgenic. No product of twentieth century biotechnology has ever lacked this causal connection to the historical evolutionary past. Before synthetic biology, every organism had ancestors connecting it to the historical processes environmentalists value.

When a synthetic biologist creates a genome from scratch, by contrast, building organisms *de novo* from bio-bricks, causal continuity with the historical evolutionary past has been severed. With synthetic biology, all trace of descent from naturally selected ancestors has been eliminated. Though they still contain the nucleic acids, the biotic artefacts created by synthetic biology borrow none of their genetic sequencing from viable products of the historical evolutionary process. A genome built from bio-bricks is as complete an artefact as any biological organism can be. This makes it possible to offer an argument that accepts hybridisation, selective breeding and late twentieth century genetic biotechnology but rejects synthetic biology. The argument hinges on the fact that synthetic biology creates a more fundamental type of biotic artefact.

The heart of this argument against synthetic biology is consistent with the worries articulated by Keekok Lee but finds them realised in a different place. Lee argued, correctly it seems, that 'the supercession of natural evolution' (Lee, 2003: 190-3) is a serious worry for environmentalists. But the supercession of natural evolution does not occur, as Lee had suggested, when humans take a genome created through natural processes and modify it. Nor does it occur when humans take a modified genome and modify *that*. It occurs when humans create new genomes from scratch. In the former cases, there remains in place a chain of viable organisms connecting the latest modification to the 3.6 billion years of the natural evolutionary process. This causal connection remains even when the last few steps in the chain have involved the active manipulation of the genome by humans. Lee was right about unnaturalness being the problem, but she drew the line in the wrong place. Contra Lee, humans do not usurp the historical evolutionary process when they simply modify an existing genome. In certain senses, by doing this humans are doing to biological organisms exactly what evolution has 'done' to them over natural history, namely, descent through modification.

But in the case of a bacterium with its DNA created through synthetic biology, there is no causal chain of viable organisms connecting the synthetic organism with the historical evolutionary process. As Lee suggested was the problem with molecular nanotechnology, synthetic biologists create biotic kinds *de novo*. It is this creation of organisms *de novo* that makes synthetic biology different from previous biotechnologies. . . .

References

Aristotle. [1941]. *Physics,* trans. R.P. Hardie and R.K. Gaye. New York: Random House.

Callicott, J. Baird. 1980. 'Animal liberation: A triangular affair'. *Environmental Ethics* **2**: 311–338.

Chopra, Paras and Akhil Kamma. 2006. 'Engineering life through Synthetic Biology'. *In Silico Biology* **6**, 0038.

Darwin, Charles, 1898. *The Origin of Species, By Means of Natural Selection,* Vol. 1. New York: Appleton and Company.

Endy, D. 2005. 'Foundations of engineering biology'. *Nature* **438**: 449–453, doi: 10.1038/nature04342.

Hargrove, Eugene. 1989. *The Foundations of Environmental Ethics.* Englewood Cliffs, NJ: Prentice Hall.

Joy, Bill. 200. 'Why the future does not need us'. *Wired Magazine* **8**(4). http://www.wired.com/wired/archive/8.04/joy.html (accessed 30 Aug 2007).

Lee, Keekok. 1999. *The Natural and the Artifactual: The Implications of Deep Science and Deep Technology for Environmental Philosophy.* New York: Lexington Books.

Lee, Keekok. 2003. *Philosophy and Revolutions in Genetics: Deep Science and Deep Technology.* Basingstoke: Palgrave MacMillan.

Leopold, Aldo. 1949. *A Sand County Almanac.* New York: Oxford University Press.

Rolston, Holmes, III. 1986. 'Can we and ought we to follow nature?' in Holmes Rolston, III, *Philosophy Gone Wild* (Buffalo, NY: Prometheus), pp. 30–52.

Rolston, Holmes, III. 1988. *Environmental Ethics: Duties to and Values in the Natural World.* Philadelphia, PA: Temple University Press.

Whitesides, George. 2001. 'The once and future nanomachine'. *Scientific American* (Sept).

POSTSCRIPT

Do the Potential Benefits of Synthetic Biology Outweigh the Possible Risks?

Much of the literature on synthetic biology is highly technical. As the debate about government oversight continues, there will be more general material, most of it available online.

The ethical issues around synthetic biology were on the agenda for the first two meetings of the President's Commission for the Study of Bioethical Issues. Transcripts from the meetings are available at http://www.bioethics.gov/.

For further reading on synthetic biology, Jonathan B. Tucker and Raymon A. Zilinskas, "The Promise and Perils of Synthetic Biology," *The New Atlantis,* is a good summary and also has a good reading list. It is available at http://www.thenewatlantis.com/publications/the-promise-and-perils-of-synthetic-biology.

Jonathan D. Moreno offers an optimistic view of synthetic biology in "Synthetic Biology Grows Up" (*Science Progress,* May 20, 2010), which is available at http://www.scienceprogress.org/2010/05/synthetic-biology-grows-up.

The Boldt and Müller article cited in the Introduction is titled "Newtons of the Leaves of Grass," *Nature Biotechnology* (April 2008).

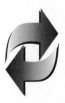

Internet References . . .

Office for Human Research Protections (OHRP)

OHRP is the government agency charged with protecting the welfare and rights of human research subjects. Its Web site contains regulations and other information on research, including prisoners.

http://www.hhs.gov/ohrp/

Tufts Center for the Study of Drug Development

This center compiles information about new drugs and the FDA approval process.

http://csdd.tufts.edu/

Human Experimentation

*T*he goal of scientific research is knowledge that will benefit society. But achieving that goal may subject humans and animals to some risks. Questions arise about not only how research should be conducted but whether or not it should be conducted at all. What, for example, are the justifications for using prisoners in research? This section contends with issues that will shape the future of experimental science.

- Should New Drugs Be Given to Patients Outside Clinical Trials?
- Does Community Consultation in Research Protect Vulnerable Groups?

ISSUE 14

Should New Drugs Be Given to Patients Outside Clinical Trials?

YES: Emil J. Freireich, from "Should Terminally Ill Patients Have the Right to Take Drugs that Pass Phase I Testing?" *British Medical Journal* (September 8, 2007)

NO: George J. Annas, from "Cancer and the Constitution—Choice at Life's End," *The New England Journal of Medicine* (July 26, 2007)

ISSUE SUMMARY

YES: Physician Emil J. Freireich believes that patients with advanced cancer and limited life expectancy should have the same privilege as all individuals in a free society.

NO: Law professor George J. Annas argues that there is no constitutional right to demand experimental interventions, and that fully open access would undermine the FDA's ability to protect the public from unsafe drugs.

At the beginning of the twentieth century, any American could manufacture a medication and sell it to the public. The era of "patent medicines" led at best to harmless but useless "cure-alls," and at worst, to illness and death. Alarmed by this practice, in 1906 the U.S. Congress enacted the Food and Drug Act, prohibiting the sale of misbranded, mislabeled, and adulterated foods and drugs in interstate commerce. In 1938, more than 100 people died as a result of taking elixir sulfanilamide, a powder that had been made into a liquid form by adding diethylene glycol, a poison used in antifreeze. In response, Congress created the Food and Drug Administration (FDA) to prevent future tragedies.

Under the current rules, drug manufacturers must submit "investigational new drug" applications to the agency and provide evidence of their safety and effectiveness before they can bring new drugs to the market. In general, drug trials involve stages of testing and data are collected from small, carefully selected groups, analyzed, and then tested in wider populations. Phase I includes a small number of patients and is designed to determine levels of toxicity (bad reactions). This process is costly and can take considerable time.

Over the years, the FDA has been criticized on grounds that it allows unsafe drugs to be marketed to the public, and in recent years several drugs have been taken off the market. It has also been criticized for its slow review process because of which promising new drugs are unavailable to people who desperately need them. In the 1980s and 1990s, HIV/AIDS activists in particular lobbied for faster access to drugs, and the FDA responded with a plan to allow access to some experimental drugs for patients with serious diseases and no other therapeutic options.

But for many people facing death, the FDA does not go far enough. They want to be able to take drugs that are in early stages of development and without being enrolled in a clinical trial, for which they may not be eligible. The Abigail Alliance, founded in 2001 by Frank Burroughs, is one of the most prominent advocates of this position. Mr. Burroughs' daughter Abigail died that year from cancer of the head and neck. He had tried unsuccessfully to obtain two drugs that were then in clinical trials, although not for her type of cancer. (One of the drugs has since been approved for that indication.) Abigail was not eligible for the clinical trials because as Mr. Burroughs said, "She had the right cells in the wrong place."

In 2003, the Alliance sued the FDA in federal district court, claiming that the agency's failure to permit the sale of investigational new drugs to terminally ill patients violated the patients' rights to privacy and due process under the Fifth Amendment of the U.S. Constitution. The three-judge panel on the first court to hear the case agreed that there was a constitutional right to such access, but 15 months later this decision was reversed by the District of Columbia Circuit Court of Appeals. In January 2008, the U.S. Supreme Court declined to hear the case.

The following selections take different views of the basic issue. Physician Emil J. Freireich asserts that dying individuals for whom all approved medications have failed should have the right to take drugs still in the investigational stage. Law professor George J. Annas believes that access to unproven drugs has to be limited to protect the public.

YES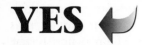

Emil J. Freireich

Should Terminally Ill Patients Have the Right to Take Drugs That Pass Phase I Testing?

Around half a million people will die from cancer-related causes in the United States this year. In the US, as in much of the Western world, patients know their diagnosis and are often given a hopeless prognosis. For most, the option of participating in phase I and phase II clinical trials of new drugs that offer some promise helps them remain optimistic. Clearly, they should have the right to take drugs that have passed phase I testing.

The problem is that most cancer patients cannot participate in phase II trials because they are either ineligible or they are unable to fulfil the financial and social requirements for participating in such trials, such as staying in the centres conducting these trials, sometimes for many weeks or months. The problem is clearly not one of safety because these drugs have completed phase I clinical trials and there is sufficient information about them to justify a phase II trial to determine efficacy.

Phase II trials are designed to give the highest probability of a positive outcome. Thus, they have patient eligibility requirements which assure that only the healthiest patients at the earliest point in their disease are entered. These decisions are not based on any reasonable evidence that patients who are ineligible would not benefit, but are strictly designed to fulfil the regulatory requirements established by bodies such as the Food and Drug Administration (FDA) and the regulatory components of industry and academia that govern these clinical trials.

Compassionate Prescribing

In the modern electronic era, most of the patients with hopeless cancer diagnoses have access through the media and the internet to information about promising new drugs that are in phase II clinical trials. These patients would like very much to receive these drugs to offer them some hope, but for the reasons mentioned above are unable to participate in those trials. So why not offer these drugs to these patients on a compassionate basis?

The first reason given is usually the safety concerns. Without knowledge about how renal function, cardiac function, age, etc. affect the action of the

From *British Medical Journal*, September 8, 2007, vol. 335, pp. 335. Copyright © 335 by BMJ Publishing Group. Reprinted by permission via Rightslink.

phase I drug, side effects might occur that could be harmful to the patient or, perhaps more importantly, the continued development of the drug. I think this objection is relatively minor since it simply states the benefit:risk ratio problem—that is, these patients are prepared to volunteer to expose themselves to increased risk because of their hopeless prognosis and because of the promise of the new drug.

The second objection is that it will interfere with the development of the drug. However, in the past, the FDA and the National Cancer Institute have allowed compassionate use of drugs and have found that it actually accelerates development. This is because when patients are offered compassionate use of an experimental drug, their doctors have to collect information as systematically as in the research protocol and submit it to the sponsor. Information is therefore available about use of the drug outside trial conditions. For example, if patients with impaired renal function not only tolerate the drug but respond, it will assist in drug development to have that knowledge collected systematically.

Drug Industry Profits

Another objection is that the drug industry might use this device to profit from investigation of a phase I drug. I believe this is a trivial objection because the usual strategy for compassionate use is that the drug is provided at cost. The last, and perhaps the most serious, objection is that expanded access would interfere with the clinical trial process. This certainly should not be the case. The clinical trial process is governed by the regulatory bodies in government, in industry, and in academic institutions. The unfortunate consequence of this is that physician scientists, who have the most experience, the most training, the most knowledge, the most productivity, and the most creativity, are completely excluded from this process. Because of the relationship between the regulatory organisations of government, industry, and academia, the academic physician scientist can only implement protocols that have been developed by the drug developer with direction from the regulatory agencies. Expanded access would bring the doctors back into the drug development process and, rather than damage the clinical trial system, would greatly expand its effectiveness and value.

In summary, patients with advanced cancer and limited life expectancy should have the same privilege as all individuals in a free society—that is, to decide their own benefit:risk ratio. It is tragic that regulatory bodies have created a circumstance where people have to live in an aura of hopelessness even though they have the will, the resources, and the ability to expose themselves to the risk of participating in investigational studies and to enjoy the potential for benefit. The solution is legislation or judicial action to permit expanded access to experimental treatments for patients with limited life expectancy.

George J. Annas 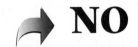 **NO**

Cancer and the Constitution— Choice at Life's End

J.M. Coetzee's violent, anti-apartheid *Age of Iron,* a novel the *Wall Street Journal* termed "a fierce pageant of modern South Africa," is written as a letter by a retired classics professor, Mrs. Curren, to her daughter, who lives in the United States. Mrs. Curren is dying of cancer, and her daughter advises her to come to the United States for treatment. She replies, "I can't afford to die in America. . . . No one can, except Americans."[1] Dying of cancer has been considered a "hard death" for at least a century, unproven and even quack remedies have been common, and price has been a secondary consideration. Efforts sponsored by the federal government to find cures for cancer date from the establishment of the National Cancer Institute (NCI) in 1937. Cancer research was intensified after President Richard Nixon's declaration of a "war on cancer" and passage of the National Cancer Act of 1971.[2] Most recently, calls for more cancer research have followed the announcement by Elizabeth Edwards, wife of presidential candidate John Edwards, that her cancer is no longer considered curable.

Frustration with the methods and slow progress of mainstream medical research has helped fuel a resistance movement that distrusts both conventional medicine and government and that has called for the recognition of a right for terminally ill patients with cancer to have access to any drugs they want to take. Prominent examples include the popularity of Krebiozen in the 1950s and of laetrile in the 1970s. As an NCI spokesperson put it more than 20 years ago, when thousands of people were calling the NCI hotline pleading for access to interleukin-2, "What the callers are saying is, 'Our mother, our brother, our sister is dying at this very moment. We have nothing to lose.'"[2] Today, families search the Internet for clinical trials, and even untested chemicals such as dichloroacetate, that seem to offer them some hope. In addition, basing advocacy on their personal experiences with cancer, many families have focused their frustrations on the Food and Drug Administration (FDA), which they see as a government agency denying them access to treatments they need.

In May 2006 these families won an apparent major victory when the Court of Appeals for the District of Columbia, in the case of *Abigail Alliance v. Von Eschenbach* (hereafter referred to as *Abigail Alliance*),[3] agreed with their argument that patients with cancer have a constitutional right of access to

From *The New England Journal of Medicine,* vol. 357, no. 4, July 26, 2007, pp. 408–413. Copyright © 2007 by Massachusetts Medical Society. All rights reserved. Reprinted by permission.

investigational cancer drugs. In reaction, the FDA began the process of rewriting its own regulations to make it easier for terminally ill patients not enrolled in clinical trials to have access to investigational drugs.[4] In November 2006, the full bench of the Court of Appeals vacated the May 2006 opinion, and the case was reheard in March 2007.[5] The decision of the full bench, expected by the fall, will hinge on the answer to a central question: Do terminally ill adult patients with cancer for whom there are no effective treatments have a constitutional right of access to investigational drugs their physicians think might be beneficial?

The Constitutional Controversy

The Abigail Alliance for Better Access to Developmental Drugs (hereafter called the Abigail Alliance) sued the FDA to prevent it from enforcing its policy of prohibiting the sale of drugs that had not been proved safe and effective to competent adult patients who are terminally ill and have no alternative treatment options. The Abigail Alliance is named after Abigail Burroughs, whose squamous-cell carcinoma of the head and neck was diagnosed when she was only 19 years old. Two years later, in 2001, she died. Before her death she had tried unsuccessfully to obtain investigational drugs on a compassionate use basis from ImClone and AstraZeneca and was accepted for a clinical trial only shortly before her death. Her father founded the Abigail Alliance in her memory.[6]

The district court dismissed the Abigail Alliance lawsuit. The appeals court, in a two-to-one opinion written by Judge Judith Rogers, who was joined by Judge Douglas Ginsburg, reversed the decision. It concluded that competent, terminally ill adult patients have a constitutional "right to access to potentially life-saving post-Phase I investigational new drugs, upon a doctor's advice, even where that medicine carries risks for the patient," and remanded the case to the district court to determine whether the FDA's current policy violated that right.[3]

The Right to Life

The appeals court found that the relevant constitutional right was determined by the due-process clause of the Fifth Amendment: "no person shall be . . . deprived of life, liberty, or property without due process of law." In the court's words, the narrow question presented by *Abigail Alliance* is whether the due-process clause "protects the right of terminally ill patients to make an informed decision that may prolong life, specifically by use of potentially life-saving new drugs that the FDA has yet to approve for commercial marketing but that the FDA has determined, after Phase I clinical human trials, are safe enough for further testing on a substantial number of human beings."[3]

The court answered yes, finding that this right has deep legal roots in the right to self-defense, and that "Barring a terminally ill patient from the use of a potentially life-saving treatment impinges on this right of self-preservation."[3] In a footnote, the court restated this proposition: "The fundamental right to take action, even risky action, free from government interference, in order to save one's own life undergirds the court's decision."[3] The court relied primarily on the *Cruzan* case,[7] in which the Supreme Court recognized the right of a competent adult to refuse life-sustaining treatment, including a feeding tube:

> The logical corollary is that an individual must also be free to decide for herself whether to assume any known or unknown risks of taking a medication that might prolong her life. Like the right claimed in *Cruzan*, the right claimed by the [Abigail] Alliance to be free of FDA imposition does not involve treatment by the government or a government subsidy. Rather, much as the guardians of the comatose [sic] patient in Cruzan did, the Alliance seeks to have the government step aside by changing its policy so the individual right of self-determination is not violated.[3]

The appeals court concluded that the Supreme Court's 1979 unanimous decision on laetrile,[8] in which the Court concluded that Congress had made no exceptions in the FDA law for terminally ill cancer patients, was not relevant because laetrile had never been studied in a phase 1 trial and because the Court did not address the question of whether terminally ill cancer patients have a constitutional right to take whatever drugs their physicians prescribe.

The Dissent

Judge Thomas Griffith, the dissenting judge, argued that the suggested constitutional right simply does not exist. He noted, for example, that the self-defense cases relied on are examples of "abstract concepts of personal autonomy," and cannot be used to craft new rights. As to the nation's history and traditions, he concluded that the FDA's drug-regulatory efforts have been reasonable responses "to new risks as they are presented."[3] Accepting his argument leaves the majority resting squarely on *Cruzan* and the laetrile case. As to *Cruzan*, the dissent argued that "A tradition of protecting individual *freedom* from life-saving, but forced, medical treatment does not evidence a constitutional tradition of providing affirmative *access* to a potentially harmful, even fatal, commercial good."[3] As to the laetrile case, the judge noted simply that the Court had agreed with the FDA that, "For the terminally ill, as for anyone else, a drug is unsafe if its potential for inflicting death or physical injury is not offset by the possibility of therapeutic benefit."[3, 8]

Finally, the dissenting judge argued that if the new constitutional right were accepted, it was too vague to be applied only to terminally ill patients seeking drugs that had been tested in phase 1 trials. Specifically, the judge asked, must the right also apply to patients with "serious medical conditions," to patients who "cannot afford potentially life-saving treatment," or to patients whose physicians believe "marijuana for medicinal purposes . . . is potentially life saving?"[3] In other words, there is no principled reason to restrict the constitutional right the majority created to either terminally ill patients or to post–phase 1 drugs.

Discussion

The facts as illustrated by stories of patients dying of cancer while trying unsuccessfully to enroll in clinical trials are compelling, and our current system of ad hoc exceptions is deeply flawed. The central constitutional issue, however, rests primarily on determining whether this case is or is not like the right-to-refuse-treatment case of Nancy Cruzan, a woman in a permanent vegetative state whose family wanted tube feeding discontinued because they believed that discontinuation was what she would have wanted. I do not think *Abigail Alliance* is like *Cruzan*. Rather, it is substantially identical to cases involving physician-assisted suicide, in which a terminally ill patient claims a constitutional right of access to physician-prescribed drugs to commit suicide.

The Supreme Court has decided, unanimously, that no right to physician-prescribed drugs for suicide exists.[9, 10] There is no historical tradition of support for this right. And although the right seems to be narrowly defined, it is unclear to whom it should apply—why only to terminally ill patients? Don't patients in chronic pain have even a stronger interest in suicide? Why is the physician necessary, and why are physician-prescribed drugs the only acceptable method of suicide? None of these questions can be answered by examining the Constitution.[11]

Similarly, in *Abigail Alliance*, the new constitutional right proposed has no tradition in the United States, and it cannot be narrowly applied. For example, why should a constitutional right apply only to people who have a particular medical status? And why should a physician be involved at all? If patients have a right to autonomy, why isn't the requirement of a government-licensed physician's recommendation at least as burdensome as the requirement of the FDA's approval of the investigational drug? And why would the Constitution apply only to investigational drugs for which phase 1 trials have been completed? Why not include access to investigational medical devices, like the artificial heart, or even to Schedule I controlled substances, like marijuana or lysergic acid diethylamide (LSD)? If it is a constitutional right, these should be available too, at least unless the state can demonstrate a "compelling interest" in regulating them.

My prediction is that after rehearing this case en banc, the full Circuit Court will reject the position of the Abigail Alliance for the same reasons that the Supreme Court rejected the "right" of terminally ill patients to have access to physician-prescribed drugs they could use to end their lives.[9, 11] To decide otherwise would entirely undermine the legitimacy of the FDA. Patients in the United States have always had a right to refuse any medical treatment, but we have never had a right to demand mistreatment, inappropriate treatment, or even investigational or experimental interventions. This will not, however, be the end of the matter. After the physician-assisted–suicide cases, the fight appropriately shifted to the states, although so far only one, Oregon, has provided its physicians with immunity for prescribing life-ending drugs to their competent, terminally ill patients.[12] In the Abigail Alliance case, the debate will continue in the forum in which it began—the FDA—and in Congress.

Congress

Congressional action also had its birth with the story of one patient with cancer and was also heavily influenced by another individual patient involved in a controversy over removal of a feeding tube. "Terri's Law" was enacted in Florida in 2003 to try to prevent the removal of a feeding tube from Terri Schiavo; the case was substantially similar to *Cruzan*. Terri's case gained national attention 2 years later.[13] In the midst of it, in March 2005, the *Wall Street Journal* asserted, in an editorial titled "How About a 'Kianna's Law'?," "If Terri Schiavo deserves emergency federal intervention to save her life, people like Kianna Karnes deserve it even more."[14] At the time, Kianna Karnes was a 44-year-old mother of four who was dying of kidney cancer. Her only hope of survival, according to the editorial, was to gain access to one of two experimental drugs in clinical trials, but neither of the two companies running the trials (Bayer and Pfizer) would make the drugs available to her on a compassionate-use basis. This was because, according to the *Wall Street Journal*, the FDA "makes it all but impossible" for the manufacturers "to provide [drugs] to terminal patients on a 'compassionate use' basis."[14]

Almost immediately after the editorial was published, both drug manufacturers contacted Kianna's physicians to discuss releasing the drugs to her. But within 2 days after publication, she was dead. The *Wall Street Journal* editorialized, "Isn't it a national scandal that cancer sufferers should have to be written about in the *Wall Street Journal* to be offered legal access to emerging therapies once they've run out of other options?"[15] It noted that Mrs. Karnes' father, John Rowe—himself a survivor of leukemia—was working with the Abigail Alliance on a "Kianna's Law." That law, formally titled the "Access, Compassion, Care, and Ethics for Seriously Ill Patients Act" or the "ACCESS Act," was introduced in November 2005 and is an attempt to make it much easier for seriously ill patients to gain access to experimental drugs.[16, 17]

The act begins with a series of congressional findings, including that "Seriously ill patients have a right to access available investigational drugs, biological products, and devices." The act permits the sponsor to apply for approval to make an investigational drug, biologic product, or device available on the basis of data from a completed phase 1 trial, "preliminary evidence that the product may be effective against a serious or life-threatening condition or disease," and an assurance that the clinical trial will continue.[17] The patient, who must have exhausted all approved treatments, must provide written informed consent and must also sign "a written waiver of the right to sue the manufacturer or sponsor of the drug, biological product, or device, or the physicians who prescribed the product or the institution where it was administered, for an adverse event caused by the product, which shall be binding in every State and Federal court."[17]

Although Congress is the proper forum to address this issue, this initial attempt has some of the same problems as the *Abigail Alliance* decision: the patients to whom it applies are ambiguously classified, and clinical research seems to be equated with clinical care. Also troubling is that the patients (and would-be subjects) are asked to assume all of the risks of the uncontrolled experiments, and current rules of research—which protect subjects by prohibiting mandatory waivers of rights—are jettisoned, with the requirement of such waivers becoming the price of obtaining the investigational agent from an otherwise reluctant drug company.

FDA Proposal

In direct response to *Abigail Alliance*, the FDA proposed amending its rules to encourage more drug companies to offer their investigational drugs through compassionate-use programs.[4] These programs first came into prominence during the early days of infection with the human immunodeficiency virus (HIV) and AIDS, when there were no effective treatments and AIDS activists insisted that they have early access to investigational drugs because, in the words of their inaccurate slogan, "A Research Trial Is Treatment Too."[18] Because the FDA could not stand the political pressure generated by the activists, the compassionate-use program was developed as a kind of political safety valve to provide enough exceptions to save their basic research rules. In early December 2006, the FDA continued this political-safety-valve approach by issuing new proposed regulations with a title that could have been taken directly from the AIDS Coalition to Unleash Power (ACT-UP): "Expanded Access to Investigational Drugs for Treatment Use."[19]

The FDA's expanded-access proposal applies to "seriously ill patients when there is no comparable or satisfactory alternative therapy to diagnose, monitor, or treat the patient's disease or condition."[4] Manufacturers are required to file an "expanded access submission," and the product must be administered or dispensed by a licensed physician who will be considered an "investigator," with all the reporting requirements that role entails.[3]

Whether or not the proposal is adopted, it will do little to increase access, since the major bottleneck in the compassionate-use program has never been the FDA. The manufacturers have no incentives to make their investigational products available outside clinical trials. This is because direct access to investigational drugs by individuals may make it more difficult to recruit research subjects, and thus to conduct the clinical trials necessary for drug approval, and could also subject the drug manufacturer to liability for serious adverse reactions. Even without a lawsuit, a serious reaction to a drug outside a trial could adversely affect the trial itself.[4, 16, 20] The drug companies are right to worry that the approaches of the judiciary, Congress, and the FDA will probably make clinical trials more difficult to conduct, because few seriously ill patients who have exhausted conventional treatments would rather be randomly assigned to an investigational drug than have a guarantee that they will receive the investigational drug their physician recommends for them. This could result in significant delays in the approval and overall availability of drugs that demonstrate effectiveness—a result no one favors. Even if patients with cancer are willing buyers, drug manufacturers are not willing sellers.

Physicians and Patients

The cover story for all the proposed changes is patients' choice. But without scientific evidence of the risks and benefits of a drug, choice cannot be informed, and for seriously ill patients, fear of death will predictably overcome fear of unknown risks. This is understandable. As psychiatrist Jay Katz, the leading scholar on informed consent, has noted, when medical science seems impotent to fight nature, "all kinds of senseless interventions are tried in an unconscious effort to cure the incurable magically through a 'wonder drug,' a novel surgical procedure, or a penetrating psychological interpretation."[21] Another *Wall Street Journal* article, entitled "Saying No to Penelope,"[22] illustrates the impossibility of limiting access to unproven cancer drugs to competent adults. The article tells the story of 4-year-old Penelope, who is dying from neuroblastoma that has proved resistant to all conventional treatments. Her parents seek "anything [that] has a prayer of saving her." In her father's words, "The chance of anything bringing her back from the abyss now is very low. But the only thing I know for sure is if we don't treat her, she will die." With Penelope hospitalized and in pain, her parents continue "searching Penelope's big brown eyes for clues as to how long she wants to continue to battle for life."

It is suggested that the requirement of a physician's recommendation can safeguard against "magical thinking" and help make informed consent real.[23] But as Katz has noted, although physicians (and, he could have added, drug companies) often justify such last-ditch interventions as simply being responsive to patient needs, the interventions "may turn out to be a projection of their own needs onto patients."[21]

Government and the Market

Another recurrent theme is the belief that government regulation is evil, a central tenet of the laetrile litigation of the 1970s. The court hearing *Abigail Alliance* was correct to note that laetrile never underwent a phase 1 trial, but every indication was that the drug, also known as vitamin B_{17}, was harmless, albeit also ineffective against cancer. Laetrile became a legal cause celebre in 1972, when California physician John A. Richardson was prosecuted for promoting laetrile. Richardson was a member of the John Birch Society, which quickly formed the Committee for Freedom of Choice in Cancer Therapy, with more than 100 committees nationwide.[24] It took another 7 years before the FDA prevailed in its case against laetrile before the Supreme Court.[8] The basic arguments against FDA regulation remain the same today: the FDA follows a "paternalistic public policy that prevents individuals from exercising their own judgment about risks and benefits. If the FDA must err, it should be on the side of patients' freedom to choose."[25]

Public Policy

The FDA will prevail again today, not only because there is no constitutional right of access to unapproved drugs but also because even if there were, the state has the same compelling interest in approving drugs as it has in licensing physicians. From a public policy view, the *Abigail Alliance* court, the Congress, and the FDA all seem to be suffering from the "therapeutic illusion" in which research, designed to test a hypothesis for society, is confused with treatment, administered in the best interests of individual patients.[21, 26, 27] Of course there is a continuum, and it is perfectly understandable that many patients with cancer, told that there is nothing conventional medicine can do for them, will want access to whatever is available in or outside the context of clinical trials. But this is a problem for patients, physicians, the FDA, and drug manufacturers. First, because terminally ill patients can be harmed and exploited, there are better and worse ways to die.[21, 26] Second, it is only through research, not "treatment," that cancer may become a chronic illness that is treated with a complex array of drugs, given either together or in a progression.[28, 29] The right to choose in medicine is a central right of patients, but the choices can and should be limited to reasonable medical alternatives, which themselves are based on evidence.

This is, I believe, good public policy. But it is also much easier said than done.[30] Death is feared and even dreaded in our culture, and few Americans are able to die at home, at peace, with our loved ones in attendance, without seeking the "latest new treatment." There always seems to be something new to try, and there is almost always anecdotal evidence that it could help. This is one reason that even extremely high prices do not affect demand for cancer drugs, even ones that add little or no survival time.[31, 32] When does caring for the patient demand primary attention to palliation rather than to long-shot, high-risk, investigational interventions? Coetzee's Mrs. Curren, who rejected new medical treatment for her cancer and insisted on dying at home, told her physician, whom she saw as "withdrawing" from her after giving her a terminal prognosis—"His allegiance to the living, not the dying"—"I have no illusions about my condition, doctor. It is not [experimental] care I need, just help with the pain."[1]

References

No potential conflict of interest relevant to this article was reported.

From the Department of Health Law, Bioethics, and Human Rights, Boston University School of Public Health, Boston.

1. Coetzee JM. Age of iron. London: Seeker & Warburg, 1990.

2. Patterson JT. The dread disease: cancer and modern American culture. Cambridge, MA: Harvard University Press, 1987.

3. Abigail Alliance v. Von Eschenbach, 445 F.3d 470 (DC Cir 2006). Vacated 469 F.3d 129 (DC Cir 2006).

4. Proposed rules for charging for investigational drugs and expanded access to investigational drugs for treatment use. Rockville, MD: Food and Drug Administration, 2006. (Accessed July 6, 2007, at http://www.fda.gov/cder/regulatory/applications/IND_PR.htm.)

5. Abigail Alliance v. Von Eschenbach, 429 F.3d 129 (DC Cir 2006).

6. Jacobson PD, Parmet WE. A new era of unapproved drugs: the case of Abigail Alliance v Von Eschenbach. JAMA 2007;297:205–8.

7. Cruzan v. Director, Missouri Dept. of Health, 497 U.S. 261 (1990).

8. United States v. Rutherford, 442 U.S. 544 (1979).

9. Washington v. Glucksberg, 521 U.S. 702 (1997).

10. Vacco v. Quill, 521 U.S. 793 (1997).

11. Annas GJ. The bell tolls for a constitutional right to assisted suicide. N Engl J Med 1997;337:1098–103.

12. Gonzales v. Oregon, 546 U.S. 243 (2006).

13. Annas GJ. "I want to live": medicine betrayed by ideology in the political debate over Terri Schiavo. Stetson Law Rev 2005;35:49–80.

14. How about a "Kianna's Law"? Wall Street Journal. March 24, 2005:A14.

15. Kianna's legacy. Wall Street Journal. March 29, 2005:Al4.

16. Groopman J. The right to a trial: should dying patients have access to experimental drugs? The New Yorker. December 18, 2006:40–7.

17. ACCESS Act (Access, Compassion, Care, and Ethics for Seriously Ill Patients), S. 1956, 109th Cong (2005).

18. Annas GJ. Faith (healing), hope and charity at the FDA: the politics of AIDS drug trials. Villanova Law Rev 1989;34:771–97.

19. FDA proposes rules overhaul to expand availability of experimental drugs: the agency also clarifies permissible charges to patients. Rockville, MD: Food and Drug Administration, December 11, 2006. (Accessed July 6, 2007, at http://www.fda.gov/bbs/topics/NEWS/2006/NEW01520.html.)

20. Prud'homme A. The cell game: Sam Waksal's fast money and false promises—and the fate of ImClone's cancer drug. New York: Harper Business, 2004.

21. Katz J. The silent world of doctor and patient. New Haven, CT: Yale University Press, 1984:151.

22. Anand G. Saying no to Penelope: father seeks experimental cancer drug, but a biotech firm says risk is too high. Wall Street Journal. May 1, 2007:A1.

23. Robertson J. Controversial medical treatment and the right to health care. Hastings Cent Rep 2006;36:15–20.

24. Culbert ML. Vitamin B17: Forbidden weapon against cancer. New Rochelle, NY: Arlington House, 1974.

25. Miller HI. Paternalism costs lives. Wall Street Journal. March 2, 2006:A15.

26. Annas GJ. The changing landscape of human experimentation: Nuremberg, Helsinki, and beyond. Health Matrix J Law Med 1992;2:119–40.

27. Appelbaum PS, Lidz CW. Re-evaluating the therapeutic misconception: response to Miller and Joffe. Kennedy Inst Ethics J 2006;16:367–73.

28. Nathan D. The cancer treatment revolution: how smart drugs and other therapies are renewing our hope and changing the face of medicine. New York: John Wiley, 2007.

29. Brugarolas J. Renal-cell carcinoma—molecular pathways and therapies. N Engl J Med 2007;356:185–6.

30. Callahan D. False hopes: why America's quest for perfect health is a recipe for failure. New York: Simon and Schuster, 1998.

31. Berenson A. Hope, at $4,200 a dose: why a cancer drug's cost doesn't hurt demand. New York Times. October 1, 2006:BU1.

32. Anand G. From Wall Street, a warning about cancer drug prices. Wall Street Journal. March 15, 2007:A1.

POSTSCRIPT

Should New Drugs Be Given to Patients Outside Clinical Trials?

In August 2008, another case involving access to experimental treatment reached the courts. While the appeals court in the Abigail Alliance case determined that there was no constitutional right to experimental drugs, Judge William J. Martini of the United States District Court in Newark ruled that 16-year-old Jacob Gunvalson, suffering from a rare and fatal form of Duchenne muscular dystrophy, should be allowed to use an experimental drug for that condition. Jacob did not meet the criteria for a clinical trial organized by the manufacturer. Jacob's mother claimed that drug company officials had led her to believe that her son would be allowed to take part in a clinical trial, but then refused to accept him. In December 2008, the U.S. Court of Appeals reversed Judge Martini's decision and ruled that PTC Therapeutics did not have to provide the experimental drug to Jacob Gunvalson.

See also Susan Okie, "Access before Approval—A Right to Take Experimental Drugs?," *The New England Journal of Medicine* (August 3, 2006); and Peter D. Jacobson and Wendy E. Parmet, "A New Era of Unapproved Drugs: The Case of *Abigail Alliance v. Von Eschenbach*," *Journal of the American Medical Association* (January 10, 2007). These articles express concerns about unregulated access to experimental drugs.

For opposing views, see Roger Pilon, "New Right to Life," *Wall Street Journal* (August 13, 2007); and A. Puckett, "The Proper Focus for FDA Regulations: Why the Fundamental Right to Self-Preservation Should Allow Terminally Ill Patients with No Treatment Options to Attempt to Save Their Lives," *SMU Law Review* (Spring 2007). Additional information about the Abigail Alliance's activities can be found at http://www.Abigail-Alliance.org. The Alliance supports the Compassionate Access Act of 2010 (H.R. 4732), introduced in March 2010, to create a new conditional approval process for drugs, biologics, and devices for seriously ill patients.

Jerome Groopman addresses the issue and its background in "The Right to a Trial: Should Dying Patients Have Access to Experimental Drugs?," *The New Yorker* (December 18, 2006). This article is available online at http://www.newyorker.com/archives.

ISSUE 15

Does Community Consultation in Research Protect Vulnerable Groups?

YES: Neal Dickert and Jeremy Sugarman, from "Ethical Goals of Community Consultation in Research," *American Journal of Public Health* (July 2005)

NO: Eric T. Juengst, from "Community Engagement in Genetic Research: The 'Slow Code' of Research Ethics?" in Bartha M. Knoppers, ed., *Populations and Genetics: Legal and Socio-Ethical Perspectives* (Koninklijke N.V., 2003)

ISSUE SUMMARY

YES: Neal Dickert and Jeremy Sugarman, physicians and ethicists, propose ethical goals for evaluating community consultation in research, which they believe will protect communities as well as individuals from harm.

NO: Philosopher Eric T. Juengst asserts that community consultation can provide researchers with cultural insights and assist in recruiting participants but not offer protection for communities.

In 2004, 41 members of the Havasupai Indians, who live in an isolated area at the bottom of the Grand Canyon, sued Arizona State University and the University of Arizona for fraud, misrepresentation, intentional infliction of emotional distress, and a host of other charges. The lawsuit alleged that researchers had used blood samples collected from 1990 to 1992 from 200 of the 650 tribe members as the basis for published articles about schizophrenia, inbreeding, and theories about population migrations from Asia to North America. The tribe claimed that they had never consented to this use of their samples, which they believed were to be used to study the tribe's high rate of diabetes. They asserted that the research on schizophrenia and inbreeding stigmatized the tribe, and the migration research conflicted with their religious beliefs about their origin.

Like all lawsuits, this case raises specific questions about the facts. But it also raises the more general question of the extent to which consulting with communities before embarking on research with its members can protect not only the individual participants but also the communities of which they are members. The current federal regulations that apply to research were put into place in 1981, and revised several times thereafter, in the wake of revelations about research abuses in the United States as well as the World War II Nazi crimes in which captives were maimed and killed in the name of medical research. The regulations focus on the individual participant, outlining his or her rights to information about the risks and benefits, consent process, and opportunity to withdraw, as well as other protections. A system of prior review through institutional review boards (IRBs) at each institution conducting research was established to ensure that the regulations are followed.

As research, particularly genetic research, began to focus on groups as well as individuals, IRBs encouraged researchers to consult with the affected communities to answer their questions about the research and to obtain their agreement to solicit participation. A distinction is frequently made in ethics between the potential for "harming" and "wronging." A person can be harmed physically or emotionally by research. Someone may have severe side effects from an experimental drug, for example, or be retraumatized by a study about prior sexual abuse. However, a person can be wronged by a study that damages his or her standing in a community, reveals personal information, or in some other way subjects him or her to an affront to dignity and respect.

The Havasupai case, for example, involved not only allegations that the members suffered severe emotional harm and distress but also that the tribe had been wronged by the unconsented-to publication of negative information about its propensity to mental illness and inbreeding. In April 2010, the case was settled when Arizona State University agreed to pay 41 members of the tribe $700,000. Some researchers fear that this outcome will block further genetic research among Native Americans and other minorities. Others look to more explicit and sensitive communications to forestall controversy.

The following selections discuss community consultation as it is currently conducted. Physicians Neal Dickert and Jeremy Sugarman assert that researchers following the ethical goals they outline in conducting consultations can help protect communities against unwarranted use of their information. Eric T. Juengst, a philosopher, likens community consultation to "slow code," a term that describes a half-hearted attempt to resuscitate a dying person. He believes that efforts at consultation, while well-meaning, are useful only as recruitment strategies.

YES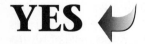

Neal Dickert and
Jeremy Sugarman

Ethical Goals of Community Consultation in Research

. . . **A**lthough ethical considerations of human subjects research have historically focused on protecting the rights, interests, and well-being of individual subjects, growing attention has been given to the importance of involving communities in research development and approval. . . . Despite an increasing sense of need for community input, difficult questions persist about how best to involve communities as partners in research. . . .

Distinguishing Community Consultation and Consent

Community consultation should not be mistaken for community consent, although the [two] are not mutually exclusive. To consult is "to seek advice or information."[1] Consulting with a community includes eliciting feedback, criticism, and suggestions; it does not include asking for approval or permission. Community consultation is designed to recognize and accommodate the relevant particularities of a given community for a specific project. . . . Conducting genetics research in an aboriginal community may necessitate discussing studies with existing political authorities and community members.[2,3]

Rather than soliciting input, community consent involves soliciting approval or permission to conduct a study within a community. Community consent may occur after community consultation and does not obviate the need for individual consent.[4,5] Rather, the community decides whether to permit investigators to solicit participation from community members. For community consent to be valid, there must be a legitimate political system in place, with representatives properly empowered to make such decisions on behalf of the community.[5,6] In many aboriginal communities, such legitimate systems exist. However, disease-based communities and many social groups typically lack a political structure, which makes community consent inappropriate.[5,6]

Although conceptually distinct, the line between community consultation and community consent is inevitably blurred in practice. It would be disingenuous to enter into a consulting arrangement where the consulting party does not intend, *ex ante*, to take the consultants' advice. If relevant consultants

From *American Journal of Public Health*, July 2005, pp. 1123–1127. Copyright © 2005 by American Public Health Association. Reprinted by permission of American Public Health Association.

have strong negative reactions or endorse particular modifications, those reactions or modifications have significant moral force and warrant respect and careful consideration, even though investigators may sometimes justifiably act contrary to such opinions. Otherwise, community consultation is merely symbolic.[7] Despite the clear conceptual distinction between consent and consultation, the degree to which consultants' support is necessary represents a persistent challenge.[8,9,10]

Challenges of Community Consultation

Potential difficulties exist at each stage of community consultation. At the outset, it can be hard to identify communities and stakeholders that have legitimate and relevant interests. Common elements exist among conceptions of community,[11] but delineating and identifying particular communities for consultation can be challenging. Identifying the community at risk for HIV, for example, can be problematic, because at-risk individuals may not believe they are a part of any such community.[12] Identifying representatives also can be difficult. Helpful procedures for identifying representatives have been suggested by The National Institute for General Medical Science,[13] but important conceptual and practical challenges remain. For example, no clear representative exists for persons who may suffer from traumatic brain injury or cardiac arrest.[14,15]

Closely related to the challenge of identifying communities is deciding when communities should be consulted (assuming they can be identified). In certain cases, there are regulatory requirements for community consultation.[16] Similarly, when research poses real risks for social stigma to well-defined communities, such as certain genetics studies in native communities, the need for community consultation is evident.[17] Yet, requiring community consultation in all research projects is unwarranted. Relevant factors to consider when deciding whether to conduct community consultation include the particular community under consideration, the nature of the research, and the likely impact of the research on that community. Further analysis is needed; however, we hope that articulating the goals of community consultation will at least be a helpful step in determining when consultation is warranted.

The type of community being considered for consultation is an important factor when determining the way in which community input is solicited. Common solicitation methods include open public forums, meetings with community advisory board members, presentations at meetings of religious or civic organizations, and radio and television call-in shows.[17-24] Devising successful methods for generating public input can be challenging, particularly in communities that lack a well-defined structure or are geographically disparate.[5,25] In many cases, multiple modalities of interaction must be employed.[17] It can also be difficult to determine when consultation efforts have been sufficient. Although insufficient consultation can be ineffective, requiring overly extensive consultation may hamper important work.

Finally, incorporating consultants' input into research plans can be challenging. Although it is undesirable to override or dismiss community objections or concerns, failure to conduct important research on the basis of objections by groups who are nonrepresentative or who have not carefully considered the issues at hand is also problematic.

Ethical Goals for Community Consultation

A clear set of ethical goals will help investigators, sponsors, institutional review boards, and regulators plan and assess community consultation methods. Additionally, such a framework will provide endpoints for measuring the adequacy of consultation methods. We propose four ethical goals of community consultation: (1) enhanced protection, (2) enhanced benefits, (3) legitimacy, and (4) shared responsibility (Table 1).

Enhanced Protection

Enhancing the protection of research participants' interests and welfare is grounded in the researchers' duty to minimize risks for research subjects. Consultation efforts should be designed and conducted to help identify risks or hazards for individuals and communities and to identify additional protections to ensure the safety of research participants.

Some risks, particularly social risks, may not be apparent at the outset to investigators, sponsors, and institutional review boards. Members of cancer advocacy groups, for example, may serve as important consultants when designing informational materials or calling attention to concerns about adverse treatment effects that may not be obvious to researchers conducting a cancer trial.[26] When research is conducted in emergency settings, community consultation may generate discussion that helps to identify groups who

Table 1

Ethical Goals of Community Consultation

Ethical Goal	Definition
Enhanced protection	Enhance protections for subjects and communities by identifying risks or hazards that were not previously appreciated and by suggesting or identifying potential protections
Enhanced benefits	Enhance benefits to participants in the study, the population for which the research is designed, or the community in which the study is conducted
Legitimacy	Confer ethical/political legitimacy by giving those parties with an interest or stake in the proposed research the opportunity to express their views and concerns at a time when changes can be made to the research protocol
Shared responsibility	Consulted communities may bear some degree of moral responsibility for the research project and may take on some responsibilities for conducting the study

are likely to want to opt out of specific studies and that suggests strategies to facilitate the identification of those groups during the study. In this sense, community consultation may be a particularly effective way for investigators to identify individuals or subgroups with particular needs or vulnerabilities that individuals outside the community may not recognize.

Community consultation also may enhance nonparticipant protections by identifying risks for community members who are not enrolled in the study. For example, studies of cancer susceptibility that were conducted among Ashkenazi Jews were opposed by some community members who were concerned that research findings might be used for eugenics or might jeopardize health coverage.[27] Although all risks are not preventable, making them explicit and minimizing them are essential goals.

Enhanced Benefits

Enhancing benefits through community consultation is consistent with researchers' general duty of beneficence toward research subjects.[28] Early HIV research illustrates how community consultation enhances benefits to individual subjects. For example, [one] community advisory board recommended that a clinical trial incorporate referral programs for participants to gain access to available ancillary services.[29] Based on this recommendation, investigators chose to incorporate such programs into their studies.

Community consultation may also enhance benefits to the community of individuals who have the condition being studied or to the larger communities to which study subjects belong. In the international setting, a common benefit of research involvement is the improvement of the research or health care delivery infrastructure. By consulting with host country researchers and others in the host community, the areas of infrastructure that need improvement can be identified.[30] Similarly, a central notion in community-based participatory research is that communities should be involved in identifying research questions and planning studies in order to conduct studies that benefit the particular communities involved.[31] In short, community consultation may enhance direct, indirect, and aspirational benefits.[32] Investigators are by no means required to provide all benefits that could conceivably be offered to participants or communities, but enhancing benefits to ensure that research efforts are mutually beneficial is an important goal.

Legitimacy

Community consultation can help to confer ethical and political legitimacy on a research project by engaging in a process in which stakeholders (those people, institutions, and groups that have an interest in the proposed research) may express their views and concerns. The opportunity to speak has significant justificatory power for imposing research risks, especially when individuals are unable to provide consent and surrogate decision makers are unavailable. In such cases, community consultation may be the only chance investigators have to assess the likely preferences of the study population. Similarly, when a study poses significant risks for a community, such as genetics research that could have potentially negative implications on the insurability of an entire population, community consultation seems essential for legitimacy.

The challenges to achieving this goal are well known. What counts as a community? Who counts as a representative? What level of community support is needed to legitimize a particular study? These are deep, conceptual questions for which we do not have well-developed answers; however, it is important to note that the goal of legitimacy refers to the process of community consultation and not the political legitimacy of consulted bodies.[5] Suggestions or concerns that are expressed during community consultations are significant, even when consultants lack the authority to provide consent on behalf of the community.

Shared Responsibility

As partners in the research process, community members may share responsibility in 2 ways. First, community consultants may assume active roles in conducting research. Community advisory board members, for example, may become involved in recruiting subjects for studies[11,23,33] and thus bear some responsibility for the success of research efforts. Second, by acknowledging the stake that community members have in the conduct of research, and by soliciting their assistance and input through a legitimate process, community consultation confers on communities a degree of moral responsibility for the research.[34]

Shared responsibility is particularly evident with cases involving HIV advocacy groups, where the advocacy groups have taken on the role of actually conducting studies,[18] and with cases involving participatory-action research or community-based participatory research, where communities are involved at every stage.[19,35,36] It is important to clarify that sharing responsibility does not constitute a shifting of blame or removal of responsibility from investigators, sponsors, and institutional review boards. On the contrary, community consultation places additional responsibility on investigators to attend to important community concerns. The degree to which responsibility can be shared is limited by the degree to which investigators and sponsors are sensitive to and accommodate those concerns.

Conclusions

As the need for identifying and incorporating community input into the design, planning, and conduct of research has become clearer, it is critical to identify the ethical goals of community consultation. Attention to the 4 ethical goals of enhancing protection, enhancing benefits, creating legitimacy, and sharing responsibility should allow for more effective assessment by communities, investigators, institutional review boards, and sponsors of particular consultation efforts. We also hope that these goals can be developed into metrics by which methods of community consultation may be systematically assessed. For example, enhanced protections can be measured by observing whether a particular consultation effort identifies additional risks previously unknown to investigators or whether it proposes new solutions for minimizing risk. There are currently few empirical data on the effectiveness of consultation strategies.[33] By identifying the goals of the process, this framework should facilitate attempts to assess different types of consultation efforts in different settings and enhance understanding of which consultation methods are appropriate in varying types of communities and types of research.

Finally, this framework draws attention to 2 important lingering issues that are beyond the scope of this article. First, an account is needed for determining when investigators may justifiably override or dismiss community concerns. Such an account must be particularly sensitive to the nature of disagreements.[37] Second, further research is needed to determine what types of studies require community consultation and what types of consultation are needed for particular research projects. In the meantime, careful attention to the 4 ethical goals we have identified should facilitate the proper incorporation of community views into research and its oversight.

References

1. *The American Heritage Collegiate Dictionary.* 3rd ed. New York, NY: Houghton Mifflin; 1993.

2. Dodson M. Indigenous peoples and the morality of the Human Genome Diversity Project. *J Med Ethics.* 1999;25:204–208.

3. The Australian Institute of Aboriginal and Torres Strait Islander Studies. *Guidelines for Ethical Research in Indigenous Studies.* Available at: http://www.aiatsis.gov.au/corp/docs/ethicsguidea4.pdf. February 7, 2005.

4. Ijsselmuiden C, Faden R. Research and informed consent in Africa— another look. *N Engl J Med.* 1992;326:830–833.

5. Weijer C, Emanuel EJ. Protecting communities in research. *Science.* 2000; 289:1142–1144.

6. Weijer C, Miller PB. Protecting communities in pharmacogenetic and pharmacogenomic research. *Pharmacogenomics J.* 2004;4:9–16.

7. Minkler M, Pies C. Ethical Issues and Practical Dilemmas in Community Organization and Community Participation. In: Minkler M, ed. *Community Organization and Community Building for Health.* 2nd ed. New Brunswick, NJ: Rutgers University Press; 2005.

8. Biros M. Research without consent: current status, 2003. *Ann Emerg Med.* 2003;42:550–564.

9. Passamani ER, Weisfeldt ML. Task force 3: special aspects of research conducted in the emergency setting: waiver of informed consent. *J Am Coll Cardiol.* 2000;35:862–880.

10. Council for International Organizations of Medical Sciences. *International Ethical Guidelines for Biomedical Research Involving Human Subjects.* Geneva, Switzerland: Council for International Organizations of Medical Sciences; 2002.

11. MacQueen KM, McLellan E, Metzger DS, et al. What is community? An evidence-based definition for participatory public health. *Am J Public Health.* 2001;91:1929–1938.

12. Grady C. *The Search for an HIV Vaccine*. Bloomington, Ind: Indiana University Press; 1995.

13. *Policy for the Responsible Collection, Storage, and Research Use of Samples from Named Populations for the NIGMS Human Genetic Cell Repository*. Available at: http://locus.umdnj.edu/nigms/comm/submit/collpolicy.html. Accessed February 7, 2005.

14. King NMP. Medical research: using a new paradigm where the old might do. In: King NMP, Henderson GE, Stein J, eds. *Beyond Regulations: Ethics in Human Subjects Research*. Chapell Hill, NC: University of North Carolina Press; 1999.

15. Browder JP. Can community consultation substitute for informed consent in emergency research: a response. In: King NMP, Henderson GE, Stein J, eds. *Beyond Regulations: Ethics in Human Subjects Research*. Chapell Hill, NC: University of North Carolina Press; 1999.

16. US Food and Drug Administration. Exception from informed consent requirements for emergency research. Title 20, Code of Federal Regulations, Section 50.24. Available at: http://www.accessdata.fda.gov/scripts/crdh/cfdocs/cfcfr/cfrsearch.cfm. Accessed April 10, 2005.

17. Foster MW, Bernsten D, Carter TH. A model agreement for genetic research in socially identifiable populations. *Am J Hum Genetics*. 1998;63:696–702.

18. Spiers HR. Community consultation and AIDS clinical trials: part L. *IRB*. 1991;13(3):7–10.

19. Quinn SC. Protecting human subjects: the role of community advisory boards. *Am J Public Health*. 2004;94:918–922.

20. Shah AN, Sugarman J. Protecting research subjects under the waiver of informed consent for emergency research: experiences with efforts to inform the community. *Ann Emerg Med*. 2003;41:72–78.

21. Santora TA, Cowell V, Trooskin SZ. Working through the public disclosure process mandated by use of 21 CFR 50.24 (exception to informed consent): guidelines for success. *J Trauma*. 1998; 45:907–913.

22. Dix ES, Esposito D, Spinosa F, Olson N, Chapman S. Implementation of community consultation for waiver of informed consent in emergency research: one institutional review board's experience. *J Invest Med*. 2004;52: 113–116.

23. Blanchard L. Community assessment and perceptions: preparations for HIV vaccine efficacy trials. In: King NMP, Henderson GE, Stein J, eds. *Beyond Regulations: Ethics in Human Subjects Research*. Chapel Hill, NC: University of North Carolina Press; 1999.

24. Strauss RP, Sengupta S, Quinn SC, et al. The role of community advisory boards: involving communities in the informed consent process. *Am J Public Health*. 2001;91:1938–1943.

25. Foster MW, Sharp RR, Freeman WL, Chino M, Bernstein D, Carter TH. The role of community review in evaluating the risks of human genetic variation research. *Am J Hum Genet*. 1999;64:1719–1727.

26. Girling DJ. Important issues in planning and conducting multi-centre randomised controlled trials in cancer and publishing their results. *Crit Rev Oncol Hematol*. 2000;36:13–25.

27. Lehrman S. Jewish leaders seek genetic guidelines. *Nature.* 1997;389:322.

28. National Commission for the Protection of Research Risks. *The Belmont Report: Ethical Principles and Guidelines for the Protection of Human Subjects of Research.* Washington, DC: Government Printing Office; 1979.

29. Valdiserri RO, Tama GM, Ho M. The role of community advisory committees in clinical trials of anti-HIV agents. *IRB.* 1988;10:5–7.

30. Participants in the 2001 Conference on Ethical Aspects of Research in Developing Countries. Enhanced: fair benefits for research in developing countries. *Science.* 2001;298:2133–2134.

31. Israel BA, Schulz AJ, Parker EA, Becker AB. Review of community-based research: assessing partnership approaches to improve public health. *Ann Rev Public Health.* 1998;19:173–202.

32. King NMP. Defining and describing benefit appropriately in clinical trials. *Am J Law, Med, Ethics.* 2000;28:332–343.

33. Morin SF, Maiorana A, Koester KA, Sheon NM, Richards TA. Community consultation in HIV prevention research: a study of community advisory boards at 6 research sites. *J Acquired Immune Defic Syndrome.* 2003;33: 513–520.

34. UNAIDS. *Ethical Considerations in Preventive HIV Vaccine Research: UNAIDS Guidance Document.* Available at: http://www.unaids.org. Accessed February 5, 2005.

35. Macaulay AC, Commanda LE, Freeman WL, et al. Participatory research maximises community and lay involvement. *BMJ.* 1999;319:774–778.

36. Lantz PM, Viruell-Fuentes E, Israel BA, Softley D, Guzman R. Can communities and academia work together on public health research? Evaluation results from a community-based participatory research partnership in Detroit. *J Urban Health.* 2001;78:495–506.

37. Gutmann A, Thompson D. *Democracy and Disagreement.* Cambridge, Mass: Belknap Press of Harvard University Press; 1996.

Eric T. Juengst   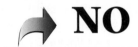 **NO**

Community Engagement in Genetic Research: The "Slow Code" of Research Ethics?

Introduction

The "slow code" is a euphemism in clinical medicine for a half-hearted attempt to resuscitate a terminally ill patient in cardiac arrest when the clinicians actually think resuscitation is futile. The practice is roundly criticized in medical ethics for subverting the purpose of "calling a code," evading the real issues at hand, and deceptively attempting to keep up the appearance of "saving the patient" when it is no longer possible to do so. As one popular clinical handbook puts it,

> The infamous "slow code," in which personnel respond slowly and without energy to an arrest, is reprehensible. It merely represents the failure to come to a timely and clear decision about a patient's resuscitation status. It is crass dissimulation.[1]

"Community engagement" has recently become an ethical watchword for population-based studies of human genetic variation. The theoretical aims of community engagement are to allow human populations[1] who are the subjects of genetic variation research some meaningful control over the initiation and conduct of that research. This goal echoes the clear obligation to secure informed consent from any human individuals being recruited for research—much as the "slow code" in dying patients echoed the clear life-saving aim of cardio-pulmonary resuscitation in other rescue situations. Conducting community engagements for genetic variation research is a delicate and hazardous business: issues of representativeness, social identity, internal politics, and cross-cultural differences abound. Slow codes were also tricky to pull off well, since they involved doing enough to look convincing to family members without actually saving the patient. In this essay, I argue that the practical difficulties of community engagement for genetic variation research are generated by the same sort of moral tension that makes slow codes difficult: there is a basic contradiction between the theoretical aims of the exercise and the actual goals it is capable of achieving.

The advocates of community engagement readily concur that the practice cannot actually secure the "consent" of a genetic population to be participants in research. When pressed, they acknowledge that community engagement as it is practiced cannot even provide much generalizable input into the ways in which studies of that genetic population are designed. In fact, I will suggest, all that community engagement *can* do at the population level is to provide researchers with cultural insights and local publicity useful to recruiting individuals from these populations. While there is nothing objectionable about that aim, it is important to note that it addresses a scientific concern—the need to enroll subjects—that has little to do with the theoretical aim of enhancing the population's control over the ways in which its members are studied.

If community engagement boils down to a recruitment strategy, it is a moral mistake to use it to reassure onlookers that "everything possible is being done" to improve group-level control over the research. Like the "slow code," even its well-intentioned invocation for that purpose involves a species of "crass dissimulation." For the "slow code," the moral tension in the practice eventually illuminated the need for clinicians to come to grips with an underlying question concerning the proper limits of the "rescue ethic" behind emergency CPR. For "community engagement," the question is similar: Are there limits to the otherwise laudable aim of enhancing group autonomy in genetic research?

The alternative to the "slow code" is to face and make explicit decisions to forego life-sustaining treatment when it is justified. Similarly, I will argue, it is time to recognize that genetic populations cannot always have a voice in, or be protected from, the recruitment of their members into genetic variation studies, and to face and make explicit decisions about when to forego efforts to involve them.

"Respect for Community" as a Principle of Research Ethics

"Community engagement" and its rhetorical siblings, "community consultation," "community review," and "community discourse," are a family of concepts that operationalize a moral concern for the interests of human groups involved in biomedical research. Advocates of this concern make three arguments. First, they argue that biomedical research projects that are framed in terms of identified human groups can have repercussions for all the groups' members, even when not all are directly enrolled in the study.[2–3] Second, they argue that people tend to identify themselves through and with the human groups to which they belong, and not as isolated existential atoms. They largely accept their groups' values and priorities as their own, and tend to be protective of their groups' interests as reflective on their own.[4] This general point gains special importance for population-based genetic variation studies, because in most cases the individual's purely private interests will be muted by the personal anonymity of the research. Unlike other gene-hunting studies, it is only through their group identity that the harms of population genomic research can come back to haunt individual subjects.[5] Third, they point that even those who envision human groups as simply free associations of atomistic contractors recognize the moral authority of many kinds of groups to make collective decisions about the best interests of their membership. After all, the very concept of autonomy, or self-governance, which we now wield in defense of individual rights, has its roots in efforts to protect the ability of particular groups to govern themselves. To the extent that it is the collective identity of the group that is the subject of scientific scrutiny, the argument goes, it is the whole group that must face any research risks involved. Therefore, a decision to incur shared risks is most appropriately made at the level of the group as a whole. Some have proposed that this moral concern be translated into a "fourth principle" for biomedical research ethics (in addition to respect for individual autonomy, beneficence, and justice), which would be called "Respect for Community."[6]

The use of the "community engagement" concept to operationalize the principle of Respect for Community is not original with genetic research. The idea has its origins in practices employed by a wide variety of research areas that recruit subjects in terms of their membership in a certain population, ranging from public health research, cultural anthropology, research on emergency medical procedures, and research with sovereign nations like Native American tribes.[7–9] They have been brought to the discussions of population genetic studies relatively recently, however, largely in response to the collapse of one of the earliest proposed sequels to the Human Genome Project, the ill-fated "Human Genome Diversity Project" (HGDP). As the research ethics and genomic research communities have worked to apply the concepts to population genomic research, they have evolved (or devolved) through three major interpretations. Each reinterpretation better reflects the realities of population genomic research, but each is also more attenuated in its ability to realize the theoretical goals of the practice. At the extreme, some examples now risk subordinating the principle of respect for community to the recruitment needs of scientific studies altogether, effectively subverting the point of the practice. . . .

Community Consultation

As the quote above suggests, the first move in this reinterpretation of community engagement is to abandon the concern for collective decision-making authority that characterized the rationale for group consent. Since genetic populations are not the sorts of groups that can claim autonomy as moral communities, it makes no sense to hinge the recruitment of their members on some corporate permission. Thus, for example, the "Points to Consider for Population-based Genetic Research" developed by the U.S. National Institutes of Health stresses that:

> Community consultation is **not** the same as consent. In the majority of cases, communities in the United States are not required to give consent or approval for research in which its members participate, nor is it reasonable to attempt to obtain community consent or approval.[10]

Instead of consent or approval, the NIH guidelines explain that "community consultation is a vehicle for hearing about the community's interests and concerns, addressing ethical issues and communicating information about the research to the community."[10] The purpose of this interchange is to solicit the study population's help in identifying any "intra-community" or "culturally specific" risks and potential benefits, so that the research can be designed in ways that best protect the group's interests.[9]

This interpretation of community engagement places much more emphasis on preserving the special values and cultural lifeways of a given population than on treating the population as a politically autonomous entity. The ethical emphasis has shifted from *respecting* the group to *protecting* their members, as research subjects vulnerable to group-related harms. Nevertheless, it continues to share with the group consent model the importance of identifying and interacting with consultants who can accurately and fairly represent the population's values. Thus, the U.S. Coriell Cell Repository's "Policy for Responsible Collection, Storage and Research Use of Samples from Identified Populations" prescribes that:

> "In advance of collection, the collector of the samples must consult with members and leaders of the community. The collector must assure that those consulted are representative of the socially identifiable population from which samples are to be obtained."[11]

As Marshall and Rotimi point out, this can be difficult:

> Despite the obvious benefits of community advisory boards, there are limits and constraints on their ability to represent the values of diverse community members. . . . In some cases community leaders on advisory boards may be politicians. Community activists represent another powerful group who might serve on such boards. Religious leaders or local celebrities also might be asked to participate on the boards. Investigators must be sensitive to the social and political agendas of members on community advisory boards and try to minimize the potential for addressing priorities that may be relevant to only a minority of the local population.[8]

Moreover, the complexities of human population structure continue to present more than local political difficulties for the community consultation of this sort. The increasing dispersion of human populations around the world means that in fact most human superfamilies no longer share common "culturally specific risks" and benefits.

This leads even the staunchest advocates of community engagement to a counterintuitive point of arguing that, for study populations like "general ethnic, racial or national populations, e.g. Ashkenazi Jews, American Indians, Puerto Ricans, etc.," the lack of distinctive common interest and structured social interaction means that "community review may not be required and even for geographically dispersed populations that share distinctive beliefs and practices, like the Amish or the Hmong, "limited social interactions between members of the study population make intra-community risks unlikely."[3]

In fact, as the range of "local" risks and benefits widens for any specific genetic population across the global spectrum of cultural, political and social environments, the utility of any specific advice becomes diluted to the vanishing point, until only the most generic biomedical design considerations become relevant to researchers. As the NIH Points to consider warn,

> Community-wide "buy-in" to the goals of the research project may improve the ability to recruit study participants. However, community consultation is not a substitute for careful, systematic preliminary studies that provide the foundation for choosing the study population, developing sampling or recruitment plans, designing protocols and measurement tools, and planning analytic strategies. A wide variety of social science methods and statistical data are available for assessing the characteristics of communities. Investigators must be cautious about relying on anecdotal information gained in the course of community consultation to guide the development of their research plans.[12]

Community Dialogue

Diverse, dispersed genetic superfamilies of the sort useful to genetic variation studies will not often enjoy the level of organisation that can make representative consultations possible. For these cases, the Coriell Repository's policy has this helpful recommendation: "If no organized groups exist at all, the investigator must identify other effective ways to consult the population."[11] Sharp and Foster suggest that all may be required is the form of community engagement they call "community dialogue": an effort to interact with the local communities and institutions at the specific site from which members of a given genetic population will be recruited, in order to acquaint them with the investigators' mission in advance of individual subject enrollment.[3]

As they describe it,

> "These discussions may be initiated by researchers or arise independently within a community after contact with researchers. Community dialogue is meant to identify collective concerns and consider ways of minimizing research-related risks, but does not provide a comprehensive review of the research in question, and often will not engage a representative sample of community members."[3]

Tellingly, since these aims do not even require that the community representatives bring any special expertise to the research design, the language shifts from "consultation" and "review," which suggest advice from peers, to terms like "dialogue," "discussion," and "engagement" more often used to describe attempts by experts to teach the uninitiated.

Instead of attempting to respect the genetic population as a moral community, or attempting to protect all its individual members from potential harm, the practice of community engagement is reinterpreted to be simply a matter of establishing a viable political collaboration with the local community in which the recruitment of individuals for DNA sampling is to take place.

Since this does not even require that the community representatives bring any special expertise to the research design, the language can shift from "consultation" and "review" to "dialogue" and "engagement": terms more often used to describe attempts to teach than to learn.

Narrowing the focus from broad study populations to localized communities does make the prospect of community engagement more plausible. Localized communities will be able to produce representatives authorized to speak for their membership more easily than unorganized populations. Local communities are more likely to face common "intra-community risks" and needs that might be usefully communicated in designing the research at that site. And to build trust and negotiate access to community members, it will be much more effective to work at the local level.

Nevertheless, by this point it is clear that we have paid a high price for this accomplishment. The kinds of study populations that are of most interest to genetic variation researchers, the international human superfamilies whose genetic variations disclose the patterns of disease susceptibilities within the species, now seem to be those least well served by the practice of community engagement. If the concern was to give those larger population groups some involvement in research that may affect them, even negotiating a full-blown "community partnership" with one localized subset of the population is as likely to be an example of the problem rather than a step toward justice: to the extent that the researcher does not confine his scientific claims to the local community at hand, that community's decisions about participation have preempted the interests of the rest of the population.

Moreover, for these same reasons, investigators cannot honestly let local communities speak for the population, and cannot promise that local research designs will protect the communities from population-related harms incurred by studies at other locales. Thus, in this most attenuated model of community engagement, even the local communities to whom the principle of "respect for community" could apply cannot be afforded a robust interpretation of that ideal.

If community engagement cannot provide a mechanism for the subjects of a population genomics study to make collective decisions about their participation, or provide a representative survey of their special concerns so that their risks can be minimized in the study design, or to respect the autonomy of local communities, why else might investigators be interested in pursuing such an exercise? The only remaining reason, which population researchers in public health and anthropological often give as the primary explanation for the practice, is a purely pragmatic one. Engaging the community in a public way is an important method of encouraging the enrollment of community members as research subjects. The NIH guidelines are remarkable for making this point nine times. At one point the guidelines explain that:

> Conducting a dialogue with the community may uncover weaknesses in the research plan. For example, the investigator may learn new information about language barriers, beliefs or concerns that would threaten the feasibility of the research or undermine the validity of measures if

they were not considered. A consultation may reveal strategies for more effectively identifying study populations. Community wide "buy-in" to the goals of the research project may improve the ability to recruit study participations. Besides being "the respectful thing to do," failure to consult with community can erode trust in scientists and in the scientific research enterprise in general, which may affect the ability of investigators to conduct future research with that community or other communities."[12]

Again, building trusting relationships with one's pool of potential research subjects in order to increase enrollment and pave the way for future studies is not in itself ethically problematic. As Marshall and Rotimi correctly point out, "ethical dilemmas are minimized when mechanisms that sustain a solid foundation of community trust are well established during the design and implementation of research protocols."[8] However, it also not the same thing as empowering the population to make its own decisions in its own terms with regard to whether entering into such relationships is ultimately in their best interests. If its utility as a recruitment strategy is all that community engagement for population genetic research can ultimately claim for itself, the practice has relatively nothing to do with the principle of "respect for community." . . .

References

1. Jonsen A, Siegler M, Winslade W. Clinical Ethics: A Practical Approach to Ethical Decisions in Clinical Medicine, 4th edition. New York: McGraw-Hill Inc., 1998.

2. Greely H. The control of genetic research: involving the 'group between'. Houston Law Review 1997; 33:1398–1430.

3. Sharp R, and Foster M. Involving study populations in the review of genetic research. The Journal of Law, Medicine, and Ethics 2000; 28(1):41–52.

4. Gostin L. Ethical principles of the conduct of human subject research: population-based research and ethics. Law, Medicine and Health Care 1991; 19:191–201.

5. Foster M, Eisenbraun AJ, Carter TH. Communal discourse as a supplement to informed consent for genetic research. Nature Genetics 1997; 17:277–279.

6. Weijer C. Protecting communities in research: philosophical and pragmatic challenges. Cambridge Quarterly of Health Care Ethics 1999; 8:501–513.

7. Dickens B. Issues in preparing ethical guidelines for epidemiological studies. Law, Medicine and Health Care 1991; 19:175–182.

8. Marshall P, and Rotimi C. Ethical challenges in community-based research. American Journal of the Medical Sciences 2001; 322:259–263.

9. Foster M, Sharp R, Freeman W, et al. The role of community review in evaluating the risks of human genetic variation research. American Journal of Human Genetics 1999; 64:1719–1727.

10. National Institutes of Health. Points to consider when planning a genetic study that involves members of named populations. Bioethics Resources on the Web, 2002. Available at: www.nih.gov/sigs/bioethics/named_populations.html.

11. Corriell Cell Repositories. Policy for the Responsible collection storage and research use of samples from identified populations for the NIGMS Human Genetic Cell Repository. Available at: http://locus.umdnj.edu/nigms/comm/submit/collpolicy.html.

12. Soo-Jinn Lee, Mountain J, Koenig B. The meanings of 'race' in the new genomics: implications for health disparities research. Yale Journal of Health Policy, Law and Ethics 2001; 1:33–75.

POSTSCRIPT

Does Community Consultation in Research Protect Vulnerable Groups?

Dena S. Davis explores one aspect of the impact of genetic research on communities in "Groups, Communities, and Contested Identities in Genetic Research," *Hastings Center Report* (November–December 2000). She points out that groups of individuals who share some aspects of identity (religion, ethnicity, genetics) may not represent the larger community, which may be stereotyped by the subgroup's behavior or characteristics.

In "The Control of Genetic Research: Involving the 'Groups Between,'" Henry T. Greely describes the intermediate group—family, set of families, disease community—as well as the individual or larger community that can be affected by genetic research. They face "the same three issues of autonomy, reputation, and commercialization" (*Houston Law Review*, 1997).

Michelle M. Mello and Leslie E. Wolf discuss the implications of the Havasupai case in "The Havasupai Indian Tribe Case—Lessons from Research Involving Stored Biologic Samples," *The New England Journal of Medicine* (July 15, 2010). They present the advantages and disadvantages of different informed-consent approaches.

To avoid problems of contacting participants, David Wendler recommends a general consent at the time of recruitment ("One-Time General Consent for Research on Biological Samples," *British Medical Journal*, March 4, 2006). He points to studies that show that most individuals support one-time general consent. He does not, however, specifically address the impact of research findings on communities.

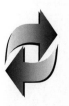

Internet References . . .

Organ Donation

This site provides current statistics and background information on the allocation of transplantable organs in the United States.

http://www.organdonor.gov

Kaiser Family Foundation

This research organization's Web site has reports and data about health care coverage in the United States, including state data.

http://www.kff.org/

World Anti-Drug Doping Agency

This international organization has information for athletes, coaches, fans, and others about the use of drugs in sports.

http://www.wada-ama.org

Bioethics and Public Policy

*I*n *its modern infancy, biomedical ethics was almost exclusively concerned with issues relating to individual doctor–patient relationships. Questions of resource allocation and public policy did occur, but mostly within the context of whether or not a patient could pay for certain kinds of care. In the past several decades, as medical care costs have skyrocketed, the issues concerning equitable distribution of scarce resources have become paramount. As medical care became more costly, it became less accessible to the uninsured and to the underinsured (people who have some employment-based health insurance but not enough to cover their own illnesses or those of their families). In this new world of market-driven health care, some old problems of resource allocation and public policy take on new urgency. How far should commercialism extend? The threat of war and bioterrorism have created new dilemmas for military doctors and policymakers as they struggle to define a balance between protecting the public's health in case of an attack and preserving the basic liberties that Americans prize so highly. This section takes up these issues.*

- Is It Fair to Require Individuals to Purchase Health Insurance?
- Should There Be a Market in Human Organs?
- Does Military Necessity Override Medical Ethics?
- Should Performance-Enhancing Drugs Be Banned from Sports?
- Should Pharmacists Be Allowed to Deny Prescriptions on Grounds of Conscience?

ISSUE 16

Is It Fair to Require Individuals to Purchase Health Insurance?

YES: Sara Rosenbaum and Jonathan Gruber, from "Buying Health Care, the Individual Mandate, and the Constitution," *The New England Journal of Medicine* (July 29, 2010)

NO: Glen Whitman, from "Hazards of the Individual Health Care Mandate," *Cato Policy Report* (September/October 2007)

ISSUE SUMMARY

YES: Law professor Sara Rosenbaum and economist Jonathan Gruber contend that the provision of the health reform legislation requiring individuals who are not covered by an employer health plan to pay a penalty if they do not buy health insurance is constitutional and the only way that access to health care can be assured for all.

NO: Economics professor Glen Whitman argues that the individual tax mandate is based on false assumptions about the level of uncompensated care and is likely to drive up costs rather than result in savings.

On March 23, 2010, President Obama signed into law the Patient Protection and Affordable Care Act (often cited as ACA), a major change in the way health care is financed and delivered in the United States. The United States remains the only industrialized country without a national health care system, despite the efforts over the past 50 years of Republican and Democratic presidents to introduce change. The ACA is intended to address two major health care problems: lack of access and high costs.

Most of the people who have health insurance today obtain it through their employers. It was not always the case, however. Employer-based insurance was introduced in World War II as an incentive to recruit and retain workers because wartime regulations restricted offering higher wages.

Even though there is no national health care system, government programs play a major role. Medicare, a federal program, was enacted in 1965 to cover people over the age of 65 and those with end-stage kidney disease.

Medicaid, introduced at the same time, is a joint federal–state program that covers people below the poverty line. There are other government-sponsored programs—TRICARE (formerly CHAMPUS) for uniformed service members, retirees, and their families; federal employees' insurance; and the Children's Health Insurance Program (CHIP) for poor children. These government-sponsored programs are administered by private insurance companies.

Even with these programs aimed at special populations, the Kaiser Commission on Medicaid and the Uninsured estimates that about 41 million nonelderly adults and 8.3 million children do not have any health insurance at all. Because of the weak job market, the number of uninsured increased by about 5 million between 2007 and 2009. Many employers also dropped or limited coverage or raised employee contributions.

Most of the adults without health insurance are in working families but have low incomes. About 60 percent have at least one full-time worker and 16 percent have only part-time workers. About 80 percent are U.S. citizens. Hospitals with emergency departments are required by law to treat patients whether they have insurance or not. "Treatment," however, is limited to stabilizing the patient, not providing follow-up care. And hospitals can still bill for the care, at a rate that is often higher than the one negotiated with health insurance plans.

The new health reform law addresses the lack of access by expanding Medicaid to cover nearly all of the nonelderly lowest-income adults. To spread this cost over the greatest number, beginning in 2014 almost every American (with a few exemptions) will be required to have health insurance or pay a fine. An individual can choose to enroll in an employer-based plan as long as it meets certain standards. Insurance will be available through new state-based insurance marketplaces called exchanges, with subsidies for low-income people. People younger than 30 will be able to satisfy the mandate by buying low-cost, high-deductible plans. In 2006, Massachusetts expanded access through a similar plan with an individual mandate provision.

This "individual tax mandate" is one of the most controversial aspects of the health reform law. It has been challenged by several states. In October 2010, a federal judge in Michigan dismissed one lawsuit, but a federal judge in Florida allowed the provision in a similar lawsuit challenging the individual tax mandate to go forward. Eventually the issue may reach the Supreme Court.

The following selections discuss the merits of individual tax mandates. Sara Rosenbaum and Jonathan Gruber assert that the key issue is whether the courts find the individual tax mandate a law that regulates economic conduct and therefore constitutional. Glen Whitman declares that individual tax mandates are based on flawed assumptions about the "free rider" problem (people who get health care without being insured) and will drive up costs.

YES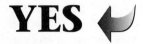

Sara Rosenbaum
and Jonathan Gruber

Buying Health Care, the Individual Mandate, and the Constitution

In *Rashomon,* a classic film that explores the concept of truth, director Akira Kurosawa presents a story about a single incident retold by four narrators, leaving the audience to figure out what is real. Litigation has a *Rashomon*-like quality to it: two sides meet in a courtroom and each presents its case, arguing not only that abstract legal principles favor its cause, but [also that it is] equally important, [and] that its version of the event that gave rise to the dispute should be the filter through which the court decides the matter.

Three separate cases raising constitutional challenges to the Affordable Care Act (ACA) are now under way,[1,2,3] and together they present issues of great legal complexity.[4] Yet although difficult legal questions must be resolved, a pivotal issue is whose version of events will serve as the judicial analytic filter. For reasons related to the very basis of Congress's constitutional power to enact health care reform, the fight is over whether the individual mandate to purchase health insurance (or pay a tax) is about regulating individuals' economic conduct or regulating their noneconomic status. Depending on which characterization of the facts prevails, the individual mandate either falls within or lies outside Congress's power to act.

The Supreme Court precedents indicate that the framers of the U.S. Constitution vested Congress with enormous powers to regulate individual economic conduct, even as they limited congressional authority over noneconomic activity. The source of this power to regulate economic activity down to the individual level is found in the Constitution's Commerce Clause (article 1, section 8, clause 3), on whose reach the legal resolution of these cases ultimately depends. This clause explicitly grants Congress the authority to regulate interstate commerce.

In *Gonzalez v. Raich,* a 2005 decision involving federal regulation of home-grown marijuana, the U.S. Supreme Court concluded that growing marijuana amounted to economic activity and interpreted the Commerce Clause as permitting Congress to reach the "consumption of commodities for which there is an established and lucrative interstate market." In other cases involving the constitutionality of federal laws sanctioning individual conduct—gun possession on school grounds (in *United States v. Lopez,* 1995) and domestic violence (in *United States v. Morrison,* 2000)—the Court concluded that the specified

From *The New England Journal of Medicine,* July 29, 2010, pp. 401–403. Copyright © 2010 by Massachusetts Medical Society. All rights reserved. Reprinted by permission.

activities did not amount to economic conduct within the definition of the Commerce Clause. To be sure, both gun possession and violence against women have economic consequences, but an indirect economic effect is insufficient to warrant congressional regulation. As a result, only states, using their police powers, can directly regulate such activity, which lies beyond the limits of Commerce Clause control.

Thus, the outcome of the battle over the individual mandate turns on whether the courts understand the ACA as a law that regulates economic conduct. Complaints recently filed by the state of Virginia and by multiple state claimants in Florida represent a direct challenge to the proposition that economic conduct is involved. In their complaint, the multistate plaintiffs argue that the law should be viewed as an attempt "to regulate and penalize Americans for choosing not to engage in economic activity." Similarly, in his June 2010 brief, the Virginia attorney general argues that the ACA must be understood as an attempt to compel individuals to undertake economic conduct by forcing them to buy health insurance. In other words, highly cognizant of the distinction drawn in *Raich* between economic and noneconomic conduct, the plaintiffs argue that health care reform is a blatant attempt to force an economic undertaking; they frame the ACA as a law about status (being uninsured) rather than about economic activity.

The U.S. government, on the other hand, frames the law as precisely about Americans' buying practices in relation to a commodity "for which there is an established and lucrative interstate market." In its briefs in the Florida and Virginia cases, the U.S. Department of Justice argues that the ACA is a quintessential economic regulatory effort because it addresses the when and how of paying for health care (a market commodity that almost all Americans will purchase at some point, either because they plan to or because of an unforeseen event). In its argument, the Justice Department lays out the congressional findings that undergird the ACA, which highlight the economic imperative of health care reform in order to save a health care system that is fundamentally failing the tens of millions of Americans who are either uninsured or faced with purchasing insurance in a dysfunctional insurance market.

From an economics standpoint, the conclusion is clear: the purpose of the ACA is to regulate how Americans buy health care, which is clearly economic conduct. Above all, the ACA's fundamental goal is to stabilize the vast U.S. market for health care services—which accounts for 17.5% of the gross domestic product, according to Congress—along with the health insurance system on which nonelderly Americans rely as a principal means for financing their health care. The law's goal is revealed through extensive legislative findings that are set forth in the ACA. The goal also can be seen in the act's provisions that collectively are aimed at making the insurance market work for millions of Americans who, because of their income, health status, or both, have been locked out of affordable, accessible, and stable coverage and must therefore try to pay for care at the point of service.

The existing system has broad economic implications for both the insured and the uninsured. Far from being passive and noneconomic, the uninsured consume more than $50 billion in uncompensated care, the costs of which are passed through health care institutions to insured Americans. Moreover, medical expenses not covered by insurance are one of the leading causes of bankruptcy in the United States, and the costs of resolving those bankruptcies are borne throughout the U.S. economy. In addition, the lack of health insurance leads to poorer health, which can, in turn, reduce workplace productivity. Even the possibility of losing health insurance makes many workers afraid to leave their jobs for more productive positions elsewhere, so the current system reduces the overall productivity of the U.S. labor force.

The changes made by the ACA to stabilize the insurance market are fundamentally economic. The legislation's core is its mandate to end pervasive discriminatory insurance practices while making care affordable. But such change is not possible without an individual mandate. If people who are in better health can opt out of the market and effectively gamble that they can pay for whatever health care they need at the point of service, prices rise for those who are in poorer health, leading to an "adverse selection" spiral that raises insurance prices for all. This is not an idle conjecture. Five states have tried to undertake reforms of the nongroup insurance market like those in the ACA without enacting an individual mandate; those five states are now among the eight states with the most expensive nongroup health insurance.

In the end, the ACA is all about altering individual economic conduct, and its importance lies in the way it changes the when and how of health care purchasing. By ensuring access to affordable coverage for most Americans, the law seeks to rationalize our economic behavior while providing the regulatory and subsidization tools to make this rationalization possible. To characterize the ACA as a law aimed at anything other than individual economic conduct is to fundamentally miss the point of the legislation.

References

1. Thomas More Law Center v. Barack Hussein Obama, Case no. 2:10-cv-11156 (E.D. Mich., 2010).
2. Commonwealth of Virginia v. Sebelius, Civil action no. 3:10cv188 (E.D. Va., 2010).
3. State of Florida v. U.S. Department of Health and Human Services, Case no.: 3:10-cv-91-RV/EMT (N.D. Fla., 2010).
4. Balkin JM. The constitutionality of the individual mandate for health insurance. N Engl J Med 2010;362:482–483.

Glen Whitman 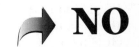 **NO**

Hazards of the Individual Health Care Mandate

$\mathbf{T}$he latest fad in health care reform is the "individual mandate"—a law that requires individuals to purchase health insurance and threatens punishment for those who don't. Massachusetts, under the governorship of presidential hopeful Mitt Romney, has already created a health care policy with an individual mandate as its centerpiece. Gov. Arnold Schwarzenegger has proposed a similar plan for California. And politicians are not alone, as analysts from across the political spectrum have jumped on board. Even analysts who usually favor markets over regulation—like economist Gary Becker, legal scholar Richard Posner, Ron Bailey of *Reason* magazine, and Robert Moffit of the Heritage Foundation—have voiced support for the individual mandate.

Their support, however, is unjustified. The individual mandate will do little, if anything, to solve the problem of "free riders" whose health expenses are paid for by the rest of us. The mandate will do nothing to decrease the actual cost of health services. Worst of all, the mandate will create a set of political incentives that will likely drive up the cost of health insurance while impeding the adoption of more effective reforms.

Is Free Riding Really the Problem?

Supporters of the individual mandate rely heavily on the problem of uncompensated care. People who lack health insurance nevertheless receive health care in this country, because hospitals and health care providers are unable or unwilling to turn them away. When recipients don't pay for their care, the rest of us end up footing the bill one way or another. Individual-mandate advocates contend, plausibly enough, that we should make the free riders pay for themselves.

But how big is the free-rider problem, really? First, we should note that not all free riders are uninsured. In fact, people with insurance consume almost a third of uncompensated care. Second, not all care received by the uninsured is paid for by others. Analysts at the Urban Institute found that the uninsured pay more than 25 percent of their health expenditures out of pocket.

So how much uncompensated care is received by the uninsured? The same study puts the number at about \$35 billion a year in 2001, or only 2.8 percent

From *Cato Policy Report*, September/October 2007. Copyright © 2007 by Cato Institute. Reprinted by permission.

of total health care expenditures for that year. In other words, even if the individual mandate works exactly as planned, it will affect at best a mere 3 percent of health care expenditures.

The Problem of Noncompliance

But, of course, the mandate will not work exactly as planned. As anyone who's ever driven over 55 mph knows, mandating something is not the same as making it happen. Realistically, some individuals will not comply.

Forty-seven states currently require drivers to purchase liability auto insurance. Do 100 percent of drivers in those states have insurance? No. For states with an auto insurance mandate, the median percentage of drivers who are uninsured is 12 percent. In some states, the figure is much higher. For example, in California, where auto insurance is mandatory, 25 percent of drivers are uninsured—more than the percentage of Californians who lack health insurance.

Of course, the number of uninsured drivers might be even higher without mandatory coverage. The point, however, is that any amount of noncompliance reduces the efficacy of the mandate. If the individual health insurance mandate succeeded in forcing half of the uninsured to get coverage, it would arguably affect a mere 1.5 percent of current health care spending (that is, half of the 3 percent of spending that covers uncompensated care for the uninsured; the precise figure would depend on which uninsured people obtained coverage).

With auto insurance, at least there is a reasonable argument that a well-enforced mandate could reduce insurance premiums. When many motorists are uninsured, those who do buy insurance need, and are sometimes required, to buy coverage for damage done to their vehicles by the uninsured. So when the uninsured become insured, others' premiums could fall. But this argument simply doesn't fly in the case of health insurance, because (as already noted) uncompensated care is such a small fraction of overall health spending. Furthermore, more than 85 percent of uncompensated care is paid for by governments, not by private insurance. That means less than 15 percent of uncompensated care—less than half a percent of all health care spending—contributes to higher private insurance premiums.

None of this means that the uninsured are not a problem. But the problem is not that they cost the rest of us too much. One reason uncompensated care is such a small fraction of health care spending is that uninsured people simply get less health care than others. (Though they do get some, health care and health insurance are not synonymous.) So if the real concern is making health insurance and health care available to those in need, we should focus on health care prices and insurance premiums.

Not all free riders are trying to take advantage of their fellow citizens. For many, health insurance premiums are just too high. Yet the individual mandate does nothing to make insurance more affordable. There do exist regulatory reforms that could make it more affordable, but those reforms are desirable independent of the individual mandate. The mandate seeks to command a better outcome—more insured people—while doing nothing to make it happen. You can't get blood from a stone.

The architects of the Massachusetts plan, recognizing the affordability problem, have already effectively admitted defeat on this front: they have exempted 20 percent of the uninsured from the tax penalties for noncompliance. That's arguably another one-fifth reduction in the already small fraction of health care spending affected by the mandate.

Furthermore, the Massachusetts plan also creates a system of public subsidies (in the form of vouchers) to help low-income people buy insurance. As far as policies to encourage more private coverage go, you could do worse—and it would be possible to have the subsidy without the mandate. But to the extent that the public has to subsidize the formerly uninsured, the free-riding problem has not been solved—it has merely been shifted. It's wrong to say we "solve" the free-rider problem if all we're doing is paying for the free riders in a different way.

To make matters worse, there is no way to ensure that subsidies will go only to people who would otherwise be uninsured. Some people who would otherwise have paid their own way will tap the subsidy. As a result, the taxpayers could actually be subject to more cost-shifting than before.

Defining the Minimum Benefits Package

If you're going to mandate something, you have to define it. Under an individual mandate, legislators and bureaucrats will need to specify a minimum benefits package that a policy must cover in order to qualify. It's not plausible to believe this package can be defined in an apolitical way. Each medical specialty, from oncology to acupuncture, will pressure the legislature to include their services in the package. And as the benefits package grows, so will the premiums.

Limiting the mandate's scope with vacuous phrases like "basic health care products and services" will not solve the problem, because what is basic to some is crucial to others. Does contraception constitute basic health care? How about psychotherapy? Dental care? Chiropractic? The phrase "medically necessary" is just as problematic, because there is no objective definition of necessity. And even if there were, it wouldn't matter, because the content of the law will be determined by the legislative process. The "basic" package might initially be minimal, but over time it will succumb to the same special-interest lobbying that affects every other area of public policy. If psychotherapy is not initially included in the package, eventually it will be, once the psychotherapists' lobby has its way. And likewise for contraception, dental care, chiropractic, acupuncture, in vitro fertilization, hair transplants, ad infinitum.

This is not mere speculation. Even now, every state in the union has a list of mandated benefits that any health insurance policy must cover. Mandated benefits have included all of the services listed above—yes, even hair transplants in some states. All states together have created nearly 1900 mandated benefits. Given that medical interest groups have found it worth their time and money to lobby 50 state legislatures for laws affecting only voluntarily purchased insurance policies, mandatory insurance will only exacerbate the problem. If the benefits package is established at the federal level, the incentive to lobby will be that much greater.

Medicare and Medicaid provide further evidence. Given the massive funds at stake in those programs, it should come as no surprise that lobbying has affected the list of covered benefits. A public outcry prevented Viagra from being covered by Medicare and Medicaid, but other drugs and services have not attracted that kind of scrutiny. In 2004, after heavy lobbying by pharmaceutical companies that make antiobesity drugs, Medicare reclassified obesity as an illness (or rather, removed language saying it was not an illness), thereby clearing the way for coverage of obesity treatments including diet pills, weight-loss programs, and bariatric surgery. Although by law Medicare can pay only for "medically necessary" services, the obesity story aptly demonstrates the subjective and ultimately political meaning of that term.

Mandated benefits drive up insurance premiums; after all, insurance companies can't make more payouts without higher revenues. Existing mandates have increased premiums by an estimated 20 to 50 percent, depending on the state. There is every reason to believe the same process will affect the minimum benefits package under an individual mandate. As a result, even more people will find themselves unable to buy insurance and decide not to comply. Others will buy the insurance, but only by relying on public subsidies. A health policy intended to rein in free riding and cost-shifting will tend to encourage more of the same.

Limiting Flexibility in Health Insurance Policies

In addition to defining a minimum benefits package, an individual mandate must also specify other features of qualifying insurance policies—such as their maximum payouts, deductibles, and copayments. The same political pressures that affect the benefits package will also affect these other characteristics. Health care providers have a strong financial incentive to assure that patients have low deductibles and copayments so that they will consume more services.

In Massachusetts, no health insurance policy with a deductible greater than $2,000 for an individual or $4,000 for a family will satisfy the mandate. In addition, qualifying policies may not have any maximum annual or per-condition payout. And this is merely the regulatory starting point for a law that has not yet gone into full effect (some aspects of the plan won't kick in until 2009). We should expect further regulations to accumulate with the passage of time.

Consequently, the individual mandate will have a deleterious impact on the flexibility of health plans. Health care buyers and insurers need the opportunity to experiment with different types of coverage. Higher deductibles and copayments, for example, give patients an incentive to weigh the potential benefits of health services against their costs—a key component of any effective plan to control health care costs. (Health Savings Accounts, or HSAs, could allow people to save tax-free dollars for out-of-pocket health expenses, with unused dollars rolling over to their retirement accounts.) Insurers might also want to experiment with other policies, such as plans that offer full coverage for only certain treatments for particular conditions, while requiring patients to cover the difference in price between covered treatments and more expensive ones. But the individual mandate's one-size-fitsall approach cuts off such innovation at the knees.

Limitations on deductibles and copayments might be justified on grounds that out-of-pocket payments deter patients from getting necessary care. But the evidence does not support that position. In a famous RAND study, patients with first dollar insurance coverage consumed 43 percent more health care than patients who had to pay a large deductible, and yet the two groups experienced indistinguishable health outcomes. The obvious conclusion is that many health services have negligible benefits, but patients will get them anyway unless they face at least some portion of the costs.

More important, health insurance plans with lower deductibles and copayments are more expensive. Regulations that mandate more generous plans drive up premiums, thereby pricing some people out of the market. The result is more uninsured people, more people insured only via public subsidy, or both.

Free Riders and Hitchhikers

Individual mandates are frequently pitched as an alternative to other forms of regulation. In practice, they will assuredly be accompanied by a package of other interventions—some desirable, most not.

As noted earlier, the Massachusetts plan creates new public subsidies for health insurance. Worse, the plan requires community rating, which means that insurance firms may not charge differential premiums based on health risks. This might seem an attractive idea (everyone should pay the same amount), but, in fact, community rating creates an incentive for lower-risk patients to go uninsured because the coverage isn't worth the price. The mandate is supposed to prevent dropouts, but compliance cannot be guaranteed.

Community rating also forces low-risk patients to subsidize high-risk patients—another form of cost-shifting. Yet the justification of the individual mandate was to reduce cost-shifting. The subsidy to higher-risk patients generates a political incentive to regulate personal lifestyles—such as diet choices or sexual behaviors—that affect health risks. We have already observed this mechanism at work: the cost of treating motorcycle accident victims has been used to justify helmet laws; the cost of Medicaid to treat cigarette smokers was used to justify lawsuits against the tobacco industry. The public is notably more willing to restrict choice when the costs are socialized—and that means individual liberty is at stake.

Governor Schwarzenegger's proposal, meanwhile, couples an individual mandate with an employer mandate: any employer with 10 or more employees would have to provide health coverage or pay an additional payroll tax. This regulation would constitute a direct tax on employment, as businesses will find it in their interest to hire fewer employees (possibly compensating with more hours per worker) to minimize health insurance costs. Meanwhile, businesses with fewer than 10 employees will have a strong incentive not to expand, as doing so could expose them to the mandate.

Effective health care reform would involve making customers more cost-conscious. The individual mandate, sadly, will tend to shield customers from costs and impede innovations that could push costs down. Rising insurance premiums, as a result of a growing mandated benefits package, will fuel greater public dissatisfaction with the health care system. Further regulations that hitchhike on the individual mandate will only make matters worse. Ironically, free markets rather than government will likely catch the blame, thus fueling demand for more intrusive interventions into the health care market.

A better approach to health reform would focus on removing, or mitigating the effect of, existing mandates that drive up insurance premiums. States that genuinely want to help the uninsured ought to repeal some or all of their mandated benefit laws, allowing firms to offer low-priced catastrophic care policies to their customers. If special-interest pressures hamper this solution, the federal government could assist by using its power—under the Constitution's interstate commerce clause—to guarantee customers the right to buy insurance policies offered in any state, not just their own. That would enable patients to patronize firms in states with fewer costly mandates. As an added bonus, state legislatures might feel pressure to ease regulations to attract more insurance business from out-of-state customers. Removing mandates would do far more to expand health care coverage than adding new mandates ever could.

POSTSCRIPT

Is It Fair to Require Individuals to Purchase Health Insurance?

To find out more about health reform and its implementation, go to the Kaiser Family Foundation Web site http://www.kff.org/ or Health Reform GPS http://www.healthreformgps.org/. Both sites are updated frequently.

Basic information about the Massachusetts Health Care Reform plan is available at http://www.kff.org/uninsured/upload/7494-02.pdf on the Web site of the Kaiser Family Foundation. In its first year, the plan enrolled over 100,000 previously uninsured people. A study by Jane Zhu and colleagues from Harvard Medical School and Harvard School of Public Health found that in its first two years the Massachusetts plan reduced cost-related barriers but did not result in improvements in self-reported health or access to a personal doctor. The authors suggest that health reform is necessary but not sufficient to achieve equity in health care (Jane Zhu, et al., "Massachusetts Health Reform and Disparities in Coverage, Access and Health Status," *Annals of General Internal Medicine* (September 2010)).

Landmark: The Inside Story of America's New Health Care Law and What It Means for Us All is a product of the staff of *The Washington Post* (2010). It covers many aspects of the health reform law.

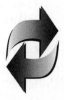

ISSUE 17

Should There Be a Market in Human Organs?

YES: Sally Satel, from "Kidney for Sale: Let's Legally Reward the Donor," *Globe and Mail* (March 10, 2010)

NO: The Institute of Medicine Committee on Increasing Rates of Organ Donation, from *Organ Donation: Opportunities for Action* (2006)

ISSUE SUMMARY

YES: Psychiatrist Sally Satel contends that a regulated and legal system of rewarding organ donors will not only save lives but also stop the illegal trafficking that offers no protections for poor people around the world.

NO: The Institute of Medicine Committee argues that a free market in organs is problematic because in live organ donation both buyers and sellers may not have complete or accurate information, and selling organs of dead people raises concerns about commodification of human bodies.

Human organ transplantation, unachievable at mid-twentieth century and still experimental a few decades ago, has now become routine. Dr. Joseph E. Murray of Brigham and Women's Hospital in Boston performed the first successful kidney transplant in 1954. By the 1980s, livers, hearts, pancreases, lungs, and heart–lungs had also been successfully transplanted. Surgical techniques, as well as methods for preserving and transporting organs, had improved over the years. But the most significant advance came from a single drug, cyclosporine, discovered by Jean Borel in the mid-1970s and approved by the Food and Drug Administration in 1983. Cyclosporine suppresses the immune system so that the organ recipient's body does not reject the transplanted organ. However, the drug does not suppress the body's ability to fight infection from other sources.

This achievement has its darker side in that there is a shortage of transplantable organs and many seriously ill people wait for months to receive one. Some die before one becomes available. In 2009 almost 7,000 people on waiting lists died while waiting to receive an organ. According to the United Network of Organ Sharing (UNOS), the national agency responsible for allocating organs, on October 11, 2010, 108,952 people were waiting for organs. Over 86,000 of these patients were waiting for kidney transplants, and over 16,000 for liver transplants. Heart transplants were the next highest category, with over 3,000 patients on the waiting list.

By contrast, the UNOS data show that in 2009 only 28,463 transplants were performed, with kidney-alone transplants leading the list at 16,829. Of the total transplants, 21,854 came from deceased donors, and 6609 from living donors. Living donors are almost always relatives of the recipient, although there have been several highly publicized cases in which the donor was not related. Like any surgery, transplantation presents risks to the donor but these are usually not grave. A person can live with one kidney, although should that kidney fail, the donor would require regular dialysis (cleansing the blood of toxic substances through a machine) or a transplant.

The shortage of transplantable organs in the United States is attributed to many factors: the reluctance of families to approve donation after death, even if the donor has indicated the desire to do so; the reluctance of medical personnel to approach families at a time of crisis; religious objections; and mistrust of the medical system. Despite many educational programs and publicity about donation, Americans seem unwilling either to move to a system of required request (mandated in a few states) or to presume that potential donors would agree to having their organs used for transplantation, unless they had explicitly consented in advance.

The shortage of organs is even more acute in other parts of the world, where cultural or religious objections to removing organs from the deceased remain strong. Organ transplantation is one area in which "technology transfer"—the export of the science and training for the procedure—has been particularly strong. Organ transplant centers have grown rapidly in areas of the world that lack even basic public health measures. However, although some countries have the technology for transplantation, they do not have enough organs to meet the demand.

In the United States, the National Organ Transplant Act (Public Law 98-507), passed in 1984, made it illegal to buy and sell organs. Violators are subject to fines and imprisonment. Congress passed this law because it was concerned that traffic in organs might lead to inequitable access to donor organs with the wealthy having an unfair advantage. (Even with the ban, the wealthy have an advantage in being able to pay for the transplant and the necessary post-transplant supportive services, and thus are more likely to be accepted for a waiting list.)

Although many countries and international medical organizations officially ban the sale of organs as well, the practice goes on. The following selections present opposing views on whether the ban should be reexamined or more aggressively implemented. Sally Satel, a psychiatrist and recipient of a kidney donated by a friend, maintains that the ban on selling organs is unfair and should be replaced by a legal system of rewarding donors with in-kind rewards, such as lifetime health insurance. The Institute of Medicine's Committee on Transplantable Organs argues that selling organs of either living or dead people raises serious questions about the commodification of human bodies.

YES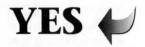

Sally Satel

Kidney for Sale: Let's Legally Reward the Donor

World Kidney Day [held every March] is part of a global health campaign meant to alert us to the impact of kidney disease. Sadly, there is little to celebrate.

According to the International Society of Nephrology, kidney disease affects more than 500 million people worldwide, or 10 per cent of the adult population. With more people developing high blood pressure and diabetes (key risks for kidney disease), the picture will only worsen.

There are nearly two million new cases of the most serious form of kidney disease—renal failure—each year. Unless patients with renal failure receive a kidney transplant or undergo dialysis—an expensive, lifelong procedure that cleanses the blood of toxins—death is guaranteed within a few weeks.

[In 2008], Australian nephrologist Gavin Carney held a press conference in Canberra to urge that people be allowed to sell their kidneys. "The current system isn't working," The Sydney Morning Herald quoted him as saying. "We've tried everything to drum up support" for organ donation, but "people just don't seem willing to give their organs away for free."

Dr. Carney wants to keep patients from purchasing kidneys on the black market and in overseas organ bazaars. As an American recipient of a kidney who was once desperate enough to consider doing that myself (fortunately, a friend ended up donating to me), I agree wholeheartedly that we should offer well-informed individuals a reward if they are willing to save a stranger's life.

If not, we will continue to face a dual tragedy: on one side, the thousands of patients who die each year for want of a kidney; on the other, a human-rights disaster in which corrupt brokers deceive indigent donors about the nature of surgery, cheat them out of payment and ignore their postsurgical needs.

The World Health Organization estimates that 5 per cent to 10 per cent of all transplants performed annually—perhaps 63,000 in all—take place in the clinical netherworlds of China, Pakistan, Egypt, Colombia and Eastern Europe.

Unfortunately, much of the world transplant establishment—including the WHO, the international Transplantation Society, and the World Medical Association—advocates only a partial remedy. They focus on ending organ trafficking but ignore the time-tested truth that trying to stamp out illicit markets either drives them further underground or causes corruption to reappear elsewhere.

For example, after China, India and Pakistan began cracking down on illicit organ markets, many patients turned to the Philippines. Last spring, after the Philippines banned the sale of kidneys to foreigners, a headline in *The Jerusalem Post* read: "Kidney transplant candidates in limbo after Philippines closes gates." (Israel has one of the lowest donation rates in the world, so the government pays for transplant surgery performed outside the country.) Similarly, patients from Qatar who travelled to Manila are "looking for alternative solutions," according to the Qatari daily *The Peninsula*.

True, more countries must develop efficient systems for posthumous donation, a very important source of organs. But even in Spain, which is famously successful at retrieving organs from the newly deceased, people die while waiting for a kidney.

The truth is that trafficking will stop only when the need for organs disappears.

Opponents allege that a legal system of exchange will inevitably replicate the sins of the black market. This is utterly backward. The remedy to this corrupt and unregulated system of exchange is a regulated and transparent regime devoted to donor protection.

My colleagues and I suggest a system in which compensation is provided by a third party (government, a charity or insurance) with public oversight. Because bidding and private buying would not be permitted, available organs would be distributed to the next in line—not just to the wealthy. Donors would be carefully screened for physical and psychological problems, as is currently done for all volunteer living kidney donors. Moreover, they would be guaranteed follow-up care for any complications.

Many people are uneasy about offering lump-sum cash payments. A solution is to provide in-kind rewards—such as a down payment on a house, a contribution to a retirement fund, or lifetime health insurance—so the program would not be attractive to people who might otherwise rush to donate on the promise of a large sum of instant cash.

The only way to stop illicit markets is to create legal ones. Indeed, there is no better justification for testing legal modes of exchange than the very depredations of the underground market.

Momentum is growing. In the *British Medical Journal,* a leading British transplant surgeon called for a controlled donor compensation program for unrelated live donors. [In 2008] the Israeli, Saudi and Indian governments have decided to offer incentives ranging from lifelong health insurance for the donor to a cash benefit. In the United States, the American Medical Association has endorsed a draft bill that would make it easier for states to offer non-cash incentives for donation.

Until countries create legal means of rewarding donors, the fates of Third World donors and the patients who need their organs to survive will remain morbidly entwined. What better way to mark World Kidney Day than for global health leaders to take a bold step and urge countries to experiment with donor rewards?

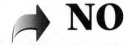

Organ Donation:
Opportunities for Action

Why a Free Market in Organs Is Problematic

Many economists begin from the position that a market is almost always the best way to allocate a scarce resource. In the standard model of a competitive market economy, markets use prices to allocate scarce resources in an automatic, decentralized fashion. In each market, the price of the good adjusts until the amount that suppliers are willing to sell at the prevailing price equals the amount that consumers are willing to pay. A higher price coaxes out more supply by making it worthwhile for producers to produce more of the good or, if the total amount of the good is fixed, by encouraging the current owners to put more of the good up for sale. On the demand side, a higher price chokes off demand, as some buyers decide that the good is not worth the new price to them.

In this model, the market outcome can be considered both efficient and equitable, provided the distribution of income and assets meets a community standard of fairness. On the demand side, price rations the good to the people who value it the most, that is, those who need it the most, where need is assessed by the people concerned rather than a regulatory body. On the supply side, the supplier is compensated for the cost of production, including a reasonable profit, and in general, resources are directed to the most productive uses. If all markets are perfectly competitive, the resulting distribution of goods is efficient, and because it is the result of voluntary trades from a fair initial distribution of income and assets, it can be argued that it is also equitable.

On the basis of this model, permitting a market in organs could be an equitable and efficient way to achieve an increase in supply that would reduce the number of people on organ transplant waiting lists. However, this conclusion is dependent on the accuracy of the strong assumptions that underlie the theoretical model. When the assumptions do not hold, the normative arguments for the desirability of markets do not hold either. A market process might still be preferable to the available alternatives as an instrument for increasing the organ supply, but the case for it must be built, brick by brick, in light of the actual circumstances. Because the application of the market model raises different issues on the supply side and the demand side, the chapter will address them separately.

The Supply Side of an Organ Market

The market model's assumptions about supply seem most plausible for living donors. In living donation, a mentally competent adult has an organ (or organ part) that can be supplied to the market at some risk and financial cost. When the person donates the organ or organ part, that is, supplies it at a zero market price, he or she suffers a loss as a result of the discomfort of the operation, the opportunity cost of the time involved, and the long-term health risks. The donor's expectation of a benefit to the recipient is some compensation for this loss, which is why some organs are supplied at a zero price. Reducing the donor's loss by making a financial payment for the organ seems fair, however, and it seems likely that more people would be willing to provide organs as a result. In an efficient market, the additional organs would come from those who require the least financial compensation for the organ and for enduring the donation process.

In evaluating a policy of allowing payment for organs from living donors, two issues that are not assumed in the standard market model become important: distributional inequity and imperfect information. Many people would agree that large, unjust disparities in income and assets exist among Americans. Poor people value extra money more highly because they need it for basic necessities, so the additional organs are likely to come from the poor, a result many find morally troubling. A common economist's response to this concern is, "True, the distribution of income and assets is not fair. But if society cannot (or will not) do anything about it, is it fair to deprive people of an opportunity that they believe would improve their situations? Competent adults should be free to make their own decisions about the medical procedures that they will undergo and the risks that they will take."

This argument is compelling superficially, but it assumes that the organ suppliers have the information and the capacity that they need to make the decision. Information about the long-term risks of donation may not be complete, and the buyers of organs have an incentive to understate the risks. In an unregulated market, organs are likely to come from people who do not fully appreciate the risks that they are taking. Avoiding this result would require the development of complete information for potential living donors and other efforts to ensure that the decisions made by living donors are fully informed, which would require planning and substantial resources. Concerns about inadequate information arise, however, even under the gift model now in place. . . .

The living-donor case is mentioned here mainly to contrast it with the far less straightforward case of obtaining organs from deceased donors. In the latter case, the organs become available only when the person dies. There is no risk to the donor at that point, but a financial payment would not provide any direct benefit to the donor either—the benefit to the donor arises from the interest that the donor had while alive in providing for the well-being of his or her family after death. In practice, the family of the donor often makes the donation decision, and market advocates usually assume that the payment would be made to the family. Essentially, this means that the family is selling a relative's body parts, which raises the issue of cultural norms surrounding the treatment of dead bodies.

Commodification of Dead Bodies

Most societies hold that it is degrading to human dignity to view dead bodies as property that can be bought and sold. . . . [B]odies are supposed to be treated with respect—with funeral rites and burial or cremation—and not simply discarded like worn out household furniture and certainly not sold by the relatives (or anyone else) to the highest bidder. These norms are very powerful. Illicit markets for bodies have existed throughout history; for example, in the 19th century, England had an illicit market in which bodies were dug up in the night by body snatchers and sold for dissection, arguably a socially useful purpose (Richardson, 2000). Buying and selling bodies for dissection was considered a despicable business, however, and even desperately poor people did not willingly sell their relatives' bodies for whatever they could get.

Organ transplantation has provided a compelling justification for using the body parts of deceased individuals, namely, the opportunity to restore life and health to someone on the brink of death. Many people see donating a person's organs for this purpose as a highly meritorious act that honors the sacredness of the body rather than degrades it. At the same time, however, many people regard the act of donating the organs for this purpose as being conceptually and morally distinct from the act of selling the organs (even when the organs are to be used for the same purpose). Currently, the sale of solid organs is prohibited, but the prohibition reflects preexisting and widely accepted cultural norms. In the context of these norms, and the attitudes underlying them, it is not at all clear that the supply of organs from deceased donors would actually increase if sales were made legal. It is possible that the reasons people have for not donating cannot be overcome by money, or that offering money induces some to provide organs while leading an equal or greater number of people who would have provided organs to decide not to. For example, family members may wish to avoid appearing to be profiting from a deceased relative's body, especially if there is any chance of appearing to have participated in a treatment decision that might have hastened death. . . .

Barriers to a Futures Market

Traditionally, the relatives of deceased individuals had the final word about whether organs would be donated, but this has been changing. Because society supports the right of individuals to control what happens to their bodies when they are alive, it is a natural extension to assume that they should also decide what happens to their bodies after death. This adds more intricacy to the application of the market model. Because money is of no use to a corpse, for financial payments to influence the donor's decision, one must introduce a futures market or a bequest motive into the picture.

A futures market is a market in which the commodity bought and sold is the right to sell organs at a future time in the event that a person dies in circumstances that permit organs to be recovered and transplanted. The person receives payment for these contingent organ sale rights while he or she is still alive. Futures markets are inherently complex. In this case, the chances of dying in the appropriate circumstances are low, death may occur far into the future, and it may not be easy to execute the right to the organ at the appropriate moment; therefore, the right to a potential organ is not worth nearly as much as an actual organ at the time of death. What if sellers want to change their minds? Can they rescind their contracts and, if so, on what terms? Also, once the rights to an individual's organs have been sold, the buyer (who would probably be an organ broker) has a financial interest in the seller's death. Some people already worry about receiving suboptimal treatment at the end of life if they are registered organ donors and adding financial interests resulting from the selling of organ rights might add to those concerns. Further, it seems unlikely that there would be enough interested investors to allow a private futures market in organ rights to develop, given the long time horizon required and the uncertainty about the size of the profits.

Alternatively, one can assume that people get satisfaction in life from the knowledge that their heirs will receive inheritances when they die. If this is so, a person could be allowed to spell out his or her wishes for the disposition of his or her body in advance (in a will or in a special organ donor registry) stating whether his or her body should be buried or cremated intact, donated all or in part to a specific organization for a specific purpose, or sold whole or in part with the proceeds forming part of the estate. To the extent that more people would agree to organ removal if they had this option, the supply of organs would increase. This is an empirical question, and as before, there is no certainty of a positive effect. Again, implementation would be complex. For example, a registry would be better than a will, because one cannot wait until the will is probated to determine whether the organs can be sold. . . .

Other Complexities

It has been assumed thus far in the discussion that paying people or their families for organs would increase the supply of organs for transplantation. However, some other complexities of the organ procurement process suggest that the creation of financial incentives for organ donation may be less important for donors and their families than it is for healthcare organizations and the participating healthcare professionals. A family does not simply make the decision to donate (or to honor the decedent's wish to donate) and then it happens automatically. First, the potential donor must be in the process of dying under the right circumstances to be eligible to donate his or her organs. Second, the medical staff must make the family aware of the possibility of organ donation. Only then does the opportunity to say yes or no to donation arise. Many people have not thought much about organ donation before the issue arises, and in any case, they are in an extremely stressful situation. How and when they are told about the opportunity for organ donation and the way in which the request is made can make a significant difference to the relatives' response. Finally, the organs must be removed, the recipients must be identified, and the organs must be transported to their final destinations. These are complex tasks that must be carried out under extreme time pressure.

Many factors—including the structure of financial incentives to the healthcare workers and organizations that carry out these organ transplant-related activities—influence the way in which the process of notification, request, removal, and conveyance to a recipient occurs. If this process is the problem, the introduction of financial payments for organs may simply raise the cost of the transplantation process without having any effect on the number of organs recovered. The efforts and successes of the Organ Donation Breakthrough Collaboratives of the Health Resources and Services Administration suggest that the process is part of the problem and, indeed, is perhaps most of it. . . . The collaboratives have demonstrated that the application of quality improvement methods to the steps in this process can significantly increase the percentage of potential organ donations that are converted into actual donations. There is also potential to increase the organ supply through medical practice changes that make more decedents medically eligible to be organ donors . . . , that is, to give more people the opportunity to consent.

The Demand Side of an Organ Market

The demand side of an organ market is also complicated. The simple market model assumes that those who benefit from the use of the good pay for the good, and this is an important element in the normative theory in favor of markets. In the case of organs, advocates for payments for organs from deceased donors generally do not expect the recipients to make the payments. Most people believe that health care is a special kind of commodity that should not be allocated strictly according to an ability to pay because of the unusual importance of health care to the well-being of all people and the uneven distribution of illness among the population. The distribution of health care, especially life-saving health care, should be determined separately from the distribution of other goods and in accord with special ethical principles. This is a major departure from the standard market model and means that even if a fair distribution of income and assets could be arranged, letting health care be determined by voluntary market trades would not yield equitable outcomes, even under the highly unrealistic assumption of the existence of a perfectly competitive market.

In the United States, the result of this societal value judgment is a complex array of private and public policies that are implicitly or explicitly intended to provide people with care that they would not receive if all health care were distributed through unregulated private markets. Unfortunately, there is no general, transparent consensus on the nature and extent of healthcare services that people should be able to receive without regard to the ability to pay and how the cost of that care should be distributed across the population. The unfortunate result is a financing system that distributes both care and cost arbitrarily in a manner that meets no rational standard of efficiency or equity.

The U.S. healthcare system does not guarantee access to life-saving treatments such as organ transplantations, and the ability to pay does play a role in the distribution of this important good. Few people pay directly for organ transplantation, which is expensive even without payment for the organs.

People in need of organs rely on public or private insurance to pay the cost of acquiring the organs and transplanting them, and a transplant is not received unless insurance coverage or access to charity care is available (the so-called green screen).

Given this system of healthcare financing (or any system that might replace it), what would the demand side of a market for organs look like? Presumably, most of the actual buyers would be the healthcare organizations that perform transplantations. They would compete with one another for the available organs, the price would settle down at the market-clearing price, and the cost of organs would become part of the total charge to a third-party payer for an organ transplant. This market would inevitably be very complex.

So far the chapter has referred to "the price" of an organ, but an actual market would have multiple prices for organs because organs are highly differentiated products. For example, hearts differ from kidneys and kidneys differ from one another along many medically significant dimensions. Organ recipients also differ from one another, and matching an organ with the right recipient is important in achieving the benefits of transplantation. This means that the kidney market or the heart market would actually be a whole set of interconnected markets for goods that are close substitutes for each other (e.g., kidneys or hearts from people of different ages, with different blood types, or different human leukocyte antigen factors). The price of a kidney would therefore actually be a price structure for all the different kinds of kidneys. This price structure would result from the interaction of the array of kidneys available with the variety of patients in need of a kidney at any point in time and the trade-offs among kidney characteristics that are medically possible for transplantation into various patients.

Of course, the original suppliers and the end users of the organs do not have the medical knowledge to make sophisticated sales and purchase decisions, and even if they did, they are hardly in the best physical condition to apply their knowledge at the time of donation or transplantation. Like the rest of the healthcare market, this market would be characterized by complicated agency relationships (situations in which decisions are made by an expert on someone else's behalf). The various potential agents here would include the transplant recipient's physician, the organ donor's physician, the healthcare organizations in which the organ recovery and the transplantation occur, a specialized organ "broker" such as the United Network for Organ Sharing (UNOS), the private and public third-party payers that pay for the transplantation-related care, and so on.

Real-world markets in which differentiated products are sold under circumstances of imperfect information and intricate agency relationships do exist, and such markets can be superior to other methods of allocation. In the case of organs, however, it is interesting to note that a nonmarket process for allocating organs to recipients and managing waiting lists has been in place since the beginning of the transplantation era. The Organ Procurement and Transplantation Network system grew up in response to a perceived need to manage the organ allocation process within the transplantation community, although it has come to have substantial government involvement. There is ongoing pressure to adjust the process to make it more efficient and equitable, with the usual difficulties in defining exactly what efficiency and equity mean in such a complicated context. There is also recognition that financial and other incentives should be aligned with ultimate goals, but little enthusiasm for relying completely on an unregulated market process exists.

In summary, in a hypothesized market for organs, the good to be sold is highly differentiated and must be matched to the final user in many ways. The process of making an organ available requires skilled labor and technology. The good is highly perishable, and recovery and transfer to the final user must be accomplished under extreme time pressure. The good has unique cultural significance that would powerfully influence the response of suppliers to market incentives, even in the absence of the existing legal constraints on their behavior. Imperfect information issues are significant, and the end user is not in a position to act as an informed buyer. The need for information, skilled labor and technology, and third-party payment means that the market transactions involve complex agency relationships. With all of these departures from the standard assumptions of the market model, organ transplantation occurs in a world of imperfect markets when it comes to evaluating efficiency. A perfectly functioning market and a fair distribution of income and assets would not likely produce equity in the current healthcare system. As a society, it is not clear what an equitable distribution of health care and its cost would look like, but it is generally agreed that the distribution of organ transplants should not be totally determined by the ability to pay.

Given all of these factors, the committee doubts that it would even be possible to have a well-functioning free market in organs from deceased donors. If such a market existed, there is no certainty that it would produce a greater supply of organs. Moreover, a free market in organs would deviate substantially from prevailing norms in the United States regarding the nature of health care and the fair distribution of organs for transplantation, norms that have been developed within various communities of stakeholders and that are now well entrenched.

POSTSCRIPT

Should There Be a Market in Human Organs?

In *When Altruism Isn't Enough: The Case for Compensating Kidney Donors* (2009), Sally Satel and other authors expand the argument for abandoning the current ban on sale of organs. Steve Farber, who received a kidney donated by his son, and Harlan Abraham describe their experience as well as another patient's in *On the List: Fixing America's Failing Organ Transplant System* (2009).

UNOS policies prohibit designating donated organs for a group—that is, limiting a donation to patients who are white, black, Catholic, male, or any other category. In "Members First: The Ethics of Donating Organs and Tissues to Groups," Timothy F. Murphy and Robert M. Veatch raise questions about the implications of the activities of LifeSharers, a voluntary organization whose members agree that their organs will be donated first to other members (*Cambridge Quarterly of Healthcare Ethics,* vol. 15, 2006). In the same issue, Barbro Bjorkman argues against selling of organs and calls instead for a "virtue ethics" approach in his article, "Why We Are Not Allowed to Sell That Which We Are Encouraged to Donate."

An intermediate approach is described in "Compensated Kidney Donation: An Ethical Review of the Iranian Model" by Alireza Bagheri (*Kennedy Institute of Ethics Journal,* vol. 16, no. 3, 2006). In this program donors receive compensation for their time taken from work, travel, and other expenses. While supporting this concept, the author warns that it does not have secure enough measures to prevent a direct monetary relationship between donors and recipients.

In the fall 2004 issue of the *American Journal of Bioethics,* David Steinberg proposes a new method for allocating organs for transplantation ("An 'Opting In' Paradigm for Kidney Transplantation"). His proposal would reward people who agree to donate their kidneys after they die by giving them preferences for a kidney should they need one while alive. Twenty-one commentaries follow the article.

As alternatives to paid organ donations, Francis Delmonico and colleagues proposed donor medals of honor, reimbursement for funeral expenses, organ exchanges, medical leaves for organ donation, and other mechanisms, in "Ethical Incentives—Not Payment—for Organ Donation," *The New England Journal of Medicine* (June 20, 2002).

From a United Kingdom perspective Charles Erin and John Harris, however, have proposed an "ethical market" in organs. In their proposal, the market would be confined to a specific area, and only citizens from that area could buy and sell organs. One purchaser, probably a government agency, would buy all organs and distribute them according to some order of medical priority.

Individuals would not be allowed to enter the market directly. See "An Ethical Market in Human Organs," *British Medical Journal* (July 20, 2002).

The most controversial consideration in the allocation of transplantable organs in the United States is whether the organs should be allocated nationally or locally. The Department of Health and Human Services (DHHS) proposed in March 1998 that current geographic disparities in the allocation of scarce organs should be addressed by creating national uniform criteria for determining a patient's medical status and eligibility for placement on a waiting list. Under the current system, local centers have first chance at organs in their region, even though patients in other areas may have greater medical need or have been on the waiting list longer.

This proposal was received enthusiastically by the large transplant centers, which attract the most ill and most affluent recipients, who can travel to the center and remain for months. However, it was criticized by smaller transplant centers, which rely on local recipients and the value of being able to tell potential donors or their families that the organs will be given to a local resident. Congress asked the Institute of Medicine (IOM), an independent agency, to study the impact of the rule. The IOM's report, issued in July 1999, agreed that organs should be allocated on the basis of medical need across wider geographical areas. A Special Section of *The Cambridge Quarterly of Healthcare Ethics* (vol. 10, 2001) contains several articles discussing this and other aspects of organ allocation in the United States.

For more information on organ transplantation, see Courtney S. Campell, "The Selling of Organs, the Sharing of Self," *Second Opinion* (vol. 19, no. 2, 1993); Stuart J. Youngner, Renee C. Fox, and Laurence J. O'Connell, eds., *Organ Transplantation: Meanings and Realities* (University of Wisconsin Press, 1996); and the title essay in Arthur Caplan, *If I Were a Rich Man, Could I Buy a Pancreas?* (Indiana University Press, 1992). In the same issue of the *Kennedy Institute of Ethics Journal* in which Gill and Sade's article appeared, Cynthia Cohen presents a critique of their arguments in "Public Policy and the Sale of Human Organs" (pp. 47–64). She believes that "public resistance to the sale of human body parts, no matter how voluntary or well informed, is ground in the conviction that such a practice would diminish human dignity."

The various reports on transplantation issued by the Institute of Medicine are available at http://www.nap.edu.

ISSUE 18

Does Military Necessity Override Medical Ethics?

YES: **Michael L. Gross**, from "Bioethics and Armed Conflict: Mapping the Moral Dimensions of Medicine and War," *Hastings Center Report* (November/December 2004)

NO: **M. Gregg Bloche and Jonathan H. Marks**, from "When Doctors Go to War," *The New England Journal of Medicine* (January 6, 2005)

ISSUE SUMMARY

YES: Political scientist Michael L. Gross argues that war brings military and medical values into conflict, and that military necessity often overwhelms a physician's other moral obligations, such as relieving suffering.

NO: M. Gregg Bloche, a physician and lawyer, and Jonathan H. Marks, a British barrister, stress that physicians remain physicians even in the military and that there is an urgent moral challenge in managing the conflict, not denying it.

As long as human beings have engaged in war, medical personnel have tended the wounded and dying. However, for centuries, the available techniques, skills, and medications were not very effective against grave battlefield wounds.

Although from the earliest times there were attempts to set limits for the proper conduct of combatants in war, serious attempts to set ethical parameters for the conduct and protection of medical personnel began in the nineteenth century. Two events are particularly important for consideration of ethical issues. First, in the United States in 1865, Captain Henry Wirz, a Confederate physician who commanded the infamous Andersonville prison in Georgia, was tried for a series of offenses alleging inhumane conduct against Union prisoners of war. He claimed in his defense that "superior orders" mitigated his behavior. Nevertheless, he was convicted and hanged.

In Europe, around the same time, Henri Dunant, a Swiss banker, was shocked by the carnage of the Battle of Solferino, which took place on June 24, 1859.

A conference Dunant helped organize in 1864 in Geneva, Switzerland, led to the creation of the International Red Cross. It also established the principle that the sick and wounded, as well as medical personnel, facilities, and transport, were to be considered neutral. This international agreement was the first Geneva Convention, and for his efforts Dunant was awarded the first Nobel Peace Prize.

In 1949, after World War II, this agreement was updated by three other international agreements collectively called the Geneva Conventions. They concern the casualties of naval warfare, the treatment of prisoners, and the protection of civilians from deportation, hostage taking, torture, and discrimination in treatment. Sixty nations, including the United States, signed. The Geneva Conventions states that medical personnel are to be regarded as "noncombatants," and are forbidden to engage in or be parties to acts of war. Furthermore, the wounded and sick of all parties must be respected, protected, treated humanely, and cared for by the belligerents. No physical or moral coercion is allowed against protected persons, in particular to obtain information from them or from third parties.

The Nuremberg Code of 1949, another influential document, followed World War II. The revelations at the Nuremberg, Germany, trial of Nazis who carried out brutal and lethal experiments on prisoners were particularly shocking because these men were physicians, sworn to heal and prevent suffering. Their experiments, such as exposing individuals to freezing water until they died, were conducted to gain knowledge that might assist the German military.

Just as medicine has changed dramatically in the past century, so has warfare. Guerrilla warfare, terrorism, unclear objectives, vastly superior weapons, the blurring of lines between civilian and military participants and targets, attacks on hospitals and ambulances—all have altered the way in which political and ideological struggles are waged. The question is, has this new type of warfare also changed the ethics of military medicine?

In 2004, this question was brought to the forefront of public and professional opinion because of revelations and allegations about mistreatment of prisoners in the U.S.-led war in Afghanistan and Iraq and in the treatment of detainees at Guantanamo Bay, Cuba, an American naval base. Widely circulated photographs of abuses at Abu Ghraib prison in Iraq showed degrading and abusive behavior by American troops. According to Steven H. Miles, a physician and human rights advocate, "Government documents show that the U.S. military medical system failed to protect detainees' human rights, sometimes collaborated with interrogators or abusive guards, and failed to properly report injuries or deaths caused by beatings."

In October 2004, the World Medical Association, a physician organization, reaffirmed its 1982 declaration that medical ethics are the same whether a nation is at war or at peace. But does this statement reflect reality? Michael L. Gross believes that it does not because war brings military and medical values into conflict and that sometimes states sacrifice the lives of many to save some intangible national asset that embodies its common vision of the good. M. Gregg Bloche and Jonathan H. Marks do not deny that a conflict exists, but stress that physicians remain physicians even in the military and that their expertise should not be used to do harm.

YES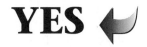

Michael L. Gross

Bioethics and Armed Conflict: Mapping the Moral Dimensions of Medicine and War

Medical ethics in time of armed conflict are identical to medical ethics in time of peace," declares the World Medical Association.[1] Were this the case, wartime and peacetime medicine would turn on the same principles and present similar dilemmas. But war fundamentally transforms the major principles and central issues that engage bioethics. A patient's rights to life and self-determination contract; human dignity strains under the barrage of military necessity; and the interests of the state and political community may outweigh considerations of patients' welfare. Also, actors and interests multiply. Combatants and noncombatants, enemies and allies, states and individuals, citizens and soldiers, prisoners of war, the wounded and the dying, those who can return to combat duty and those who cannot—all of these litter the battlefield.

Armed conflict augments the general principles of bioethics with those peculiar to the conduct of war. For instance, states are obliged to recognize noncombatant immunity, minimize collateral damage, and adhere to a principle of proportionality when fighting threatens to take the lives of civilians and destroy their property. If difficult bioethical dilemmas arise when fundamental moral principles conflict, war adds novel dimensions of its own, as competing bioethical principles must contend not only with one another, but also with the overriding "reason of state" and military necessity that animate any issue of military ethics and may overwhelm other fundamental moral obligations.

Medical ethics in war are not identical to medical ethics in times of peace. Moreover, the nature of war is itself changing as conflicts between nation-states and sub-state actors—guerillas, insurgent ethnic groups, and international terrorist organizations—replace conventional war between sovereign nations. The changing modes of warfare create difficulties for the established conventions of war. They also create new dilemmas for medical personnel, who may be called upon to lend their expertise to the prosecution of war rather than simply to relieve the suffering it causes.

Medical and Military Ethics

In contrast to medical ethics, a wide range of agents, interests, and principles characterize military ethics. Whereas bioethics turns its attention to the patient, either as an individual or class of individuals, military ethics focuses on the rights and interests of three distinct actors: combatants, noncombatants, and the state. The 1949 Geneva Conventions define noncombatants as "persons taking no active part in the hostilities." These include civilians— "people who do not bear arms"—as well as prisoners of war and wounded soldiers. Combatants, on the other hand, bear arms and belong to military organizations that oversee compliance with international law; they include uniformed soldiers, irregulars, members of militia, and guerillas. This definition excludes terrorists who defy international law by intentionally targeting civilian populations.

Alongside individual actors stands the nation-state or political community with interests of its own. Nationstates are internationally recognized sovereign bodies, while political communities reflect the underlying linguistic, historical, ethnic, or religious groups that state or sub-state actors may represent. Representing a "collective way of life" or national ethos, states and political communities are "super-personalities" with a range of interests not necessarily identical to, and possibly in conflict with, the interests of their members.

In spite of divergent actors and interests, the ethics of medicine and armed conflict share norms anchored in the right to life, autonomy, dignity, and utility. The right to life, a central feature of contemporary political theory, grounds a state's obligation to safeguard the lives of its citizens, while liberty interests secure political self-determination and its close cousin, medical autonomy. Dignity is of more recent political interest than either the right to life or self-determination, although it is certainly an integral part of Kant's discussion of autonomy and an enduring aspect of medical ethics. Enshrined in post-war humanitarian law, dignity turns on the inherent worth of any person by virtue of being human. First among Rawls's primary goods, dignity is a correlate of self-esteem, a function of the value and confidence one places in one's own life plans, and the respect others accord their fellow men and women as they pursue their vision of the good.[2] Degradation, humiliation, ill-treatment, and debasement invariably cripple self-esteem and make it impossible for individuals to formulate, much less realize, the goals that will make them better people.

Despite the supreme value we attach to life, liberty, and dignity, they sometimes conflict. One way of avoiding these conflicts is to invoke a "utility maximizing" principle, according to which one should act so as to bring about the outcome that best promotes human welfare. Bioethics, which has largely resigned itself to the difficulties of using multiple first principles, places utility maximization alongside other principles. Military ethics, on the other hand, elevates utility in a way that may run roughshod over other fundamental principles, as utility allows military necessity to trump other moral constraints on military action.

The Right to Life in Medicine and War

Most countries hold that the right to life obligates the state to protect its citizens' life and well-being, and that this entails, among other things, the provision of medical care, particularly acute care. Liberty interests and the right to self-determination also secure the right to medical care, since access to adequate and basic medical care is necessary if a person is to exercise liberty. The sick, after all, make poor citizens. The state's duty to protect life is not absolute, however, and contemporary medical practice generally allows individuals to withdraw or withhold life-sustaining care when the quality of life deteriorates badly.

War fundamentally abridges an individual's right to life together with the state's concomitant duty to protect life. Combatants lose their right to life as they gain the right to kill. Whether they pose an immediate threat or man a desk, fight for a just cause or engage in open aggression, soldiers are perpetually at risk. Noncombatants, too, find their lives subject to the constraints of permissible harm, as the principle of noncombatant immunity provides only limited protection from the destruction and devastation of armed conflict.

Just as war impinges on one's right to life, it undermines each actor's right to medical care. Enemy soldiers' right to medical care is a function of the threat they pose. Deprived of their right to life, enemy combatants have no intrinsic right to medical care. Once wounded and no longer a threat, however, they regain their right to life and to medical care. This is the moral significance of *hors de combat* (literally "out of combat"), the special status accorded combatants who are no longer a threat. Yet once wounded enemy soldiers recover sufficiently to pose a threat, their status reverts again to that of enemy combatant.

If the enemy's right to medical treatment is contingent upon the threat they pose, the right of one's own wounded soldiers to receive medical care is contingent upon their "salvage value"—that is, the likelihood that they will return to duty. "Salvage," a criterion of medical care unique to war, largely replaces "quality of life."[3] During war, medical personnel do not treat individual soldiers as discrete patients, but as components of a fighting force, a living collective entity. To maintain this force, medical personnel bear an obligation to salvage soldiers and return as many to duty as quickly as possible. Salvage speaks to a specific and *objective* measure of quality of life distinct from the patient's own, subjective evaluation. Salvageable soldiers may not invoke quality of life to refuse treatment, however painful or onerous, if it will return them to military duty. Those beyond salvage, on the other hand, may not appeal to any right to life to secure medical care when resources are scarce. Combatants who are critically wounded and unlikely to return to duty revert to a noncombatant status and lose their privileged claim to scarce medical resources.

War significantly restricts noncombatants' rights as well. Although civilians are generally immune from the ravages of combat, they remain vulnerable to "collateral harm," that is, to unintended but proportionate harm that noncombatants suffer as the unavoidable outcome of a legitimate military operation. This is the original context of the much-vaunted doctrine of double effect, which prohibits adversaries from intentionally harming non-combatants.[4] Though it is subject to considerable controversy and conflicting interpretation, the doctrine subordinates a noncombatant's right to life, and access to medical care, to the imperatives peculiar to war, most notably those concerning military necessity and scarcity of resources.

In the final analysis, each set of actors—enemy wounded, unsalvageable friendly soldiers, and civilians—has a fundamentally different claim to medical treatment contingent on the threat they pose, their salvage value, and military necessity, respectively. Further, the status of each actor is not stable, and constant shifting from one status to another plays havoc with medical ethics.

During war, neither combatants nor noncombatants enjoy the same right to life as ordinary patients. Moreover, the state has a life of its own and will wage war to preserve its right to life and common good. Sometimes the common good reflects the welfare of many citizens, but during war the state rarely sacrifices a few lives to save many. Instead, it sacrifices the lives of many to save some intangible national asset that embodies its common vision of the good life and the collective goods that it believes are worth saving.

Autonomy and Self-Determination in Medicine and War

As ordinary citizens, patients command the right of political and medical self-determination. The former embraces such commonly accepted political rights as representation, movement, and free speech, while the latter encompasses the well-known principles of autonomy and patient self-determination: informed consent, privacy, and confidentiality. War complicates and attenuates these principles. Regardless of a nation's state of war, military service limits, if not alters, the nature of autonomy. Autonomy no longer denotes "self-rule"—that is, rule of one's self for the good of oneself—for the good of the self is not a concern of anyone in the military. Rather, autonomy gives way to benign paternalism as others (officers, for example) rule one's self for the good of the state and its armed forces.

As a consequence, civil liberties—be they freedom of speech, movement, or assembly—face distinct limits, and autonomy in medical decisionmaking largely disappears. Informed consent, confidentiality, and privacy are all curtailed, and as a result, bioethical questions largely settled during peacetime emerge with renewed vigor during war.

Noncombatants find that war tears their liberties apart in a similar manner. During war, nations will often abridge civil liberties, including the rights of free speech, assembly, and representation, to safeguard national security and protect the state's sovereignty and territorial integrity. The patient rights of noncombatants, on the other hand, should remain secure and intact. An occupying power, for example, must provide medical care to civilian populations under its control. Exigencies may occasionally prevent this, but there is nothing to indicate that military medical personnel are relieved of their duty to guarantee informed consent, privacy, and confidentiality. On the contrary, developments since World War Two render it imperative to take particular care with the medical rights of occupied peoples to prevent the kind of abuses that characterized Nazi medical experimentation. This, of course, was the intent of the Geneva Conventions and the post-war Nuremberg Code.[5] These prohibit medical experiments contrary to a person's medical interests. Interestingly enough, wartime medicine brings the principles of autonomy and self-determination to the fore far more urgently than peacetime medicine. The same is true for human dignity and self-esteem.

Dignity and Self-Esteem During War

While war curtails the right to life and autonomy of all but the state itself, human dignity should remain unaffected by the vagaries of armed conflict. Dignity entails respect for personhood and a commitment to non-humiliation. For most medical practitioners, neither principle is particularly controversial. However, dignity and self-esteem are among the first casualties of armed conflict. Humanitarian law embraces absolute rights untouched by war, the threat of war, or any other public emergency, and prohibits humiliation, torture, slavery, cruel and inhuman treatment, crushing poverty, ignorance, and political impotence.[6] During armed conflict there is a great temptation to inflict all this and more upon one's enemy, and humanitarian law exists to insure that human rights do not go the way of civil liberties in time of war.

Human rights are inviolable, however, only insofar as they do not conflict, and during war it is not difficult to imagine conflicts between holders of competing rights. Freedom from ill-treatment may conflict with the right to life, leading a state to consider sacrificing the dignity of some to protect the lives of others. This is the hard problem of interrogational torture, and it often draws medical personnel into its web.[7] While torture is an extreme example, tension between life and dignity and the costs of maintaining each are at the heart of many bioethical dilemmas in war.

War exacerbates these tensions because individual and collective interests are often incommensurable and difficult to reconcile. There is, then, during times of war a tendency to turn to the principle of utility and maximize the interests of state above all else. . . .

Bioethics *or* Armed Conflict?

As citizens evaluate the arguments surrounding patient rights, neutrality, and unconventional warfare, and more generally assess the moral implications of going to war, they may quickly confront conflicting duties. Familial duties, small group loyalties, and professional obligations are all thrown off track when states go to war, impose military service, and partake in armed violence. Individuals often identify with a nation's reasons for going to war and subordinate their other moral obligations to their civic duties. Often, indeed, they seem willing to risk their own lives and take those of others. They will desist, if at all, only when higher moral principles compel them to pursue conscientious objection or civil disobedience when they perceive wars to be unjust.

In times of war every citizen, regardless of profession, has the same obligation to weigh reason of state and evaluate humanitarian principles. Nevertheless, one is sometimes tempted to ask whether medical personnel have a unique obligation to resolve dilemmas during war in a way that is consistent with their professional obligations. While one might not expect an individual's professional obligations to assume overriding importance as one contemplates the intractable ethical and moral questions of war, a medical practitioner's duties seem, to many, to be different. In each case above, it appears at first glance that physicians have a special duty to avoid some non-caregiving uses of medical expertise, even if these are militarily justified. Although international law permits certain types of nonlethal weapons, and assuming one could provide reasonable grounds to justify the policy of the Egyptian government, medical personnel must nonetheless refuse to develop these weapons systems because their professional obligation to "do no harm" requires them to use their expertise solely to promote human good. Similarly, health care professionals may be expected to uphold patient rights and medical neutrality regardless of military necessity.

But this conclusion, if correct, seems to push medicine into a moral class of its own. It allows medical personnel to invoke professional duties in order to avoid causing harm while ordinary citizens must subordinate their professional duties to reason of state when conditions merit. Those who believe medicine answers a "higher calling" may find this conclusion attractive. Yet it confuses professional duties with humanitarian obligations. When the WMA prohibited medical participation in chemical and biological warfare, it declared: "It is the privilege of the medical doctor to practice medicine in the service of humanity, to preserve and restore bodily and mental health without distinction as to persons, to comfort and ease the suffering of his or her patients. The utmost respect for human life is to be maintained even under threat, and no use made of any medical knowledge contrary to the laws of humanity."[8]

The WMA, however, uses the word "humanity" in two distinct senses, and this, perhaps, sums up the difficulty facing the medical profession during war. "Service of humanity" refers to beneficence and the imperative to preserve and restore human health. This is a professional obligation and, in principle, no different from those duties that obligate other professions that serve different human needs and that may fall before reason of state during war. The "laws of humanity," in contrast, invoke humanitarian law and respect for human rights. They are inviolable insofar as they do not conflict with one another, and, in spite of the tendency sometimes to conflate the laws of humanity and medicine's professional duty of beneficence, the two are not synonymous. Preserving this distinction is important. While one would not expect a physician or anyone else to use his or her knowledge contrary to the laws of humanity, there is sometimes room to ask whether any individual, physicians included, may violate another person's "bodily and mental health." This is the question we all face in the shadow of armed conflict.

References

1. *World Medical Association Regulations in Time of Armed Conflict*, amended by the 35th World Medical Assembly, Venice Italy, October 1983.

2. J. Rawls, *A Theory of Justice* (Cambridge, Mass.: Harvard University Press, 1971): 440.

3. *Emergency War Surgery NATO Handbook,* part 3, chapter 12. . . . Ordinary triage classifies the wounded so all will receive optimum care, while mass casualty triage treats the injured according to salvage value when the injured overwhelm available medical facilities and not all can be treated.

4. A. McIntyre, "Doing Away with Double Effect," *Ethics* 111 (2001): 219–55; W.S. Quinn, "Actions, Intentions and Consequences: The Doctrine of the Double Effect," *Philosophy and Public Affairs* 18 (1989): 334–51; J. McMahan, "Revising the Doctrine of Double Effect," *Journal of Applied Philosophy* 11, 2 (1994): 201–212.

5. First and Second Geneva Convention, common article 12, Third Geneva Convention, article 13, Fourth Geneva Convention, article 32; Geneva, 1949. These prohibit medical experiments contrary to a person's medical interests. Requirements stipulating informed consent did not enter international law until 1966. United Nations, "International Covenant on Civil and Political Rights," article 7. Adopted and opened for signature, ratification, and accession by General Assembly resolution 2200A (XXI) of December 16, 1966, entry into force March 23, 1976. . . . Also, L.C. Green, *The Contemporary Law of Armed Conflict*, Second Edition (Manchester, England: University of Manchester Press, 2000): 234–39.

6. United Nations, "International Covenant on Civil and Political Rights." The only non-derogable rights during war or public emergency are the right to life; freedom from torture, slavery, servitude, and retroactive legislation; freedom of conscience; the right to recognition before the law; and the right not to be imprisoned for breach of contract.

7. M.L. Gross, "Doctors in the Decent Society: Medical Care, Torture and Ill-Treatment," *Bioethics* 18, 2 (2004): 181–203.

8. World Medical Association, *Declaration on Chemical and Biological Weapons.*

M. Gregg Bloche and
Jonathan H. Marks

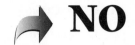 **NO**

When Doctors Go to War

When military forces go into combat, they are typically accompanied by medical personnel (physicians, physician assistants, nurses, and medics) who serve in noncombat roles. These professionals are bound by international law to treat wounded combatants from all sides and to care for injured civilians. They are also required to care for enemy prisoners and to report any evidence of abuse of detainees. In exchange, the Geneva Conventions protect them from direct attack, so long as they themselves do not become combatants.

Recently, there have been accounts of failure by U.S. medical personnel to report evidence of detainee abuse, even murder, in Iraq and Afghanistan.[1] There have also been claims, less well supported, that medics and others neglected the clinical needs of some detainees. The Department of Defense says it is investigating these allegations, though no charges have been brought against caregivers.

But Pentagon officials deny another set of allegations: that physicians and other medical professionals breached their professional ethics and the laws of war by participating in abusive interrogation practices. The International Committee of the Red Cross (ICRC) has concluded that medical personnel at Guantanamo Bay shared health information, including patient records, with army units that planned interrogations.[2] The ICRC called this "a flagrant violation of medical ethics" and said some of the interrogation methods used were "tantamount to torture."[2] The Pentagon answered that its detention operations are "safe, humane, and professional" and that "the allegation that detainee medical files were used to harm detainees is false."[2]

Our own inquiry into medical involvement in military intelligence gathering in Iraq and Guantanamo Bay has revealed a more troublesome picture. Recently released documents and interviews with military sources point to a pattern of such involvement, including participation in interrogation procedures that violate the laws of war. Not only did caregivers pass health information to military intelligence personnel; physicians assisted in the design of interrogation strategies, including sleep deprivation and other coercive methods tailored to detainees' medical conditions. Medical personnel also coached interrogators on questioning technique.

Physicians who did such work tend not to see these practices as unethical. On the contrary, a common understanding among those who helped to plan interrogations is that physicians serving in these roles do not act as physicians and are therefore not bound by patient-oriented ethics. In an interview, Dr. David Tornberg, Deputy Assistant Secretary of Defense for Health Affairs, endorsed this view. Physicians assigned to military intelligence, he contended, have no doctor–patient relationship with detainees and, in the absence of life-threatening emergency, have no obligation to offer medical aid.

Most people we interviewed who had served or spent time in detention facilities in Iraq or Guantanamo Bay reported being told not to talk about their experiences and impressions. Dr. David Auch, commander of the medical unit that staffed Abu Ghraib during the time of the abuses made notorious by soldiers' photographs, said military intelligence personnel told his medics and physician assistants not to discuss deaths that occurred in detention. Physicians who cared for so-called high-value detainees were especially hesitant to share their observations.

Yet available documents, the consistency of multiple confidential accounts, and confirmation of key facts by persons who spoke on the record make possible an understanding of the medical role in military intelligence in Iraq and Guantanamo. They also shed light on how those involved tried to justify this role in ethical terms.

In testimony taken in February 2004, as part of an inquiry into abuses at Abu Ghraib (and recently made public under the freedom of Information Act and posted on the Web site of the American Civil Liberties Union [ACLU] . . ., Colonel Thomas M. Pappas, chief of military intelligence at the prison, described physicians' systematic role in developing and executing interrogation strategies. Military intelligence teams, Pappas said, prepared individualized "interrogation plans" for detainees that included a "sleep plan" and medical standards. "A physician and a psychiatrist," he added, "are on hand to monitor what we are doing."

What was in these interrogation plans? None have become public, though Pappas's testimony indicates that he showed army investigators a sample, including a sleep deprivation schedule. However, a January 2004 "Memorandum for Record" (also available on the ACLU Web site) lays out an "Interrogation and Counter-Resistance Policy" calling for aggressive measures. Among these approaches are "dietary manipulation—minimum bread and water, monitored by medics"; "environmental manipulation—i.e., reducing A.C. [air conditioning] in summer, lower[ing] heat in winter"; "sleep management—for 72-hour time period maximum, monitored by medics"; "sensory deprivation—for 72-hour time period maximum, monitored by medics"; "isolation—for longer than 30 days"; "stress positions"; and "presence of working dogs."

Physicians collaborated with prison guards and military interrogators to put such approaches into practice. "Typically," said Pappas, military intelligence personnel give guards "a copy of the interrogation plan and a written note as to how to execute [it]. . . . The doctor and psychiatrist also look at the files to see what the interrogation plan recommends; they have the final say as to what is implemented." The psychiatrist would accompany interrogators to the prison and "review all those people under a management plan and provide feedback as to whether they were being medically and physically taken care of," said Pappas. These practices, he conceded, were without precedent. "The execution of this type of operation . . . is not codified in doctrine," he said. "Except for Guantanamo Bay, this sort of thing was a first."

At both Abu Ghraib[3] and Guantanamo,[2] "behavioral science consultation teams" advised military intelligence personnel on interrogation tactics. These teams, each of which included psychologists and a psychiatrist, functioned more formally at Guantanamo; staff shortages and other administrative difficulties reduced their role at Abu Ghraib.

A slide presentation prepared by medical ethics advisors to the military as a starting point for internal discussion poses a hypothetical case that, we were told, is a "thinly veiled" account of actual events. A physician newly deployed to "Irakistan" must decide whether to post physician assistants and medics behind a one-way mirror during interrogations. A military police commander tells the doctor that "the way this worked with the unit here before you was: We'd capture a guy; the medic would screen him and ensure he was fit for interrogation. If he had questions he'd check with the supervising doctor. The medic would get his screening signed by the doc. After that, the medic would watch over the interrogation from behind the glass."[4]

Interrogation facilities at Abu Ghraib included a one-way mirror, according to internal FBI documents obtained and made public by the ACLU in December. Draft rules of conduct, now under review, would permit army medical personnel to attend interrogations but would give them a right to refuse on ethical grounds.

Military intelligence interrogation units also had access to detainees' medical records and to clinical caregivers in both Iraq and Guantanamo Bay. "They couldn't conduct their job without that info," Tornberg told us. Caregivers, he said, have only a limited doctor–patient relationship with detainees and "make it very clear to the individuals that their medical information will not be protected . . . To the extent it is military-relevant . . ., that information can be used."

In helping to plan and execute interrogation strategies, did doctors breach medical ethics? Military physicians and Pentagon officials make a case to the contrary. Doctors, they argue, act as combatants, not physicians, when they put their knowledge to use for military ends. A medical degree, Tornberg said, is not a "sacramental vow"—it is a certification of skill. When a doctor participates in interrogation, "he's not functioning as a physician," and the Hippocratic ethic of commitment to patient welfare does not apply. According to this view, as long as the military maintains a separation of roles between clinical caregivers and physicians with intelligence-gathering responsibilities, assisting interrogators is legitimate.

Military physicians point to civilian parallels, including forensic psychiatry and occupational health, in arguing that the medical profession sometimes serves purposes at odds with patient welfare. They argue, persuasively in our view, that the Hippocratic ideal of undivided loyalty to patients fails to capture the breadth of the profession's social role. This role encompasses the legitimate needs of the criminal and civil justice systems, employers' concerns about workers' fitness for duty, allocation of limited medical resources, and protection of the public's health.

But the proposition that doctors who serve these social purposes don't act as physicians is self-contradictory. Their "physicianhood"—encompassing technical skill, scientific understanding, a caring ethos, and cultural authority— is the reason they are called on to assume these roles. The forensic psychiatrist's judgments about personal responsibility and competence rest on his or her moral sensibility and grasp of mental illness. And the military physician's contributions to interrogation—to its effectiveness, lawfulness, and social acceptance in a rights-respecting society—arise from his or her psychological insight, clinical knowledge, and perceived humanistic commitment.

In denying their status as physicians, military doctors divert attention from an urgent moral challenge—the need to manage conflict between the medical profession's therapeutic and social purposes. The Hippocratic ethical tradition offers no road map for resolving this conflict, but it provides a starting point. The therapeutic mission is the profession's primary role and the core of physicians' professional identity. If this mission and identity are to be preserved, there are some things doctors must not do. Consensus holds, for example, that physicians should not administer the death penalty, even in countries where capital punishment is lawful. Similarly, when physicians are involved in war, some simple rules should apply.

Physicians should not use drugs or other biologic means to subdue enemy combatants or extract information from detainees, nor should they aid others in doing so. They should not be party to interrogation practices contrary to human rights law or the laws of war, and their role in legitimate interrogation should not extend beyond limit setting, as guardians of detainees' health.[5] This role does not carry patient care responsibilities, but it requires physicians to tell detainees about health problems they find and to make treatment available. It also demands that physicians document abuses and report them to chains of command. By these standards, military medicine has fallen short.

The conclusion that doctors participated in torture is premature, but there is probable cause for suspecting it. Follow-up investigation is essential to determine whether they helped to craft and carry out the counter-resistance strategies—e.g., prolonged isolation and exposure to temperature extremes— that rise to the level of torture.

But, clearly, the medical personnel who helped to develop and execute aggressive counter-resistance plans thereby breached the laws of war. The Third Geneva Convention states that "[n]o physical or mental torture, nor any other form of coercion, may be inflicted on prisoners of war to secure from them information of any kind whatever." It adds that "prisoners of war who refuse to answer [questions] may not be threatened, insulted, or exposed to any unpleasant or disadvantageous treatment of any kind." The tactics used at Abu Ghraib and Guantanamo were transparently coercive, threatening, unpleasant, and disadvantageous. Although the Bush administration took the position (rejected by the ICRC) that none of the Guantanamo detainees were "prisoners of war," entitled to the full protections of the Third Geneva

Convention, it has acknowledged that combatants detained in Iraq are indeed prisoners of war, fully protected under this Convention.

The Surgeon General of the U.S. Army has begun a confidential effort to develop rules for health care professionals who work with detainees. Such an initiative is much needed, but it ought not to happen behind a veil of secrecy. Ethicists, legal scholars, and civilian professional leaders should participate, and the process should address role conflict in medicine more generally. An Institute of Medicine study committee, broadly representative of competing concerns (including the military's), would be a more suitable venue. To their credit, some military physicians in leadership roles have tried to involve outside ethicists in discussion of duties toward detainees. The Pentagon's civilian leadership has blocked these efforts.

Military physicians, nurses, and other health care professionals have served with courage in Iraq and other theatres of war since September 11, 2001. Some have received serious wounds, and some have died in the line of duty. By most accounts, they have delivered superb care to U.S. soldiers, enemy combatants, and wounded civilians alike. We owe them our gratitude and respect. We would affirm their honor, not besmirch it, by acknowledging the tensions between their Hippocratic and national service commitments and by working with them to map a course between the two.

References

1. Miles SH. Abu Ghraib: its legacy for military medicine. Lancet 2004; 364:725–9.
2. Lewis NA. Red Cross finds detainee abuse in Guantanamo. New York Times. November 30, 2004:A1.
3. Joint Interrogation & Debriefing Center. Abu Ghraib, Iraq. 2004. . . .
4. Medics, detainee: muddy waters. Presented at the USU Faculty Workshop on Military Healthcare Ethics, 14 October 2004.
5. Principles of medical ethics relevant to the role of health personnel, particularly physicians, in the protection of prisoners and detainees against torture and other cruel, inhuman, or degrading treatment or punishment. Adopted by U.N. General Assembly resolution 37/194 of 18 December 1982. . . .

POSTSCRIPT

Does Military Necessity Override Medical Ethics?

Several investigations into abuses of prisoners were launched after Abu Ghraib incidents came to light. In August 2004, the U.S. Army released a report, known as the Fay Report, after one of its chief investigators Maj. Gen. George Fay. The report implicated 27 members of a military intelligence unit in the abuses, in addition to the seven reservist military police previously charged. Among the failures detailed were those of medics who failed to report abuses. Gen. Paul Kern, who supervised the inquiry, said that the report laid out "serious misconduct and a loss of moral values," but stressed that the abusers were a tiny minority of the military personnel.

The debate was joined in 2006 by three authors. Michael Gross expanded this issue into a book, *Bioethics and Armed Conflict: Moral Dilemmas of Medicine and War* (MIT Press). John Yoo, a former assistant attorney general in the U.S. Justice Department, goes even further in his assertion that the Geneva Conventions are outmoded and that presidential authority to counter terrorism is essentially unlimited, in *War by Other Means: An Insider's Account of the War on Terror* (Atlantic Monthly Press). On the other hand, in *Oath Betrayed: Torture, Medical Complicity, and the War on Terror* (Random House, 2nd Edition, 2009), Steven Miles, a physician, argues that the medical profession's participation in torture and abuses are grossly unethical.

Articles on the conflict between military and medical ethics include Jerome Amir Singh, "American Physicians and Dual Loyalty Obligations in the 'War on Terror,'" *BMC Medical Ethics* (August 1, 2003, http://www.biomedcentral.com); Giovanni Maio, "History of Medical Involvement in Torture—Then and Now," *The Lancet* (May 19, 2001); Leonard S. Rubenstein, "The Medical Community's Response to Torture," *The Lancet* (May 3, 2003); and Edmund G. Howe, "Dilemmas in Military Medical Ethics Since 9/11," *Kennedy Institute of Ethics Journal* (June 2003).

In September 2008, the American Psychological Association voted to bar its members from participating in interrogations at Guantanamo Bay, Cuba, and other military detention sites. An update from Marks and Bloche ("The Ethics of Interrogation—The U.S. Military's Ongoing Use of Psychiatrists," *The New England Journal of Medicine*, September 11, 2008) claims, on the basis of U.S. Army documents, that the Department of Defense continues to resist the positions taken by professional organizations.

The American Medical Association's policy on torture is available at: http://www.ama-assn.org. It is Report 10-A-06 of the Council on Ethical and Judicial Affairs. The Geneva Conventions are available at http://www.genevaconventions.org. The World Medical Association policy on torture is available at http://www.wma.net/en/20activities/20humanrights/40torture/index.html.

ISSUE 19

Should Performance-Enhancing Drugs Be Banned from Sports?

YES: **Thomas H. Murray,** from "Making Sense of Fairness in Sports," *Hastings Center Report* (March–April 2010)

NO: **Julian Savulescu, Bennett Foddy, and Megan Clayton,** from "Why We Should Allow Performance Enhancing Drugs in Sport," *British Journal of Sports Medicine* (December 2004)

ISSUE SUMMARY

YES: Social psychologist Thomas H. Murray contends that the ban on performance-enhancing drugs should continue because it furthers the true meaning of sports—which is to compare athletes on their natural talent and abilities.

NO: Philosopher Julian Savulescu and research colleagues Bennett Foddy and Megan Clayton argue that legalizing drugs in sport may be fairer and safer than banning them.

In sports, there are winners and losers. But for many athletes, winning is not enough. Elite athletes want to set records or exceed their prior performances. Athletes of less than elite status aspire to reach that higher level. And even ordinary competitors who know they will never jump as high as Michael Jordan or hit a hockey puck as precisely as Wayne Gretsky want to go farther than their natural talent and motivation might take them. The potential rewards are enormous, not just in personal gratification but also in prestige, career opportunities, and financial success.

For all these different types of sports figures, there is a strong temptation to enhance their performance through the use of drugs. And increasingly they can find some drugs that may help them do it. Drug use in sports is not a new phenomenon. Athletes in the original Greek Olympics are believed to have used mushrooms and herbs to make them stronger and faster. In the nineteenth century, French cyclists drank Vin Mariani, a combination of wine and coca leaf extract called "the wine of athletes." Coca leaf, the source of cocaine, made it easier for them to endure the prolonged exertion of cycling.

These potions, however, were mild compared to the modern pharmacopeia available to athletes. In addition to natural substances, prescription drugs used in megadoses, and illegal substances like cocaine and marijuana, there are synthesized forms of human hormones and "designer drugs" for particular purposes.

Concern about drug use in sports in modern times is relatively recent. Steroid use first emerged in the 1964 Olympics. Anabolic androgenic steroids are compounds synthesized from the hormone testosterone, which is present in normal amounts in males. ("Anabolic" means "to build," and "androgenic" means "masculinizing.") Physicians prescribe such steroids to repair damaged tissue, but the doses that athletes use are many times greater than therapeutic ones. Because anabolic steroids build muscle mass, weight lifters, hammer throwers, and other athletes whose performance depends on muscle power are most likely to use them. In females, the results may be not just muscle mass but masculinizing features. In the Montreal Olympics in 1976, East German women swimmers were able to swim faster than other competitors, but they also had deep voices and body hair.

Stimulants such as amphetamines serve a different purpose; they give athletes unusually high levels of alertness, energy, and aggressiveness, characteristics particularly appealing to football players. Other kinds of medical intervention to enhance performance include "blood doping"—storing some of a cyclist's own blood and injecting it before a race to give the maximum number of oxygen-carrying red blood cells. A synthetic substance—erythropoetin (EPO), prescribed to treat anemia in cancer patients—can also be used in this way.

What has been the response of official sports organizations to this growing use of drugs? The World Anti-Doping Agency, an offshoot of the International Olympic Committee, has a nine-page list of banned substances (available at http://www.wada-ama.org). The major categories are anabolic agents, hormones and related substances (such as EPO and human growth hormone), beta-2 agonists (substances that relieve breathing stress, except for athletes who have asthma), agents with antiestrogenic activity (substances that enhance feminine characteristics), and diuretics and other agents that might mask the presence of drugs by depleting the body of urine. In addition, blood doping, chemical and physical manipulation, and gene doping—a new addition to the armamentarium—are prohibited. Some substances are prohibited in competitions, including stimulants, narcotics, cannabinoids (marijuana and hashish), and other steroids. Certain sports prohibit alcohol or beta-blockers (drugs that lower blood pressure).

Is all this antidrug activity warranted, or is it an unacceptable invasion of privacy and a losing battle? Why should adults for whom sports is a primary value not be allowed to do whatever they choose to enhance their performance? Can drugs and sport coexist? The two following selections take opposite views. Thomas H. Murray contends that drug use violates the integrity of sport and deprives it of its essential value and meaning. Julian Savulescu, Bennett Foddy, and Megan Clayton, on the other hand, argue that there is nothing inherently wrong in athletes' using drugs to perform at higher levels, and it would be better for all if drug use were legalized and controlled for athletes' safety.

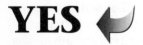
Thomas H. Murray

Making Sense of Fairness in Sports

From the steroid scandals of major league baseball to analysis of Oscar Pistorius's cheetahs to the sex-verification test of Caster Semenya, questions today about what constitutes fairness in sports are wide-ranging and varied.

It's easier to see what's unfair in sports. Suppose that the judges award the Olympic figure skating gold medal in Vancouver because of the skaters' wacky costumes—all feathers, sequins, and teasing glimpses of skin. Or that they choose based on their views on the skaters' countries of origin, or because they were bribed, or by tossing a coin.

All these are unfair (and some have been documented, or at least suspected, in past competitions). How do we know they're unfair? Because everyone who understands figure skating—or alpine skiing, or bobsledding, or, for that matter, baseball, cycling, or any other competitive sport—knows what's supposed to separate winners from also-rans. Among the countless differences between competitors, from eye color to favorite food, only certain differences are meant to be highlighted in each particular sport.

Successful short-track speed skaters possess explosive strength, finely honed technique, and the courage to face the possibility of serious injury from razor-sharp blades. Nordic skiers must have astonishing stamina. Each sport calls upon its particular mix of physical talents. Every sport requires the commitment to perfect those talents and to learn how to employ them skillfully and strategically. It may not be easy to say exactly what fairness means, but the ease with which we can call out unfairness suggests that the task is worthwhile and far from hopeless.

A match that should never happen is a one-on-one basketball game between LeBron James and me. When LeBron trounces me—as he assuredly will—it may be uninteresting, probably comical, perhaps even YouTubeable, but it will not be unfair. He is simply a superior player, not merely to me but probably to every other person living on this planet. (Kobe Bryant is likely to disagree.) The playing field, or court, is level. Talent and dedication determine the winner.

Then there are times when we choose to level the playing field by multiplying it. In the 2008 Paralympics there were thirteen distinct finals for the men's one-hundredmeter dash, twelve for the women's. The varieties and degrees of impairment among Paralympians in no way detract from the talents and dedication that competitors bring to the games. But the variety also requires that the playing field be made level so that every athlete is competing against people with similar levels of impairment. In that way, talent and the many things we admire about dedicated athletes are on display and shape each athlete's performance.

The first thing to note is that a fair sports competition does not require that athletes be equal in every imaginable respect. Some basketball players are taller, stronger, quicker, or more agile than others. No one—well, almost no one—regards such differences in natural talents as unjust or unfair. Some have better coaches or more favorable training environments. At what point such differences cross the line from inevitable and acceptable to iniquitous and deplorable is something to be debated and settled by the people who participate in, understand, and love that sport—not by distant and disinterested philosophers. Debates such as this go on regularly in sports over new equipment, rules, strategies, and the like. Take the recent kerfuffle over the super-slippery, buoyant full-body swimsuits. After initial dithering, the Fédération Internationale de Natation (FINA)—the international governing body for swimming—[in 2009] banned many suits on the grounds that they changed the nature of the sport by allowing bulky athletes to float on top of the water rather than having to push through it. Whatever one thinks of FINA's ruling, it was right to focus on the meaning of the sport and on what characteristics lead to excellence and success.

Then again, the most gifted, hardest-working athlete or team does not always win. A random bounce, a slip, a hesitation can give victory to the side that might lose nine of ten matches. That's why we play the game.

When it comes to performance-enhancing drugs, gene doping, and the panoply of manipulations banned widely in sports, the challenge is less about fairness than about meaning. If the rules ban performance-enhancing drugs, then using those drugs to gain an advantage over athletes who refuse to cheat is unfair. Simple enough. Antidoping skeptics, however, often proclaim that the problem isn't with the drugs, but with the ban on drugs. It would be fairer, they argue, to give all competitors access to the same drugs. If everyone had ample supplies of anabolic steroids, erythropoietin, growth hormone, or whatever drugs boosted performance in their sport, then—they claim—unfairness would be eliminated along with the nuisances of drug testing, adjudication, and enforcement.

One response to the skeptics is to ask a different question: Is it not unfair to put the athletes who want to compete without drugs or gene doping at a competitive disadvantage by permitting everything—to tilt the playing field in favor of the drug users?

Any serious ethical commentary on the uses of performance-enhancing technology in sports must confront two compelling realities. First, sports science has provided a great deal of information about how to optimize training and performance. It has also led to a plethora of technologies and methods to enhance performance, from altitude chambers that allow athletes to gain the benefits of "training low, living high," to ice-filled vests runners can wear before a long race to cool their core temperatures, to esoteric measurements of muscle and organ function. Why, the skeptics ask, should we distinguish between these technologies of performance enhancement on the one hand and drugs like steroids on the other?

Part of the answer to this challenge is to recognize that sports are about what can be accomplished under specific limitations. Soccer players, other than goal tenders, may not use their hands or arms to direct the ball, even when that would be far more convenient and accurate than one's foot or head. Golf imposes strict limits on balls and clubs. Marathon runners may not use wheels, whether attached to their shoes or, as Rosie Ruiz did, to subway cars.

The other piece of the answer requires an understanding of what that particular sport values. What makes a great weight lifter does not make a great distance runner. Bodies that possess massive explosive strength are rarely the lithe, sinewy bodies best suited to run great distances. The limitations each sport chooses for itself reflect a shared understanding of what that sport is meant to display and reward. The rules of sports are arbitrary in the sense that they could be otherwise, and, in practice, sports modify their rules in response to changes in equipment, tactics, and athletes' abilities. But in another sense, the rules and the changes wrought in them are far from arbitrary: they must pass muster with the community of those who play and love that sport. The community must be satisfied that the new rules keep alive what it values, what natural talents enable athletes to excel, and what, in the end, is meaningful about participating and winning.

The second reality is the ineluctably comparative nature of sports. Athletes compete against other athletes. Winners and losers may be separated by fractions of a second. A drug that gives a 1 or 2 percent performance boost can be decisive. When some athletes use such technologies, all athletes feel the pressure to use them, merely to avoid losing ground. So the notion that we should just leave it up to each athlete to decide whether to use drugs is naive. When the lid is blown off, all athletes will feel the pressure to dope.

One proposed solution is to continue to ban some drugs—those deemed to be particularly harmful—but allow athletes free reign to use all others. Consider what is likely to happen. We'll continue to need drug testing and enforcement to deter athletes from using the substances on the banned list, so all the complaints about the inconvenience and intrusiveness of testing will remain. And now athletes will feel pressured to take ever more drugs, often at higher dosages, in untested and possibly dangerous combinations. It's hard to see that scenario as progress.

Whether performance-enhancing drugs or gene doping should be permitted in sports is, in the end, a matter to be decided by the communities of athletes and those who understand and love each sport. The dynamics of competition mean that, if doping were permitted, athletes would confront a terrible choice: refrain from drugs and give up an edge that will often be decisive, or join in an ever-rising spiral of drug use. I fear a public health catastrophe in the making if we choose the second path. I also would grieve for all those athletes who desire to compete without doping but who will mostly lose to their pharmacologically amped competitors.

Opening the doors of sports to drug use will also accelerate the dominance of doping gurus over the athletes who succumb to their sales pitches. An athlete's performance will become more and more a function of expert manipulations, and less of the athlete's talents or dedication. I cannot see that as a good thing for athletes, for sports, or for all of us who care about them.

Julian Savulescu, Bennett
Foddy, and Megan Clayton

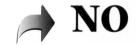 **NO**

Why We Should Allow Performance Enhancing Drugs in Sport

In 490 BC, the Persian Army landed on the plain of Marathon, 25 miles from Athens. The Athenians sent a messenger named Feidipides to Sparta to ask for help. He ran the 150 miles in two days. The Spartans were late. The Athenians attacked and, although out-numbered five to one, were victorious. Feidipides was sent to run back to Athens to report victory. On arrival, he screamed "We won" and dropped dead from exhaustion.

The marathon was run in the first modern Olympics in 1896, and in many ways the athletic ideal of modern athletes is inspired by the myth of the marathon. Their ideal is superhuman performance, at any cost.

Drugs in Sport

The use of performance enhancing drugs in the modern Olympics is on record as early as the games of the third Olympiad, when Thomas Hicks won the marathon after receiving an injection of strychnine in the middle of the race.[1] The first official ban on "stimulating substances" by a sporting organisation was introduced by the International Amateur Athletic Federation in 1928.[2]

Using drugs to cheat in sport is not new, but it is becoming more effective. In 1976, the East German swimming team won 11 out of 13 Olympic events, and later sued the government for giving them anabolic steroids.[3] Yet despite the health risks, and despite the regulating bodies' attempts to eliminate drugs from sport, the use of illegal substances is widely known to be rife. It hardly raises an eyebrow now when some famous athlete fails a dope test.

In 1992, Vicky Rabinowicz interviewed small groups of athletes. She found that Olympic athletes, in general, believed that most successful athletes were using banned substances.[4]

Much of the writing on the use of drugs in sport is focused on this kind of anecdotal evidence. There is very little rigorous, objective evidence because the athletes are doing something that is taboo, illegal, and sometimes highly dangerous. The anecdotal picture tells us that our attempts to eliminate drugs from sport have failed. In the absence of good evidence, we need an analytical argument to determine what we should do.

From *British Journal of Sports Medicine*, vol. 38, issue 6, December 2004, pp. 666–667, 670.

Condemned to Cheating?

We are far from the days of amateur sporting competition. Elite athletes can earn tens of millions of dollars every year in prize money alone, and millions more in sponsorships and endorsements. The lure of success is great. But the penalties for cheating are small. A six month or one year ban from competition is a small penalty to pay for further years of multimillion dollar success.

Drugs are much more effective today than they were in the days of strychnine and sheep's testicles. Studies involving the anabolic steroid androgen showed that, even in doses much lower than those used by athletes, muscular strength could be improved by 5–20%.[5] Most athletes are also relatively unlikely to ever undergo testing. The International Amateur Athletic Federation estimates that only 10–15% of participating athletes are tested in each major competition.[6]

The enormous rewards for the winner, the effectiveness of the drugs, and the low rate of testing all combine to create a cheating "game" that is irresistible to athletes. Kjetil Haugen[7] investigated the suggestion that athletes face a kind of prisoner's dilemma regarding drugs. His game theoretic model shows that, unless the likelihood of athletes being caught doping was raised to unrealistically high levels, or the payoffs for winning were reduced to unrealistically low levels, athletes could all be predicted to cheat. The current situation for athletes ensures that this is likely, even though they are worse off as a whole if everyone takes drugs, than if nobody takes drugs.

Drugs such as erythropoietin (EPO) and growth hormone are natural chemicals in the body. As technology advances, drugs have become harder to detect because they mimic natural processes. In a few years, there will be many undetectable drugs. Haugen's analysis predicts the obvious: that when the risk of being caught is zero, athletes will all choose to cheat.

The recent Olympic games in Athens were the first to follow the introduction of a global anti-doping code. From the lead up to the games to the end of competition, 3000 drug tests were carried out: 2600 urine tests and 400 blood tests for the endurance enhancing drug EPO.[8] From these, 23 athletes were found to have taken a banned substance—the most ever in an Olympic games.[9] Ten of the men's weightlifting competitors were excluded.

The goal of "cleaning" up the sport is unattainable. Further down the track the spectre of genetic enhancement looms dark and large.

The Spirit of Sport

So is cheating here to stay? Drugs are against the rules. But we define the rules of sport. If we made drugs legal and freely available, there would be no cheating.

The World Anti-Doping Agency code declares a drug illegal if it is performance enhancing, if it is a health risk, or if it violates the "spirit of sport."[10]

They define this spirit as follows.[11] The spirit of sport is the celebration of the human spirit, body, and mind, and is characterised by the following values:

- ethics, fair play and honesty
- health
- excellence in performance
- character and education
- fun and joy
- teamwork
- dedication and commitment
- respect for rules and laws
- respect for self and other participants
- courage
- community and solidarity[11]

Would legal and freely available drugs violate this "spirit"? Would such a permissive rule be good for sport?

Human sport is different from sports involving other animals, such as horse or dog racing. The goal of a horse race is to find the fastest horse. Horses are lined up and flogged. The winner is the one with the best combination of biology, training, and rider. Basically, this is a test of biological potential. This was the old naturalistic Athenian vision of sport: find the strongest, fastest, or most skilled man.

Training aims to bring out this potential. Drugs that improve our natural potential are against the spirit of this model of sport. But this is not the only view of sport. Humans are not horses or dogs. We make choices and exercise our own judgment. We choose what kind of training to use and how to run our race. We can display courage, determination, and wisdom. We are not flogged by a jockey on our back but drive ourselves. It is this judgment that competitors exercise when they choose diet, training, and whether to take drugs. We can choose what kind of competitor to be, not just through training, but through biological manipulation. Human sport is different from animal sport because it is creative. Far from being against the spirit of sport, biological manipulation embodies the human spirit—the capacity to improve ourselves on the basis of reason and judgment. When we exercise our reason, we do what only humans do.

The result will be that the winner is not the person who was born with the best genetic potential to be strongest. Sport would be less of a genetic lottery. The winner will be the person with a combination of the genetic potential, training, psychology, and judgment. Olympic performance would be the result of human creativity and choice, not a very expensive horse race.

Classical musicians commonly use blockers to control their stage fright. These drugs lower heart rate and blood pressure, reducing the physical effects of stress, and it has been shown that the quality of a musical performance is improved if the musician takes these drugs.[12] Although elite classical music is arguably as competitive as elite sport, and the rewards are similar, there is no stigma attached to the use of these drugs. We do not think less of the violinist or pianist who uses them. If the audience judges the performance to be improved with drugs, then the drugs are enabling the musician to express him or herself more effectively. The competition between elite musicians has rules—you cannot mime the violin to a backing CD. But there is no rule against the use of chemical enhancements.

Is classical music a good metaphor for elite sport? Sachin Tendulkar is known as the "Maestro from Mumbai." The Associated Press called Maria Sharapova's 2004 Wimbledon final a "virtuoso performance."[13] Jim Murrary[14] wrote the following about Michael Jordan in 1996:

> You go to see Michael Jordan play for the same reason you went to see Astaire dance, Olivier act or the sun set over Canada. It's art. It should be painted, not photographed.
> It's not a game, it's a recital. He's not just a player, he's a virtuoso. Heifetz with a violin. Horowitz at the piano.

Indeed, it seems reasonable to suggest that the reasons we appreciate sport at its elite level have something to do with competition, but also a great deal to do with the appreciation of an extraordinary performance.

Clearly the application of this kind of creativity is limited by the rules of the sport. Riding a motorbike would not be a "creative" solution to winning the Tour de France, and there are good reasons for proscribing this in the rules. If motorbikes were allowed, it would still be a good sport, but it would no longer be a bicycle race.

We should not think that allowing cyclists to take EPO would turn the Tour de France into some kind of "drug race," any more than the various training methods available turn it into a "training race" or a "money race." Athletes train in different, creative ways, but ultimately they still ride similar bikes, on the same course. The skill of negotiating the steep winding descent will always be there. . . .

Test for Health, Not Drugs

The welfare of the athlete must be our primary concern. If a drug does not expose an athlete to excessive risk, we should allow it even if it enhances performance. We have two choices: to vainly try to turn the clock back, or to rethink who we are and what sport is, and to make a new 21st century Olympics. Not a super-Olympics but a more human Olympics. Our crusade against drugs in sport has failed. Rather than fearing drugs in sport, we should embrace them.

In 1998, the president of the International Olympic Committee, Juan-Antonio Samaranch, suggested that athletes be allowed to use non-harmful performance enhancing drugs. This view makes sense only if, by not using drugs, we are assured that athletes are not being harmed.

Performance enhancement is not against the spirit of sport; it is the spirit of sport. To choose to be better is to be human. Athletes should be given this choice. Their welfare should be paramount. But taking drugs is not necessarily cheating. The legalisation of drugs in sport may be fairer and safer.

References

1. House of Commons, Select Committee on Culture, Media and Sport. 2004. Seventh Report of Session 2003–2004, UK Parliament, HC 499–1.

2. House of Commons, Select Committee on Culture, Media and Sport. 2004. Seventh Report of Session 2003–2004, UK Parliament, HC 499–1.

3. Longman J. 2004. East German Steroids' toll: 'they killed Heidi', *New York Times* 2004 Jan 20, sect D:1.

4. Rabinawicz V. Athletes and drugs: a separate pace? *Psychol Today* 1992;25:52–3.

5. Hartgens F, Kuipers H. Effects of androgenic-anabolic steroids in athletes. *Sport Med* 2004;34:513–54.

6. IAAF, 2004. . . .

7. Haugen KK. The performance-enhancing drug game. *Journal of Sports Economics* 2004;5:67–87.

8. Wilson S. *Boxer Munyasia fails drug test in Athens.* Athens: Associated Press, 2004 Aug 10.

9. Zinser L. With drug-tainted past, few track records fall. *New York Times* 2004 Aug 29, Late Edition, p. 1.

10. WADA. World Anti-Doping Code, Montreal. World Anti-Doping Agency, 2003:16.

11. WADA. World Anti-Doping Code, Montreal. World Anti-Doping Agency, 2003:3.

12. Brantigan CO, Brantigan TA, Joseph N. Effect of beta blockade and beta stimulation on stage fright. *Am J Med* 1982;72:88–94.

13. Wilson S. *Sharapova beats Williams for title. Associated Press,* 2004 Jul 3, 09:10am.

14. Murray J. It's basketball played on a higher plane. *Los Angeles Times* 1996 Feb 4 1996, sect C:1.

POSTSCRIPT

Should Performance-Enhancing Drugs Be Banned from Sports?

In July 2008, Marion Jones, who won five medals in track and field at the 2000 Sydney Olympics, became the highest profile American to become tarnished by a doping scandal. After admitting that she had used steroids and had lied to federal investigators, the International Olympics Committee stripped her of her medals. The Beijing Olympics in August 2008 passed without a major doping scandal, although in October, Olympic officials announced that it would use a new test for CERA, a new form of EPO (erythropoietin, an oxygen-enhancing steroid), to analyze 1,000 blood samples collected during the Beijing games. See D.H. Catlin, K.D. Fitch, and A. Ljungqvist, "Medicine and Science in the Fight Against Doping in Sport," *Journal of Internal Medicine,* August 2008, for a review of current testing regimens.

Internationally, the Olympics and professional cycling have the toughest drug testing rules and penalties. Until recently, major American sports have not acknowledged the problem. In 2005, Major League Baseball Commissioner Bud Selig announced a tougher policy for drug use, with suspensions of increasing times for violations. This action averted congressional action, but Joseph M. Saka argues that Congress can still address performance-enhancing drugs if voluntary action fails ("Back to the Game: How Congress Can Help Sports Leagues Shift the Focus from Steroids to Sports," *Journal of Contemporary Health Law and Policy,* 2007).

In December 2007, a committee chaired by former Senate Majority Leader George Mitchell issued a report asserting that Major League Baseball has a "serious drug culture" in which steroid use is "widespread." The drugs of choice include steroid and increasingly human growth hormone, which cannot be detected by standard urine tests. Mitchell named many current and former well-known baseball players, including Roger Clemens, Miguel Tejada, Andy Pettitte, and Barry Bonds. The report blames all levels of baseball management and players' unions, as well as club owners, for ignoring the problem.

The first global treaty against doping in sports became effective February 2007, after 30 nations ratified an international agreement. (The United States ratified the agreement in 2008.) The treaty allows governments to take action against the illegal manufacture and supply of doping substances, among other provisions. More information is available at http://www.unesco.org/en/antidoping.

Many articles on drugs and sports can be found in newspapers and magazines. For a fuller exposition of Thomas H. Murray's views, see his chapter, "The Ethics of Drugs in Sport," in *Drugs & Performance in Sports,* edited by Richard H. Strauss, M.D. (W. B. Saunders, 1987). Norman Fost, a pediatrician, says appeals to ban drugs are paternalistic and caused more by a displeasure at the loss of innocence in sports than by actual harm ("Banning Drugs in Sports: A Skeptical View," *Hastings Center Report,* August 1986). An unsigned "Opinion" essay in *The Economist* (August 5, 2004) argues that an inflexible anti-doping attitude is unsustainable in a society that uses performance-enhancing drugs so freely for other reasons. See also Gary Wadler and Brian Hainline, *Drugs and the Athlete* (F.A. Davis, 1989) and David R. Mottram, ed., *Drugs in Sport,* 3rd ed. (Routledge, 2002).

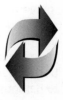

ISSUE 20

Should Pharmacists Be Allowed to Deny Prescriptions on Grounds of Conscience?

YES: Donald W. Herbe, from "The Right to Refuse: A Call for Adequate Protection of a Pharmacist's Right to Refuse Facilitation of Abortion and Emergency Contraception," *Journal of Law and Health* (2002/2003)

NO: Julie Cantor and Ken Baum, from "The Limits of Conscientious Objection—May Pharmacists Refuse to Fill Prescriptions for Emergency Contraception?" *The New England Journal of Medicine* (November 4, 2004)

ISSUE SUMMARY

YES: Law student Donald W. Herbe asserts that pharmacists' moral beliefs concerning abortion and emergency contraception are genuinely fundamental and deserve respect. He proposes that professional pharmaceutical organizations lead the way to recognizing a true right of conscience, which would eventually result in universal legislation protecting against all potential ramifications of choosing conscience.

NO: Julie Cantor, a lawyer, and Ken Baum, a physician and lawyer, reject an absolute right to object, as well as no right to object, to these prescriptions but assert that pharmacists who cannot or will not dispense a drug have a professional obligation to meet the needs of their customers by referring them elsewhere.

Under U.S. law and practice, a person who objects on grounds of conscience or religious belief to performing certain acts has considerable protections. To force someone to perform an act totally forbidden by his or her religion would be a profound violation of ethical and human rights. But there are limits to exercising this right. Right now there is no military draft in the United States; however, all young men must register with the Selective Service Agency on their eighteenth birthday. If there were to be a military draft, a conscientious objector would have to demonstrate that he has a strongly held religious or moral belief, not just a political one, against participation in the military. Conscientious objectors could request alternative community service, such as caring for the elderly, or serving in the military as a noncombatant, for example, as a medic. In the Vietnam War, some conscientious objectors were jailed for their refusal to serve.

Conscientious objection has ethical implications for medical personnel as well. Physicians, for example, may refrain from performing procedures that are legal but repugnant to them on moral grounds. Just as in the military example, there are limits. Physicians cannot ethically refuse to provide life-saving or emergency treatment to a person on the grounds that the individual is a murderer or has committed an act that violates the physician's religion. They can refuse to perform abortions on grounds of conscience, but ethical codes require them to refer patients to another provider. Nurses have less discretion than physicians because they are employees of hospitals and are subject to disciplinary action. Nevertheless, they too can establish grounds for refusing to assist in an abortion procedure, sterilization, or the withdrawal of life-sustaining treatment.

The issue is murkier, however, when it comes to pharmacists, who are generally self-employed, or pharmacy employees. They do not directly participate in the acts they find objectionable, but they make those acts possible by dispensing medications. What are their options and obligations?

Birth control pills and emergency contraception medications, which are basically high doses of regular birth control pills taken to prevent pregnancy after unprotected sexual intercourse, have been on the market for years. Some pharmacists object to dispensing these medications. The issue became much more controversial when in September 2000 the Food and Drug Administration (FDA) approved the drug mifepristone as safe and effective. This drug, formerly known as RU-486 after Russel Uclaf, its initial French manufacturer, had been marketed in Europe for several years. Mifepristone is a synthetic steroid that blocks progesterone, preventing an implanted fertilized egg from developing. It must be taken within 49 days of conception and followed within 48 hours by a second drug, misoprostol, related to the hormone prostaglandin. Taken together, the two drugs act as a chemical form of early abortion. Emergency contraception, on the other hand, is not a form of abortion, since no conception has taken place.

And it is here that some pharmacists have drawn the line. Believing strongly that abortion is immoral, they want the legal right to exercise their religious beliefs and ethical right by refusing to dispense the drugs for this purpose and to be protected from losing their jobs, or other repercussions. Should they be allowed to do so and without referring women to another, more willing pharmacist?

The following selections present different points of view. Donald Herbe sees the exercise of conscientious objection as fundamental to pharmacists' human rights and calls for legislation to protect them from any kind of repercussions or discrimination. While recognizing that pharmacists have a legitimate interest in avoiding conflicts of conscience, Julie Cantor and Ken Baum believe that because pharmacists are licensed and have a professional obligation to serve the public, they must make alternative options available to customers who seek legal prescription drugs they find objectionable.

YES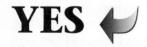

Donald W. Herbe

The Right to Refuse: A Call for Adequate Protection of a Pharmacist's Right to Refuse Facilitation of Abortion and Emergency Contraception

Introduction

The ability to convince an individual, through the art of honest persuasion, of the righteousness of a belief is celebrated; however, in failure of such persuasion, compelling that person to act contradictory to their retained ideal is detestable. The free will to reject a movement or disagree with a practice is the sort of liberty this Nation was founded upon, yet today the potential exists that many in the pharmaceutical profession will be forced into behaviors repugnant to their basic standards of goodness and morality. The proliferation of abortive and contraceptive drug therapies has thrust many pharmacists into roles as facilitators of practices they oppose on fundamental levels without a corresponding ability to opt out of such action.

When a patient desires drug therapies that, in the eyes of the pharmacist, are likely to destroy an unborn human life, the pro-life pharmacist is left in an unsettling position: accommodate the patient and breach basic moral principles *or* adhere to conscience and risk liability and disciplinary action.

Section I: Anti-Reproduction Pills and the Pharmacist's Role

The Pills

On September 28, 2000, the Food and Drug Administration (FDA) approved the drug mifepristone, formerly known as RU-486, for use in the United States as an abortifacient. Mifepristone had previously been approved and is currently used in some European countries, including France, England, and Sweden. Although mifepristone has other potential uses, such as postcoital contraception and daily-use birth control, its FDA approved use is as an early pregnancy abortifacient.

From *Journal of Law and Health*, vol. 17, issue 1, 2002/2003, excerpts from 77–103. Copyright © 2003 by Donald W. Herbe. Reprinted by permission of the author.

Mifepristone acts as an anti-hormone and precludes a woman's uterus from retaining an *implanted* fertilized egg. The drug blocks progesterone, an essential hormone in the acceptance and retention of an implanted egg within a woman's uterus; and, when taken in concurrence with misoprostol, induces a spontaneous abortion. The fact that the mifepristone abortion regimen acts to destroy an implanted egg as opposed to a fertilized yet not implanted egg, is what distinguishes it from emergency contraception.

Drugs used post-coitally with the intent to prevent the development of a pregnancy are referred to as emergency contraception. This labeling as emergency contraception is a bit conclusory, as the definition of whether use of such drugs is contraception or abortion lies at the heart of the controversy over them. However, for purposes of convenience and clarity, this Note will refer to drug regimens consumed post-intercourse for the purpose of preventing the onset or continuance of pregnancy as emergency contraception (EC), as that is the term that has been attached to them in modern medical, social, and political arenas.

Notwithstanding this controversy, the physical and biological effects of orally administered EC, often referred to as the morning-after pill, are not in dispute. EC may prevent the development of a pregnancy by inhibiting any of four successive biological events, either pre or post fertilization, necessary to establish and maintain a pregnancy. EC works before fertilization by either suppressing ovulation, like regular birth-control pills, or preventing fertilization of an egg by inhibiting the movement of the sperm or the egg. If an egg becomes fertilized, then EC may disrupt transport of the fertilized egg to the uterus or, if the transport through the fallopian tube is complete, prevent the implantation of the fertilized egg in the woman's uterus. EC is most effective when used up to seventy-two hours after unprotected intercourse and becomes completely ineffective after implantation occurs, usually six or seven days after intercourse.

The Pharmacist's Role

During the past twenty years emergency contraception pills (ECPs) have been available to and used by American women. During this time frame non-emergency oral contraceptives (those taken as a daily pre-intercourse regimen) were used off-label as emergency contraception and were distributed as such "primarily in hospital emergency rooms, reproductive health clinics, and university health centers." These medical facilities would repackage oral contraceptives for use as emergency contraception; pharmacies associated with certain clinics would repackage oral contraceptives into EC regimens and label them as such; and private physicians would instruct patients to take a larger dosage of their regular birth control pills as EC.

In 1998 the FDA approved the Preven Emergency Contraceptive Kit, an EC based on the Yuzpe regimen. In 1999, the FDA also approved Plan B, another EC regimen. While different regimens of oral contraceptives had been distributed and used before 1998 as emergency contraceptives, Preven and Plan B are the first regimens specifically approved by the FDA as safe and effective emergency contraceptives, to be packaged and marketed as such. Additionally, modified doses of oral contraceptives, not specifically packaged for use as an EC, can still be prescribed in doses that would effect emergency contraception if doctor and patient desire such a method.

Emergency contraception pills are classified as prescription drugs, and "states are delegated the power and responsibility of determining which health care professionals . . . have prescriptive authority." Currently, many states have authorized collaborative practices that have expanded the role of pharmacists. These collaborative practices generally authorize greater independence of the pharmacist to initiate drug therapies not specifically prescribed by a patient's physician or other authorized health care professional. In other words, some patients may not require a prescription from their doctor before being distributed certain medications or drugs from a pharmacist. However, with the exception of Washington, California, and Alaska, states do not authorize this expanded pharmacist role in the distribution of ECPs. Pharmacists are generally limited to dispensing ECPs specifically prescribed by some other authorized health care professional. Other general duties of a pharmacist in the distribution of ECPs may include counseling and educating women on EC use at the time the prescription is filled.

In Washington, California, and Alaska, pharmacists have the dual authority to prescribe *and* dispense ECPs under each state's respective collaborative practices. Generally speaking, the pharmacist may dispense ECPs in accordance with "standardized procedures or protocols developed by the pharmacist and an authorized prescriber[.]" Thus, a woman need not receive authorization from her doctor prior to buying ECPs; the pharmacist acts not as a third party or indirect provider of ECPs, but as a direct provider in accordance with a general collaborative protocol.

If pro-choice groups and the American Medical Association have their way, pharmacists will have no future role in ECPs. This is because these groups support an FDA reclassification of ECPs as over-the-counter (OTC) drugs, rather than prescription. Many pro-choice groups claim as a top goal the persuasion of the FDA to reclassify ECPs as OTC. If OTC status were granted, then "women would be able to get ECPs without encountering any type of health care provider."

OTC status for ECPs is not generally supported by pharmacists however, and is not likely in today's political climate. Advocates on both sides of the issue believe the Bush administration, with its influence on the FDA, will delay or negate a switch in classification from prescription to OTC. The behavioral and social policy concerns raised by ECPs "may make switching ECPs to OTC status a politically unpopular move." In any event, ECPs are currently available only by prescription.

Many restrictions have been imposed by the FDA in the use and distribution of mifepristone. First, the drug can only be used during the first forty-nine days after a woman's last menstrual cycle. Also, the drug is distributed to women directly from doctors and certain health clinics. Mifepristone "is not and will not be available in pharmacies[.]" Thus, under the current FDA restrictions, pharmacists have no role in mifepristone-induced abortions.

While current mifepristone use is much lower than expected since its FDA approval and subsequent availability to the public, some signals suggest that future use or access may become more widespread. A survey of doctors by the Kaiser Family Foundation discovered that twenty-three percent of doctors said they were "likely" to offer mifepristone in 2002; up from the seven percent that actually provided the drug since its approval. Also, health centers offering mifepristone have reported a ninety-nine percent rate of abortion in women who have taken the drug. An expected increase in availability, a near perfect rate of achieving the desired ends of abortion, together with continued efforts by pro-choice groups, such as Planned Parenthood, to increase accessibility to abortion, could be the impetus to pharmaceutical distribution of mifepristone in the future.

FDA approval of mifepristone and ECPs, such as Preven and Plan B, has made drug related reproductive therapy a real and potentially widespread option for women. Marketing campaigns by women's and abortion-rights groups and the drug manufacturers themselves will further introduce these drug options to women. This drug therapy revolution of sorts has expanded the pharmacist's role in the provision of emergency contraception, and perhaps, in the future, the provision of mifepristone.

The more women that are aware of and desire EC, the more involved and important pharmacists will become in the contraception process. One can imagine that if more and more states adopt the liberal EC distribution procedures of Washington and California, then pharmacists would become the primary providers of ECPs. And if mifepristone distribution restrictions are relaxed, pharmacists could feasibly become key players in the furnishing of abortion drugs as well. Whether they like it or not, pharmacists are being thrust into the role of common, everyday providers of controversial reproductive medications, and this position may put some pharmacists in the predicament of having to choose between their moral convictions regarding EC and abortion and the patient's wishes. . . .

The Pharmacist's Professional Ethical Obligations

Pharmacy is a profession, and much like the professions of medicine and law, entails a duty to assure and promote the patient's best interests. As professionals, pharmacists are expected to give priority to the patient's interests over their own immediate interests. As key players in the implementation of drug therapies, pharmacists are expected to withhold drugs "from those who have no authority to use them" and not to withhold "medications from those who do have authority to use them."

The patient's best interests are the pharmacist's primary commitment and concern. Among other things, pharmacists are expected to "help individuals achieve optimum benefit from their medications, to be committed to their welfare, and to maintain their trust"; to place "concern for the well-being of the patient at the center of professional practice" taking into consideration the "needs stated by the patient"; and to hold "the patient's welfare paramount." Further, patient autonomy and "personal and cultural differences among patients" must be respected by the pharmacist. These professional duties, and others, encompass the "collective conscience" of the pharmaceutical profession, and their implementation by each pharmacist is considered a moral obligation.

When presented with a validly authorized prescription for a legal medication, by a patient aware of the risks involved in taking the medication, and for whom the medication would be reasonably safe, the aforementioned principles and expectations leave the pharmacist with an ethical duty to fill and dispense the prescription. The duty to dispense in these circumstances may give rise to a serious conflict between the pharmacist's personal conviction concerning abortion and her professional duty to the patient.

In 1998, the American Pharmaceutical Association (APhA), and subsequently various other pharmaceutical organizations, eased the conflict between personal and professional morals by adopting policies recognizing a pharmacist's right to refuse dispensing medications based on the pharmacist's personal beliefs. However, if the pharmacist exercises her right of conscience and refuses to fill the prescription, the duty to the patient is not extinguished, and could be fulfilled by referring the patient to another pharmacist or distributor. In any event, "the patient should not be required to abide by the pharmacist's personal, moral decision." For many pharmacists, a referral would be no more than passive participation in the activity they initially refused to actively assist. Thus the dilemma, while transformed into whether to refer or not, is equally troublesome to the pharmacist.

Section II: The Potential Ramifications of Choosing Conscience

The pharmacist who ultimately decides that her moral convictions regarding abortion outweigh her professional obligation to the patient may refuse to fill the prescription and refer the patient to another pharmacist; or, the pharmacist with conscientious objection may refuse to dispense and refuse to refer. While the former decision will, in practical terms, shield the pharmacist from most negative consequences, the latter decision could have serious implications for the pharmacist, including employment termination or demotion, civil tort liability, or disciplinary action from the state pharmacy board. . . .

Legal protection must serve two purposes in order to appropriately ensure a pharmacist's right of conscientious refusal: 1) prevent and deter detrimental recriminatory action against the pharmacist; and 2) provide adequate remedies in the case that the pharmacist is sued or disciplined. The most efficient and effective means to these ends is the enactment of state and federal legislation.

The first step to successful enactment of pharmacist conscience legislation in each state and the United States is the cooperation of local, regional, and national pharmaceutical associations. The American Pharmaceutical Association took a large positive step when it adopted its pharmacist conscience clause. However, in the same pronouncement it rejected adoption of a policy encouraging enactment of state and national legal protection of the right of conscience. If pharmacists themselves, as represented by their professional associations and organizations, do not call for state and national legislative action, the road to adequate protection will be more difficult.

In any event, an effective conscience statute should take into consideration many complex issues including broad protection against recriminatory action, efficient administration of pharmacies, and accommodation of patients. First and foremost the conscience clause should serve its purpose stating clearly that no pharmacist shall be required to dispense abortion or EC drugs, nor shall any pharmacist be required to refer to another pharmacist who will dispense abortion or EC drugs. Although pharmacists currently have no role in the distribution of mifepristone, the abortion language should nonetheless be included as the potential for future pharmaceutical access exists. Next, the conscience statute should prohibit discrimination, civil liability, and professional disciplinary action that result from exercising the aforementioned rights of refusal. The statute should also encompass provisions prohibiting discrimination in the hiring process so as to preclude pharmacy-employers from screening applicants to avoid hiring pro-life pharmacists in the first place. Finally, the statute should provide adequate methods of deterrence. Employment discrimination could be deterred through its criminalization or by providing an express cause of action in tort as a remedy to the discriminatory hiring, firing, demotion, or promotion of pharmacists.

Employer and patient considerations should also exist in a pharmacist conscience clause. Prior notification of a pharmacist's beliefs regarding abortion and EC should be disclosed to the employer so as to enable efficient administration of the pharmacy. Further, patients should be put on notice in advance regarding when pharmacists with moral objections to abortion and EC will be on duty. For example, schedules could be posted conspicuously within a pharmacy as to when abortion and EC drugs will and will not be available to customer-patients. This will enable patients to avoid the hassle of going to a pharmacy and having their prescription refused. In any event, matters such as the aforementioned should be considered when drafting a pharmacist conscience clause.

Conclusion

Pharmacists, like other professionals such as physicians and attorneys, have a general duty to ensure their client's best interests, and thus must put the health of patients above all other considerations. Thus, it would seem to follow, when a pharmacist is presented with a valid prescription of what is safe for the patient to consume, the drugs should be distributed without dispute. However, to require that a pharmacist, or any professional, participate in what she would equate to the taking of a human life should never be a principle of professional ethics.

Certain issues, because of their inherent complexity and ambiguity, must be resolved, with guidance from religion, philosophy, and science, in the heart and mind of each individual. The commencement of human life and the relative sanctity of unborn life are issues that fall within this category of subjective individual determination. The thoughtful decision should be respected and free from vilifying recrimination. If a pharmacist, in her heart of hearts, concludes that accommodating prescriptions for abortive and EC medications is akin to directly facilitating the destruction of a precious human life, a refusal to accommodate such prescriptions should be protected under the law and within the profession. A safeguard of the right to refuse is imminently necessary as abortive drugs and EC become more widespread and risk of liability and loss of employment may compel many pharmacists to disregard their sacred beliefs or reap the consequences of their objections. Proactive acceptance of a pharmacist's conscientious objection to abortion and EC within the pharmaceutical community would pave the way to legislative protection already afforded doctors and nurses.

Julie Cantor and
Ken Baum

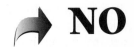 NO

The Limits of Conscientious Objection—May Pharmacists Refuse to Fill Prescriptions for Emergency Contraception?

Health policy decisions are often controversial, and the recent determination by the Food and Drug Administration (FDA) not to grant over-the-counter status to the emergency contraceptive Plan B was no exception. Some physicians decried the decision as a troubling clash of science, politics, and morality.[1] Other practitioners, citing safety, heralded the agency's prudence.[2] Public sentiment mirrored both views. Regardless, the decision preserved a major barrier to the acquisition of emergency contraception—the need to obtain and fill a prescription within a narrow window of efficacy. Six states have lowered that hurdle by allowing pharmacists to dispense emergency contraception without a prescription.[3-8] In those states, patients can simply bypass physicians. But the FDA's decision means that patients cannot avoid pharmacists. Because emergency contraception remains behind the counter, pharmacists can block access to it. And some have done just that.

Across the country, some pharmacists have refused to honor valid prescriptions for emergency contraception. In Texas, a pharmacist, citing personal moral grounds, rejected a rape survivor's prescription for emergency contraception.[9] A pharmacist in rural Missouri also refused to sell such a drug,[10] and in Ohio, Kmart fired a pharmacist for obstructing access to emergency and other birth control.[11] This fall, a New Hampshire pharmacist refused to fill a prescription for emergency contraception or to direct the patron elsewhere for help. Instead, he berated the 21-year-old single mother, who then, in her words, "pulled the car over in the parking lot and just cried."[12] Although the total number of incidents is unknown, reports of pharmacists who refused to dispense emergency contraception date back to 1991[13] and show no sign of abating.

Though nearly all states offer some level of legal protection for health care professionals who refuse to provide certain reproductive services, only Arkansas, Mississippi, and South Dakota explicitly protect pharmacists who refuse to dispense emergency and other contraception.[14] But that

From *The New England Journal of Medicine*, November 4, 2004, pp. 2008–2012. Copyright © 2004 by Massachusetts Medical Society. All rights reserved. Reprinted by permission.

list may grow. In past years, legislators from nearly two dozen states have taken "conscientious objection"—an idea that grew out of wartime tension between religious freedom and national obligation[15] and was co-opted into the reproductive-rights debate of the 1970s[16]—and applied it to pharmacists. One proposed law offers pharmacists immunity from civil lawsuits, criminal liability, professional sanctions, and employment repercussions.[17] Another bill, which was not passed, would have protected pharmacists who refused to transfer prescriptions.[18]

This issue raises important questions about individual rights and public health. Who prevails when the needs of patients and the morals of providers collide? Should pharmacists have a right to reject prescriptions for emergency contraception? The contours of conscientious objection remain unclear. This article elucidates those boundaries and offers a balanced solution to a complex problem. Because the future of over-the-counter emergency contraception is in flux, this issue remains salient for physicians and their patients.

Arguments in Favor of a Pharmacist's Right to Object

Pharmacists Can and Should Exercise Independent Judgment

Pharmacists, like physicians, are professionals. They complete a graduate program to gain expertise, obtain a state license to practice, and join a professional organization with its own code of ethics. Society relies on pharmacists to instruct patients on the appropriate use of medications and to ensure the safety of drugs prescribed in combination. Courts have held that pharmacists, like other professionals, owe their customers a duty of care.[19] In short, pharmacists are not automatons completing tasks; they are integral members of the health care team. Thus, it seems inappropriate and condescending to question a pharmacist's right to exercise personal judgment in refusing to fill certain prescriptions.

Professionals Should Not Forsake Their Morals as a Condition of Employment

Society does not require professionals to abandon their morals. Lawyers, for example, choose clients and issues to represent. Choice is also the norm in the health care setting. Except in emergency departments, physicians may select their patients and procedures. Ethics and law allow physicians, nurses, and physician assistants to refuse to participate in abortions and other reproductive services.[14, 20] Although some observers argue that active participation in an abortion is distinct from passively dispensing emergency contraception, others believe that making such a distinction between active and passive participation is meaningless, because both forms link the provider to the final outcome in the chain of causation.

Conscientious Objection Is Integral to Democracy

More generally, the right to refuse to participate in acts that conflict with personal ethical, moral, or religious convictions is accepted as an essential element of a democratic society. Indeed, Oregon acknowledged this freedom in its Death with Dignity Act,[21] which allows health care providers, including pharmacists, who are disquieted by physician-assisted suicide to refuse involvement without fear of retribution. Also, like the draftee who conscientiously objects to perpetrating acts of death and violence, a pharmacist should have the right not to be complicit in what they believe to be a morally ambiguous endeavor, whether others agree with that position or not. The reproductive-rights movement was built on the ideal of personal choice; denying choice for pharmacists in matters of reproductive rights and abortion seems ironic.

Arguments Against a Pharmacist's Right to Object

Pharmacists Choose to Enter a Profession Bound by Fiduciary Duties

Although pharmacists are professionals, professional autonomy has its limits. As experts on the profession of pharmacy explain, "Professionals are expected to exercise special skill and care to place the interests of their clients above their own immediate interests."[22] When a pharmacist's objection directly and detrimentally affects a patient's health, it follows that the patient should come first. Similarly, principles in the pharmacists' code of ethics weigh against conscientious objection. Given the effect on the patient if a pharmacist refuses to fill a prescription, the code undermines the right to object with such broadly stated objectives as "a pharmacist promotes the good of every patient in a caring, compassionate, and confidential manner," "a pharmacist respects the autonomy and dignity of each patient," and "a pharmacist serves individual, community, and societal needs."[23] Finally, pharmacists understand these fiduciary obligations when they choose their profession. Unlike conscientious objectors to a military draft, for whom choice is limited by definition, pharmacists willingly enter their field and adopt its corresponding obligations.

Emergency Contraception Is Not an Abortifacient

Although the subject of emergency contraception is controversial, medical associations,[24] government agencies,[25] and many religious groups agree that it is not akin to abortion. Plan B and similar hormones have no effect on an established pregnancy, and they may operate by more than one physiological mechanism, such as by inhibiting ovulation or creating an unfavorable environment for implantation of a blastocyst.[26] This duality allowed the Catholic Health Association to reconcile its religious beliefs with a mandate adopted by Washington State that emergency contraception must be provided to rape survivors.[27] According to the association, a patient and a provider who aim only to prevent conception follow Catholic teachings and state law. Also, whether one believes that pregnancy begins with fertilization or implantation, emergency contraception cannot fit squarely within the concept of abortion because one cannot be sure that conception has occurred.

Pharmacists' Objections Significantly Affect Patients' Health

Although religious and moral freedom is considered sacrosanct, that right should yield when it hinders a patient's ability to obtain timely medical treatment. Courts have held that religious freedom does not give health care providers an unfettered right to object to anything involving birth control, an embryo, or a fetus.[28, 29] Even though the Constitution protects people's beliefs, their actions may be regulated.[30] An objection must be balanced with the burden it imposes on others. In some cases, a pharmacist's objection imposes his or her religious beliefs on a patient. Pharmacists may decline to fill prescriptions for emergency contraception because they believe that the drug ends a life. Although the patient may disapprove of abortion, she may not share the pharmacist's beliefs about contraception. If she becomes pregnant, she may then face the question of abortion—a dilemma she might have avoided with the morning-after pill.

Furthermore, the refusal of a pharmacist to fill a prescription may place a disproportionately heavy burden on those with few options, such as a poor teenager living in a rural area that has a lone pharmacy. Whereas the savvy urbanite can drive to another pharmacy, a refusal to fill a prescription for a less advantaged patient may completely bar her access to medication. Finally, although Oregon does have an opt-out provision in its statute regulating assisted suicide, timing is much more important in emergency contraception than in assisted suicide. Plan B is most effective when used within 12 to 24 hours after unprotected intercourse.[31] An unconditional right to refuse is less compelling when the patient requests an intervention that is urgent.

Refusal Has Great Potential for Abuse and Discrimination

The limits to conscientious objection remain unclear. Pharmacists are privy to personal information through prescriptions. For instance, a customer who fills prescriptions for zidovudine, didanosine, and indinavir is logically assumed to be infected with the human immunodeficiency virus (HIV). If pharmacists can reject prescriptions that conflict with their morals, someone who believes that HIV-positive people must have engaged in immoral behavior could refuse to fill those prescriptions. Similarly, a pharmacist who does not condone extramarital sex might refuse to fill a sildenafil prescription for an unmarried man. Such objections go beyond "conscientious" to become invasive. Furthermore, because a pharmacist does not know a patient's history on the basis of a given prescription, judgments regarding the acceptability of a prescription may be medically inappropriate. To a woman with Eisenmenger's syndrome, for example, pregnancy may mean death. The potential for abuse by pharmacists underscores the need for policies ensuring that patients receive unbiased care.

Toward Balance

Compelling arguments can be made both for and against a pharmacist's right to refuse to fill prescriptions for emergency contraception. But even cogent ideas falter when confronted by a dissident moral code. Such is the nature of belief. Even so, most people can agree that we must find a workable and respectful balance between the needs of patients and the morals of pharmacists.

Three possible solutions exist: an absolute right to object, no right to object, or a limited right to object. On balance, the first two options are untenable. An absolute right to conscientious objection respects the autonomy of pharmacists but diminishes their professional obligation to serve patients. It may also greatly affect the health of patients, especially vulnerable ones, and inappropriately brings politics into the pharmacy. Even pharmacists who believe that emergency contraception represents murder and feel compelled to obstruct patients' access to it must recognize that contraception and abortion before fetal viability remain legal nationwide. In our view, state efforts to provide blanket immunity to objecting pharmacists are misguided. Pharmacies should follow the prevailing employment-law standard to make reasonable attempts to accommodate their employees' personal beliefs.[32] Although neutral policies to dispense medications to all customers may conflict with pharmacists' morals, such policies are not necessarily discriminatory, and pharmacies need not shoulder a heightened obligation of absolute accommodation.

Complete restriction of a right to conscientious objection is also problematic. Though pharmacists voluntarily enter their profession and have an obligation to serve patients without judgment, forcing them to abandon their morals imposes a heavy toll. Ethics and law demand that a professional's morality not interfere with the provision of care in life-or-death situations, such as a ruptured ectopic pregnancy.[29] Whereas the hours that elapse between intercourse and the intervention of emergency contraception are crucial, they do not meet that strict test. Also, patients who face an objecting pharmacist do have options, even if they are less preferable than having the prescription immediately filled. Because of these caveats, it is difficult to demand by law that pharmacists relinquish individual morality to stock and fill prescriptions for emergency contraception.

We are left, then, with the vast middle ground. Although we believe that the most ethical course is to treat patients compassionately—that is, to stock emergency contraception and fill prescriptions for it—the totality of the arguments makes us stop short of advocating a legal duty to do so as a first resort. We stop short for three reasons: because emergency contraception is not an absolute emergency, because other options exist, and because, when possible, the moral beliefs of those delivering care should be considered. However, in a profession that is bound by fiduciary obligations and strives to respect and care for patients, it is unacceptable to leave patients to fend for themselves. As a general rule, pharmacists who cannot or will not dispense a drug have an obligation to meet the needs of their customers by referring them elsewhere. This idea is uncontroversial when it is applied to common medications such as antibiotics and statins; it becomes contentious, but is equally valid, when it is applied to emergency contraception. Therefore, pharmacists who object should, as a matter of ethics and law, provide alternatives for patients.

Pharmacists who object to filling prescriptions for emergency contraception should arrange for another pharmacist to provide this service to customers promptly. Pharmacies that stock emergency contraception should ensure, to the extent possible, that at least one nonobjecting pharmacist is on duty at all times. Pharmacies that do not stock emergency contraception should give clear notice and refer patients elsewhere. At the very least, there should be a prominently displayed sign that says, "We do not provide emergency contraception. Please call Planned Parenthood at 800-230-PLAN (7526) . . . for assistance." However, a direct referral to a local pharmacy or pharmacist who is willing to fill the prescription is preferable. Objecting pharmacists should also redirect prescriptions for emergency contraception that are received by telephone to another pharmacy known to fill such prescriptions. In rural areas, objecting pharmacists should provide referrals within a reasonable radius.

Notably, the American Pharmacists Association has endorsed referrals, explaining that "providing alternative mechanisms for patients . . . ensures patient access to drug products, without requiring the pharmacist or the patient to abide by personal decisions other than their own."[33] A referral may also represent a break in causation between the pharmacist and distributing emergency contraception, a separation that the objecting pharmacist presumably seeks. And, in deference to the law's normative value, the rule of referral also conveys the importance of professional responsibility to patients. In areas of the country where referrals are logistically impractical, professional obligation may dictate providing emergency contraception, and a legal mandate may be appropriate if ethical obligations are unpersuasive.

Inevitably, some pharmacists will disregard our guidelines, and physicians—all physicians—should be prepared to fill gaps in care. They should identify pharmacies that will fill patients' prescriptions and encourage patients to keep emergency contraception at home. They should be prepared to dispense emergency contraception or instruct patients to mimic it with other birth-control pills. In Wisconsin, family-planning clinics recently began dispensing emergency contraception, and the state set up a toll-free hotline to help patients find physicians who will prescribe it.[34] Emergency departments should stock emergency contraception and make it available to rape survivors, if not all patients.

In the final analysis, education remains critical. Pharmacists may have misconceptions about emergency contraception. In one survey, a majority of pharmacists mistakenly agreed with the statement that repeated use of emergency contraception is medically risky.[35] Medical misunderstandings that lead pharmacists to refuse to fill prescriptions for emergency contraception are unacceptable. Patients, too, may misunderstand or be unaware of emergency contraception.[36] Physicians should teach patients about this option before the need arises, since patients may understand their choices better when they are not under stress. Physicians should discuss emergency contraception during office visits, offer prescriptions in advance of need, and provide education through pamphlets or the Internet. Web sites . . . allow users to search for physicians who prescribe emergency contraception by ZIP Code, area code, or address, and Planned Parenthood offers extensive educational information . . . , including details about off-label use of many birth-control pills for emergency contraception.

Our principle of a compassionate duty of care should apply to all health care professionals. In a secular society, they must be prepared to limit the reach of their personal objection. Objecting pharmacists may choose to find employment opportunities that comport with their morals—in a religious community, for example—but when they pledge to serve the public, it is unreasonable to expect those in need of health care to acquiesce to their personal convictions. Similarly, physicians who refuse to write prescriptions for emergency contraception should follow the rules of notice and referral for the reason previously articulated: the beliefs of health care providers should not trump patient care. It is difficult enough to be faced with the consequences of rape or of an unplanned pregnancy; health care providers should not make the situation measurably worse.

Former Supreme Court Chief Justice Charles Evans Hughes called the quintessentially American custom of respect for conscience a "happy tradition"[37]—happier, perhaps, when left in the setting of a draft objection than when pitting one person's beliefs against another's reproductive health. Ideally, conflicts about emergency contraception will be rare, but they will occur. In July, 11 nurses in Alabama resigned rather than provide emergency contraception in state clinics.[38] As patients understand their birth-control options, conflicts at the pharmacy counter and in the clinic may become more common. When professionals' definitions of liberty infringe on those they choose to serve, a respectful balance must be struck. We offer one solution. Even those who challenge this division of burdens and benefits should agree with our touchstone—although health professionals may have a right to object, they should not have a right to obstruct.

References

1. Drazen JM, Greene MF, Wood AJJ. The FDA, politics, and Plan B. N Engl J Med 2004;350:1561–2.
2. Stanford JB, Hager WD, Crockett SA. The FDA, politics, and Plan B. N Engl J Med 2004;350:2413–4.
3. Alaska Admin. Code tit. 12, § 52.240 (2004).
4. Cal. Bus. & Prof. Code § 4052 (8) (2004).
5. Hawaii Rev. Stat. § 461-1 (2003).
6. N.M. Admin. Code § 16.19.26.9 (2003).
7. Wash. Rev. Code § 246-863-100 (2004).
8. Me. Rev. Stat. Ann. tit.32, §§ 13821-13825 (2004).
9. Pharmacist refuses pill for victim. Chicago Tribune. February 11, 2004:C7.
10. Simon S. Pharmacists new players in abortion debate. Los Angeles Times. March 20, 2004:A18.

11. Sweeney JF. May a pharmacist refuse to fill a prescription? Plain Dealer. May 5, 2004:E1.

12. Associated Press. Pharmacist refuses to fill morning after prescription.

13. Sauer M. Pharmacist to be fired in abortion controversy. St. Petersburg Times. December 19, 1991:1B.

14. State policies in brief: refusing to provide health services. New York: Alan Guttmacher Institute, September 1, 2004.

15. Seeley RA. Advice for conscientious objectors in the armed forces. 5th ed. Philadelphia: Central Committee for Conscientious Objectors, 1998:1–2.

16. 42 U.S.C. § 300a-7 (2004).

17. Mich. House Bill No. 5006 (As amended April 21, 2004).

18. Oregon House Bill No. 2010 (As amended May 11, 1999).

19. Hooks Super X, Inc. v. McLaughlin, 642 N.E. 2d 514 (Ind. 1994).

20. Section 2.01. In: Council on Ethical and Judicial Affairs. Code of medical ethics: current opinions with annotations. 2002–2003 ed. Chicago: American Medical Association, 2002.

21. Oregon Revised Statute § 127.885 § 4.01 (4) (2003).

22. Fassett WE, Wicks AC. Is pharmacy a profession? In: Weinstein BD, ed. Ethical issues in pharmacy. Vancouver, Wash.: Applied Therapeutics, 1996:1–28.

23. American Pharmacists Association. Code of ethics for pharmacists: preamble.

24. Hughes EC, ed. Obstetric-gynecologic terminology, with section on neonatology and glossary of congenital anomalies. Philadelphia: F.A. Davis, 1972.

25. Commodity Supplemental Food Program, 7 C.F.R. § 247.2 (2004).

26. Glasier A. Emergency postcoital contraception. N Engl J Med 1997; 337:1058–64.

27. Daily reproductive health report: state politics & policy: Washington governor signs law requiring hospitals to offer emergency contraception to rape survivors. Menlo Park, Calif.: Kaisernetwork, April 2, 2002.

28. Brownfield v. Daniel Freeman Marina Hospital, 208 Cal. App. 3d 405 (Cal. Ct. App. 1989).

29. Shelton v. Univ. of Medicine & Dentistry, 223 F.3d 220 (3d Cir. 2000).

30. Tribe LH. American constitutional law. 2nd ed. Mineola, N.Y.: Foundation Press, 1988:1183.

31. Brody JE. The politics of emergency contraception. New York Times. August 24, 2004:F7.

32. Trans World Airlines v. Hardison, 432 U.S. 63 (1977).

33. 1997–98 APhA Policy Committee report: pharmacist conscience clause. Washington, D.C.: American Pharmacists Association, 1997.

34. Politics wins over science. Capital Times. May 13, 2004:16A.

35. Alford S, Davis L, Brown L. Pharmacists' attitudes and awareness of emergency contraception for adolescents. Transitions 2001;12(4):1–17.

36. Foster DG, Harper CC, Bley JJ, et al. Knowledge of emergency contraception among women aged 18 to 44 in California. Am J Obstet Gynecol 2004;191:150–6.

37. United States v. Macintosh, 283 U.S. 605, 634 (1931) (Hughes, C.J., dissenting).

38. Elliott D. Alabama nurses quit over morning-after pill. Presented on All Things Considered. Washington, D.C.: National Public Radio, July 28, 2004 (transcript). *Copyright © 2004 Massachusetts Medical Society.*

POSTSCRIPT

Should Pharmacists Be Allowed to Deny Prescriptions on Grounds of Conscience?

In November 2004, the FDA announced a labeling change for mifepristone. Because the FDA and the manufacturer Danco Laboratories had received reports of serious side effects, the warning label was changed to reflect this new information.

As of 2005, the federal government and 47 state governments had laws protecting conscientious objectors in health care. The Illinois Health Care Right of Conscience Act is the most detailed and protects physicians, health care personnel, health care facilities, and health care payers who refuse to participate in services that are contrary to their conscience. In April 2005, however, Gov. Rod Blagojevich issued an emergency rule requiring pharmacies to fill prescriptions for birth control and mifepristone "without delay." Bills have been introduced that specifically include pharmacists in the Health Care Right of Conscience Act.

Four states (South Dakota, Mississippi, Arkansas, and Georgia) have laws specifically recognizing a pharmacist's right of conscientious objection, while in 2005 California enacted a law requiring pharmacists to dispense these drugs. Considerable activity on both sides of the issue is going on in the states. The National Conference of State Legislatures monitors these bills. See http://www.ncsl.org/programs/health/conscienceclauses.htm.

A national survey of physicians found that physicians who were male, religious, and had moral objections to controversial but legal procedures like administering terminal sedation in dying patients or prescribing birth control to teenagers without parental approval were less likely to report that doctors must disclose information or refer patients for these medical procedures (Farr A. Curlin et al., "Religion, Conscience, and Controversial Clinical Practices," *The New England Journal of Medicine,* February 8, 2007).

In "Pharmacies, Pharmacists, and Conscientious Objection," Mark R. Wicclair argues that the health needs of patients and the professional obligations of pharmacists limit the extent to which they may refuse to assist patients who have lawful prescriptions for medically indicated drugs (*Kennedy Institute of Ethics Journal,* vol. 16, no. 3, 2006). On the other hand, Brian P. Knestout asserts that "conscience clauses" protect medical professionals who do not wish to perform or assist in procedures related to abortion, sterilization, or euthanasia ("An Essential Prescription: Why Pharmacist-Inclusive Clauses Are Necessary," *Journal of Contemporary Health Law and Policy,* Spring 2006).

Adrienne Asch compares conscientious objections to health care practices to similar behavior in times of war and offers limited support for these exceptions to professional responsibility ("Two Cheers for Conscience Exceptions," *Hastings Center Report,* November–December 2006).

Contributors to This Volume

EDITOR

CAROL LEVINE joined the United Hospital Fund in New York City in October 1996 where she directs the Families and Health Care Project. This project focuses on developing partnerships between health care professionals and family caregivers, who provide most of the long-term and chronic care to elderly, seriously ill, or disabled relatives. She founded the Orphan Project: Families and Children in the HIV Epidemic in 1991. She was director of the Citizens Commission on AIDS in New York City from 1987 to 1991. As a senior staff associate of The Hastings Center, she edited the *Hastings Center Report*. In 1993 she was awarded a MacArthur Foundation Fellowship for her work in AIDS policy and ethics. She has written several articles and books, most recently *Always On Call: When Illness Turns Families into Caregivers* (Vanderbilt University Press, 2004); with Thomas H. Murray, *The Cultures of Caregiving: Conflict and Common Ground among Families, Health Professionals, and Policy Makers* (Johns Hopkins University Press, 2004); and with Geoff Foster and John Williamson, *A Generation at Risk: The Global Impact of HIV/AIDS on Orphan and Vulnerable Children* (Cambridge University Press, 2005).

AUTHORS

MARCIA ANGELL, MD, is a senior lecturer in the department of social medicine at Harvard Medical School and the former editor-in-chief of *The New England Journal of Medicine.*

GEORGE J. ANNAS, ID, is the Edward R. Utley Professor of Health Law and chairman of the Health Law Department at the Boston University School of Public Health in Boston, Massachusetts. He is also the cofounder of Global Lawyers & Physicians and the Patients' Rights Project.

PAUL ANTONY, MD, is the chief medical officer of the Pharmaceutical Research and Manufacturers of America (PhRMA).

ROBERT M. ARNOLD, MD, is the director of the Palliative Care Service at the University of Pittsburgh's Medical Center.

JOSEPH E. BALOG, PhD, teaches in the Department of Health Science, College at Brockport, State University of New York.

MARGARET P. BATTIN, PhD, is the Distinguished Professor of Philosophy and Adjunct Professor of Internal Medicine, Division of Medical Ethics, at the University of Utah, Salt Lake City.

KEN BAUM is a physician and attorney at the firm of Wiggin and Dana, New Haven, CT.

DEENA BERKOWITZ, MD, MPH, is an assistant professor of pediatrics at Georgetown University School of Medicine and Health Sciences in Washington, DC.

LESLIE J. BLACKHALL, MD, is an associate professor of medicine and an associate professor of medical education at the University of Virginia. She is a medical director at the Center for Geriatric and Palliative Care and coordinator for research at the Center for Biomedical Ethics.

M. GREGG BLOCHE is a professor of law at Georgetown University and an adjunct professor at the Bloomberg School of Public Health, Johns Hopkins University.

JULIE CANTOR is an attorney at Yale University School of Medicine.

MEGAN CLAYTON is a research associate at the Oxford Centre for Applied Ethics, Oxford University, England.

NEAL DICKERT, MD, is with the Phoebe R. Berman Bioethics Institute, Johns Hopkins University, Baltimore, MD.

ANGELA FAGERLIN, PhD, is an experimental psychologist and member of the Center for Bioethics and Social Sciences in Medicine at the University of Michigan Health System, Ann Arbor, MI.

BENNETT FODDY is a research associate at the Oxford Centre for Applied Ethics, Oxford University, England.

KATHLEEN M. FOLEY holds The Society of Memorial Sloan-Kettering Cancer Center chair in pain research. She is a professor of neurology and pharmacology at the Weill Medical College of Cornell University and attending neurologist in the Pain and Palliative Care Service at Memorial Sloan-Kettering, New York City.

GELYA FRANK is a professor of occupational science and occupational therapy and anthropology in the department of occupational science and occupational therapy at the University of Southern California, in Los Angeles, CA.

EMIL J. FREIREICH, MD, is a professor of Special Medical Education at the MD Anderson Cancer Center, Houston, TX.

ROBERT P. GEORGE is McCormick Professor of Jurisprudence at Princeton University and the director of the James Madison Program in American Ideals and Institutions.

LAWRENCE O. GOSTIN is a professor of law at Georgetown University, a professor of public health at the Johns Hopkins University, and the director of the Center for Law and the Public's Health at Johns Hopkins and Georgetown Universities.

MICHAEL L. GROSS is codirector of the Graduate Program in Applied and Professional Ethics, Division of International Relations, School of Political Science, University of Haifa, Israel.

JONATHAN GRUBER, PhD, is a health economist at the Massachusetts Institute of Technology, Cambridge, MA.

BERNARD J. HAMMES is the director of medical humanities at Gundersen Lutheran Medical Foundation and Medical Center, LaCrosse, WI.

DONALD W. HERBE is a law student at Cleveland State University.

SUSAN E. HICKMAN, PhD, is associate professor, Department of Environments for Health, Indiana University School of Nursing, Indianapolis.

GAIL JAVITT, JD, MPH, is the law and policy director at the Genetics and Public Policy Center in Washington, DC. She is also a research scientist at the Berman Institute of Bioethics at Johns Hopkins University in Baltimore, Maryland.

ERIC T. JUENGST is Professor of Bioethics and Director of the Center for Genetic Research Ethics and Law within the Department of Bioethics at the Case Western Reserve University School of Medicine in Cleveland, Ohio.

GREGORY E. KAEBNICK is the editor of *The Hastings Center Report* and a research scholar at The Hastings Center, Garrison, NY.

DAVID A. KESSLER, MD, is a professor of medicine at the University of California, San Francisco, and a former commissioner of the Food and Drug Administration.

MARK KUCZEWSKI is a philosopher and director of the Neiswanger Institute for Bioethics and Health Policy at the Stritch School of Medicine, Loyola University, in Chicago.

PATRICK LEE is an associate professor of philosophy at the Franciscan University in Steubenville, OH. He is the author of *Abortion and Unborn Life* (1996).

DOUGLAS A. LEVY, JD, teaches in the School of Medicine, University of California, San Francisco, CA.

CHARLES W. LIDZ is a professor of psychiatry at the University of Pittsburgh. Currently, he is on leave from the University of Pittsburgh and works at the University of Massachusetts Medical School, where he is the director of the Center for Mental Health Services Research.

MARGARET OLIVIA LITTLE is a philosopher at the Kennedy Institute of Ethics, Georgetown University. Her research interests focus on the intersection of ethics, feminist theory, and public policy.

JONATHAN H. MARKS is a barrister at Matrix Chambers, London, and Greenwall Fellow in Bioethics at Georgetown University Law Center and Bloomberg School of Public Health, Johns Hopkins University.

PATRICK J. McCRUDEN is the vice president of mission and ethics at St. Joseph's Mercy Health Center in Hot Springs, AR.

VICKI MICHEL is an adjunct professor at Loyola Law School in Los Angeles, CA.

ALVIN H. MOSS, MD, is a professor of medicine and director of the Center for Health Ethics and Law at the Robert C. Byrd Health Sciences Center of West Virginia University, Morgantown, WV.

SHEILA MURPHY is an associate professor at the Annenberg School for Communication and the department of psychology at the University of Southern California, in Los Angeles, CA.

THOMAS H. MURRAY is the president of The Hastings Center in Garrison, NY. He was formerly a professor of biomedical ethics and director of the Center for Biomedical Ethics in the School of Medicine at Case Western Reserve University in Cleveland, OH.

ONORA O'NEILL is the principal of Newnham College, Cambridge University, England. She has chaired the Nuffield Council on Bioethics and is currently chair of the Nuffield Foundation. She has written widely on political philosophy and ethics, international justice, and the philosophy of Immanuel Kant.

LYNN M. PALTROW is an attorney and executive director of National Advocates for Pregnant Women.

CHARLES PETERS is an associate professor of clinical pediatrics in the division of hematology–oncology and blood and marrow transplantation at the University of Minnesota Medical School in Minneapolis, MN.

CHRISTOPHER J. PRESTON, PhD, is an environmental ethicist at the University of Montana Missoula, MT.

SARA ROSENBAUM, JD, is a professor of health policy, School of Public Health and Health Services, George Washington University Medical Center, Washington, DC.

LAINIE FRIEDMAN ROSS is an assistant professor of pediatrics in the McLean Center for Clinical Medical Ethics, Department of Medicine, at the University of Chicago in Chicago, IL. She is also the director of the Ethics Case Consultation Service and codirector of the Multidisciplinary Ethics Lecture Series at the university.

MICHAEL J. SANDEL teaches political philosophy at Harvard University, where he is the Anne T. and Robert M. Bass Professor of Government.

SALLY SATEL, MD, is a psychiatrist and lecturer at the Yale University School of Medicine. She is a resident scholar at the American Enterprise Institute in Washington, DC.

TERESA A. SAVAGE, PhD, RN, is the associate director, Donnelley Family Disability Ethics Program, Rehabilitation Institute of Chicago, and the assistant professor—research, Department of Maternal-Child Nursing, University of Illinois at Chicago College of Nursing.

JULIAN SAVULESCU, PhD, is the Uehiro Professor of Practical Ethics, Oxford University, and the director of the Oxford Uehiro Centre for Practical Ethics.

CARL E. SCHNEIDER, JD, is the Chauncey Stillman Professor for Ethics, Morality, and the Practice of Law at the University of Michigan Law School, Ann Arbor, MI. He is also a professor of internal medicine at the medical school.

SARAH E. SHANNON, PhD, RN, is an associate professor, biobehavioral nursing and health systems, University of Washington, Seattle.

JEREMY SUGARMAN, MD, is with the Phoebe R. Berman Bioethics Institute, Johns Hopkins University, and the Department of Medicine, Johns Hopkins University, Baltimore, MD.

JEAN TOAL is a justice of the South Carolina Supreme Court.

SUSAN W. TOLLE, MD, is a professor of general internal medicine and geriatrics at Oregon Health & Science University and the cofounder and director of the University's Center for Ethics in Health Care, Portland, OR.

HOWARD TRACHTMAN, MD, is a physician at Schneider Children's Hospital, New Hyde Park, NY.

ROBERT F. WEIR is the director of the Program in Biomedical Ethics and Medical Humanities in the College of Medicine at the University of Iowa. A professor of pediatrics, he is also on the faculty of the university's School of Religion.

GLEN WHITMAN is an associate professor of economics at California State University, Northridge, CA.